Practising Colonial Medicine

Practising Colonial Medicine

The Colonial Medical Service in British East Africa

Anna Crozier

I.B. TAURIS

LONDON · NEW YORK

Published in 2007 by I.B. Tauris & Co Ltd
6 Salem Road, London W2 4BU
175 Fifth Avenue,
New York, NY 10010
www.ibtauris.com

In the United States of America and in Canada
distributed by St Martins Press, 175 Fifth Avenue, New York NY 10010

ISBN 978 84511 459 6

A full CIP record for this book is available from the British Library
A full CIP record for this book is available from the Library of Congress

Library of Congress catalog card: available

Printed and bound in Great Britain by TJ International Ltd, Padstow, Cornwall
From camera-ready copy edited and supplied by the author

Contents

List of Figures

Acknowledgements

This research that forms the basis of this monograph was made possible through a Wellcome Trust Studentship from October 2001 to October 2004. Travel to archives within England was funded by the Wellcome Trust Centre for the History of Medicine at University College London. Research at the Kenya National Archives was funded by the Royal Historical Society, University College London Graduate School and the Department of Anatomy and Development Biology, University College London. I thank these sources for allowing me to travel so usefully. My particular thanks are extended to my former PhD supervisors Bill Bynum and Anne Hardy, as well as my PhD examiners Michael Worboys and Felix Driver. I also thank David Greenwood, Tony Kirk-Greene and Alex McKay for their very useful comments on earlier drafts of this work. Thanks too to Lester Crook, Liz Friend-Smith and Elizabeth Galloway at IB Tauris for their support and guidance and to João Rangel de Almeida for his generous help and many hours patience to help prepare camera-ready copy. Tom Rodwell is also thanked for his help with some horrible formatting issues. Of course, any shortfalls or inaccuracies are my own. Finally, I thank a very good husband, Ivan. He, along with our new son, Otto, makes it all worthwhile.

Preface

The Colonial Medical Service was the branch of the Colonial Service responsible for healthcare provision in the British overseas territories. This book profiles Colonial Medical Officers (MOs) serving in Kenya, Uganda and Tanzania from the beginnings of British colonial rule to the start of World War Two.

The work is divided into two substantive parts: entering the Colonial Medical Service and experiencing the colonial medical career. The first looks at how doctors joined the Service, what the objective and subjective criteria for recruitment were and how these criteria influenced the types of individuals that were recruited. Then reasons for entering the Service are analysed, particularly looking at explanations from officers as well as examining broader contextual factors that may have stimulated recruitment. The second part of the work focuses upon the experiences specific to being a MO once arrived in East Africa. It outlines job descriptions and typical duties as well as the common experiences Officers were likely to have and how these changed over time. Special attention is paid to the way colonial life demanded particular characteristics, ones stressed during the recruitment process and by the appointees themselves as defining the job as a particularly different choice for medical graduates. This reflection upon the shared professional encounters moves to an argument for the development of a distinct colonial medical identity, arguing that the sense of common mission and the shared experiences of the colonial medial cohort bound Officers together symbolically in a progressive British (political and medical) project. This formation of distinct colonial identities relied upon various (although also unifying) factors of race, situation, employer, profession and medical interests. The resulting sense of kinship both determined, and also to some degree regulated, colonial medical attitudes and behaviour. These colonial subjectivities embodied the cultural values that were an intrinsic part of the colonising enterprise. They disciplined the actions, attitudes and ideologies of the participants, thus making a uniform cohort of representatives of Empire.

This study is no apologist's account. It does not aim to resurrect colonial officers as 'misunderstood'; it does not deny that certain medical policies were ill-conceived, or even oppressive. In fact, it makes no particular comment on these aspects, which have already formed the basis of much scholarly investigation. The aim is to seek a greater understanding of the European perspective: the creation of the Colonial civil servant. By examining recruitment policy (Chapters 2 and 3), motives for joining the Medical Service (Chapters 4 and 5), common career experiences (Chapters 6 and 7) and the features of a colonial medical identity (Chapters 8 and 9), important aspects of European colonial history are placed within their proper cultural context.

Explanatory Notes

Although 'East Africa' includes Zanzibar, Nyasaland (British Central Africa, 1891–1907; Nyasaland 1907–64; now Malawi) and British Somaliland (part of modern-day Somalia), it is used in this book as a general descriptor referring only to the largest three territories that form the basis of this study: Kenya, Tanzania and Uganda. I do not examine Somaliland, despite its inclusion in some contemporary definitions of British East Africa, largely because it is geographically separate from the three countries that inform this research. Long on-going border disputes with Italy placed British Somaliland at the Northern edge of the Kingdom of Ethiopia (modern-day Ethiopia) making it necessarily isolated from the other major East African countries. Furthermore, the number of MOs allocated there was extremely small: at the end of the period comprising only five officers.[1] Similarly, Nyasaland had only a comparatively small Medical Service (12 staff in 1914 compared with those of Kenya (31) and Uganda (26) in the same year).[2] In the Colonial Office mentality at least, the regional 'block' to which Nyasaland belonged was prone to change: although it was sometimes included in descriptions of East Africa, it was as often grouped together with Northern Rhodesia as part of Central Africa.[3] Finally, this research has excluded the Sultanate of Zanzibar. Although interesting in its own right, the colonial medical organisation of the island is more likely to show divergence rather than similarities to the countries I have chosen to consider. Zanzibar became a protectorate in 1890 (and was transferred from the Foreign Office to the Colonial Office in 1913), but retained a distinct political and social organisation due to the heavily Muslim influences on the island. Its Medical Service therefore did not have the typical administrative structure of officers answerable to a Governor with supreme power. Rather, until 1913, the Sultan maintained his dominance over the island.

Finally, the choice of Kenya, Uganda and Tanzania supplements and invites comparison with the work of Ann Beck who has written the only monograph to date on the medical administrative history of the area.[4] It seems appropriate, even though her focus is pointedly different that of this monograph, to compare like with like.

At the time Tanzania was referred to as Tanganyika Territory; Kenya as British East Africa, East Africa Protectorate or Kenya Colony; and Uganda as Uganda Protectorate. Because the names changed within the period I have used the modern-day name for each country to avoid confusion. Sometimes I have referred to the three countries collectively as 'colonies' — although this is not strictly correct (Kenya was a Colony and Protectorate, Uganda a Protectorate and Tanzania a mandated territory). This seems to be acceptable given the contemporary perception that 'from the administrative point of view...the distinction is of little or no practical importance'.[5]

Lastly, for easier reading, I do not disrupt the narrative by giving place and dates of service for each MO at each mention. This information can be found in Appendix 2. Additionally, the preferred given name (if known) of any MO is used rather than their full birth name (e.g. Colin Carothers rather than John Colin Dixon Carothers; Bagster Wilson rather than Donald Bagster Wilson). Although some women MOs made up the cohort, the gender specific 'he' is sometimes used for stylistic purposes.

Chapter 1: Introduction

[A] body of men whose collective experience far outsteps [*sic.*] the bounds of any single Dependency.[1]

Arthur Williams, a former Colonial Medical Officer (MO), summed up his reasons for joining the Colonial Service concisely: although his family had no particular connections with the African continent, he had been 'captivated and drawn by the idea of East Africa'.[2] This self-professed sense of captivation points directly to the central argument of this book, namely that at the very heart of the Colonial Medical Service career was a desire to enrol into a certain lifestyle. Participation in this life symbolised something markedly different from that offered by medical careers back at home. Working in Africa evoked potent images of adventure and allowed medical graduates, sometimes of quite modest backgrounds, to combine good works with an active participation in governance. For doctors particularly it was intimately associated with the practice of tropical medicine and offered scope, as one MO put it, for 'clinical practice and epidemiological research undreamed of…in the UK.'[3] Choosing the colonial medical career allowed for the formation not only of a professional, but also a social, political and cultural identity, based on race, Britishness, and the new tropical medicine.

From the end of the nineteenth century when British presence in Africa became officially established, the Colonial Service offered one of the first practical opportunities for those who did not want to be missionaries to work there. The Empire beckoned to many people with its long associations with a Victorian tradition of adventure, while also affording active participation in a modern political project that was popularly — almost uniformly before 1939 — conceived as being a good thing, 'destined to last forever'.[4] Colonial medical careers in this context were loaded with powerful associations, uniquely combining a reverence for tradition with a desire to play a part in modernity. Although pay was poor, tours of service long, and health risks considerable, doctoring in Africa provided a prospect to escape the workaday concerns of home. The perceived trials and risks actually further demarcated the job as interesting and alluringly different.

    This book is an exploration of the career experiences of the 424 Colonial
Service doctors who served in Kenya, Uganda and Tanzania under British rule
before 1939. It makes no claims to offer a history of East African medical policy
or procedure, although the findings naturally touch upon both.[5] Rather, this is a
cultural-historical enquiry into a particular government cohort: it profiles the
cadre; asks how were they recruited, and how they presented themselves in
relation to their careers. Central to this analysis is the investigation of personal
experiences, through participant memoirs and papers, contemporaneous
commentaries on the Service within the medical literature, and the official files of
the Colonial Office patronage and personnel divisions. The aim has been to
project the career's attractions and experiences against its relevant context and to
contribute to an emergent field within medical history that has recently begun to
emphasise the intricate relationship between medicine, identity and colonialism.[6]
The study argues that a distinct colonial medical identity developed, shaped by a
sense of common mission and shared experiences as well as recruitment policies,
compliance with certain attitudes and behaviours, membership of the medical
profession and the rise of tropical medicine as a new discipline. This emergence of
the colonial subject within medicine places the doctors in contrast to the
indigenous Africans whom they colonised, with all of the power relations such a
position entails. But the same colonial subjectivity also disciplined the identities of
the individual doctors who were a part of the Colonial Service. It is anticipated
that many of the themes identified may not just be typical of East Africa or of
medical workers, but may provide a cultural-historical template with which to
view the colonial experience in general.

Historical Background

The Colonial Service constituted the staff of those British imperial territories that
were administered first by the Foreign Office and later, after departmental
organisations in the early 1900s, by the Colonial Office. While the Colonial Office
officially oversaw the Colonial Service, the two organisations were nevertheless
distinct. Simply put, the Colonial Service was the government department that
oversaw the local administration of those British territories whose civil services
were not otherwise administered separately. [7] Although they technically worked
towards the same political ends, Colonial Office interests in the metropolitan
ruling centre often clashed with the concerns of those who bore direct
administrative responsibility abroad.[8]

    Colonial Service personnel (apart from subordinate posts) were
predominantly recruited in London, but once appointed officers were paid by, and
immediately responsible to, the individual colonial governments they served. It
was assumed that Britain's colonies should be largely self-supporting, principally
through funds collected by local taxation imposed upon indigenous populations.
Unsurprisingly, this led to frequent complaints from Colonial Service members
that their pay, pensions and benefits were not equal to those of civil servants
employed centrally by the Colonial Office.[9] In most respects, however, the relative
independence that the Colonial Service enjoyed from central command was fêted
rather than mourned. It was only in matters of extreme political importance, or in

the case of very senior appointments, that Colonial Office approval had to be specifically sought. Mergers between the Colonial Office and the Colonial Service were discussed throughout the period, but perhaps because both parties tacitly acknowledged the benefits of independence, these plans never materialised.[10]

Although the Secretary of State for the Colonies and the Colonial Office had ultimate responsibility for the Colonial Service, the Governor of each colony had a powerful role. He was normally assisted by an advisory body called the Executive Council and a legislative body called the Legislative Council. These two Councils formulated policies and regulations for each territory.[11] The Medical Department was one of the major departments of each colony; others included the Treasury, the Legal Department, the Customs Department, the Education Department, the Agricultural Department and the Public Works Department.[12] The head of each department was usually a member of the profession that they represented; the head of the Medical Department therefore was always a doctor.

Although the Colonial Service had been in existence since 1838, it was the appointment of Joseph Chamberlain (1836–1914) as Secretary of State in 1895 that marks the moment when the Colonial Service really began to become organised into an important career.[13] Before Chamberlain's investiture, the Colonial Office was not considered an important branch of government, especially in comparison to the prestigious India Office that administered the affairs of the Raj. Famously, Chamberlain's leading theory for imperial governance was 'constructive imperialism' and his initiatives on behalf of the Colonial Service were an integral part of this ideological framework that sought to draw the different parts of the Empire closer together for purposes of defence and commerce. Under his influence the control of most of the African territories was transferred from the Foreign Office to the Colonial Office. The power and remit of the Colonial Office was thus expanded and an immediate need was created for the administrative, legal and medical staff to be effectively organised.

In order to streamline the bureaucracy of Empire, one of Chamberlain's first acts was to re-assess the extent and condition of the vaguely-defined Colonial Service that he had inherited. He commissioned a survey under the guidance of Lord Selborne, the then Parliamentary Under-Secretary of State. Selborne's report (completed in 1899, returned to Chamberlain in 1900), indicated that there were substantial organisational problems inherent in the Service; not least large discrepancies between the various colonies themselves, which lacked coordination and standardisation. Chamberlain consequently set to work reorganising the administrative infrastructure, a task that particularly impacted the Medical Service which, it was estimated, comprised nearly a third of the Colonial Service.[14]

In Africa especially, where health problems loomed large, successful medical colonisation was recognised as one of the fundamental springboards by which to establish political objectives. Chamberlain accordingly paid unprecedented attention to medical matters in connection with the colonial project. He appointed Patrick Manson (1844–1922), widely regarded as the most important doctor in the tropical medical field, as the first Consulting Physician for the Colonial Office and together they commenced plans to coordinate the training of MOs for the first time. As early as 1888, Chamberlain addressed the General Medical Council and the Deans of the principal medical schools in Britain putting forward his suggestion that all MOs in the Colonial Service should undertake a specialist course of study before embarkation abroad.[15] It took over ten years for the plan to materialise, with the opening of the London and Liverpool Schools of Tropical Medicine in 1899. Principally because it was the brainchild of Chamberlain and Manson, the London School of Tropical Medicine was always more closely associated with the Colonial Medical Service career. Although the Liverpool School was also to offer a Diploma in Tropical Medicine to perspective MOs, its ethos was driven more by commercial interests than the political ideals of the British Government.[16] It was from the London base that the first official organisation of a specific training facility for Colonial MOs was conceived. Other centralising features occurred later on, but this marks the true beginning for structured Colonial Medical Service careers.

Tropical medicine was at this time growing in stature. As early as 1895, Manson had initiated at St George's Hospital a course of twenty lectures on tropical diseases designed specifically for graduates who sought a career in the tropical world.[17] Chamberlain, meanwhile, viewed common medical training as an integral part of his wider campaign to reform and modernise the Colonial Service and laid increasing emphasis upon internal regulation. Medical consultants began to be regularly used to offer advice on Medical Service matters, such as recruitment or the way the Service was to be structured. Medical advisers with expertise in tropical medical matters were appointed in London, Liverpool, Edinburgh and Dublin, although it was not until 1926 that the official post of Chief Medical Adviser to the Colonial Office was established. With one exception, all Chief Medical Advisers were former Colonial MOs, drawing on their in-field experiences to help guide central government practice.[18]

The Colonial Medical Service, although frequently referred to as one body, was in fact run country by country with each colony having its own Medical Service, often with slightly different terms and conditions of Service. Transfers, even between geographically contiguous territories were difficult to manage administratively, as pensions or leave entitlement had to be re-calculated. One of the earliest attempts to remedy this problem occurred in 1902 with the establishment of the unified West African Medical Staff (WAMS). This initiative united the medical services of Nigeria, Gold Coast, Sierra Leone and Gambia together under the management of one regional governing body. This scheme was a response to recruitment problems for West Africa, which had a notoriously unhealthy reputation. It was a resounding success: appointments rose from 120 in 1905 to 170 in 1909. Indeed, the West African model became to be so highly revered that it was soon regarded as the template to which all Medical Services should aspire.[19] Despite this, the East African service continued in its old ways for nearly twenty years. Although the Tropical African Services Committee in 1910 and the Egerton Committee in 1919 considered the idea of creating a unified Service, it was regarded as rather premature. Pay scales and conditions of service among colonial servants were considered to be too variable from territory to territory. Moreover, the exigencies of World War One made moves towards greater unification increasingly difficult. Although the time was not ripe for the formation of a unified Colonial Medical Service, the Egerton Committee concluded that an East African Medical Service (EAMS) would be one of the best ways for enhancing Colonial Service prestige overall and, as a direct result of this enquiry, a united East African Medical Service was eventually created in 1921.[20] The committee also saw the need for centralised guidance for the medical services and suggested that a medical Director-General be appointed to oversee the regional services.[21] This came to fruition with the appointment of Thomas Stanton as the first Chief Medical Adviser to the Secretary of State in 1926.[22]

The real turning point in Colonial Service history, however, occurred in 1930 when the Warren Fisher Committee met to discuss all aspects of the Colonial Services including recruitment, training and structure. Medical Service recruitment was specifically affected (see Chapter 2), but it changed the face of the whole Service by establishing a single unified Colonial Service with different vocational branches.[23] The Colonial Administrative Service was first established in 1932; the Colonial Medical Service two years later. By 1949 there were twenty branches of the unified British Colonial Service, including: the Colonial Legal Service; the Colonial Police Service; the Colonial Administrative Service; the Colonial Veterinary Service, the Colonial Education Service and the Colonial Agricultural Service.[24]

Throughout the development of the Colonial Service the administration was working towards greater ideological unity and institutional uniformity. Great emphasis was put upon the merits of standardisation and this served to increasingly bind officers together and reinforce their professional similarities over and above their individual differences.[25] How these administrative developments towards centralisation were played out in the regions can be appreciated by considering the early development of the Colonial Medical Service in East Africa.

The Colonial Medical Service in East Africa

More Colonial Service entrants were posted to Africa than to any other colony, so the continent consistently took the majority of candidates entering government service overseas. The largest vocational group recruited into the Colonial Service in tropical Africa were Administrative Officers who represented British rule and order in the localities. Doctors were the second largest group. Although some had been to East Africa as individual pioneers, or with expedition parties, medicine as a colonial career in East Africa effectively began in 1888.[26] This was the year that the Imperial British East Africa Company (IBEAC), received its royal charter to trade in the region, bringing with it administrators, commercial managers, and the first government doctors to attend to the medical needs of British residents. Before the establishment of the Imperial British East Africa Company, the sparse European medical presence mainly consisted of missionaries. In particular, the base set up by the Church Missionary Society (CMS) at Mengo, Uganda, which was synonymous with the work of Albert and (to a lesser extent) Howard Cook, and became very important regionally.

The early government doctors worked for the Imperial British East Africa Company until the individual countries were officially incorporated into the British Empire. Uganda became a British Protectorate in 1893 and Kenya (British East Africa, East Africa Protectorate or after 1920, Kenya Colony) became a Colony in 1895. Both passed from Foreign Office to Colonial Office control in

1905. The mandate for Tanganyika Territory (modern-day Tanzania) was not granted until 1919 and was not effective until 1920 (it had been a German territory until the end of the war). With the formalisation of British government rule, in 1895, the Imperial British East Africa Company was officially disbanded and many company doctors made the smooth transition from company employment to government service. The doctors that participated in this transition — Archibald Mackinnon, James MacPherson, Walter MacDonald and Robert Moffat — became the first East African Colonial MOs.[27] Titles changed, as did accountability, but in general the transition from one organisational body to another was seamless. The Imperial British East Africa Company staff was supplemented by a few local recruits to the newly-formed Colonial Medical Service; for example, by William Ansorge who had arrived in Kampala in 1894, looking for work in the area.[28]

The new administration had only just formed when the region experienced a revolt among the Sudanese in Uganda. This war put great strains on the Medical Department during its formative years, creating an immediate need for more personnel and diverting energies to containing the rebellion, at the expense of longer-term medical policies. [29] By 1898, however, the uprising was largely suppressed and Robert Moffat was appointed as the first Principal Medical Officer (PMO) of Uganda. The medical administration of the region became divided along colonial borders between Moffat in Uganda and Walter MacDonald, an ex-Imperial British East Africa Company official, in charge of Kenya since 1895. During the early years of British rule the distinction between military and civil personnel, continued to be blurred. Military doctors had often been the first to lay the foundations of a medical infrastructure and in the transition to civil rule many simply transferred to civil posts. Some effectively had both civil and military obligations, but by the end of the first decade of the twentieth century military commands had almost completely receded in favour of civil rule.[30]

Another factor that changed the face of the country and also shaped the constitution of the early Colonial Medical Service was the building, between 1895 and 1901, of the Uganda railway that ran from Mombasa, Kenya to Port Florence, Uganda. The railway company had its own medical staff under a separate Principal Medical Officer (Dr Sieveking), but on completion of the railway in 1901 medical staff were absorbed into the Colonial Medical Service. Some Colonial Service doctors, including Drs Waters and Paget, came to the career via this route.[31]

Plainly, the early histories of the medical services in Kenya and Uganda were much intertwined. The Imperial British East Africa Company and the railway company had been responsible for both territories. Even when the countries were established as separate entities, the relationship between the two remained remarkably fluid. This sinuous association culminated in the formal amalgamation of the two medical departments under the guidance of a single Principal Medical Officer (Robert Moffat and then James Will) between 1903–8, with the headquarters and the sole regional laboratory in Nairobi.[32] The appointment of James Will in 1904 marked an important milestone in the organisational development of the Colonial Medical Service. Will had been originally seconded from the Royal Army Medical Corps (RAMC) where he had gained a broad experience in dealing with medical organisation. His successor, Dawson Milne, described him as a man who in the course of his short career 'did much to engender that spirit [sic.] de corps without which no administration can be a success.'[33] It was in 1904, for example, that the grading of senior ranks with differentiated emoluments began and the first important departmental structures where put into place. Under Will the post of Deputy Principal Medical Officer (DPMO) was instituted and he made the first inroads into public health administration by appointing a Medical Officer of Health (MOH) for the Port of Mombassa, thereby establishing the rudiments of an early sanitation branch.[34] During Will's tenure the first European Hospital was opened in Nairobi, plans for the first mental hospital were put in place, and the first laboratory facilities, dispensaries and native hospitals were opened. By the time he retired in 1909 the EAMS had rapidly grown, with a combined regional staff of 37 MOs, plus numerous support staff.[35] After 1908 the EAMS split once more into two distinct territorial medical services, each with characteristic ambitions and foci. Aubrey Hodges took the headship of the Uganda Medical Service in autumn of 1908 and Will continued administering the Kenyan branch until Arthur Milne succeeded to the position in 1909.

Since most of the early doctors came from the Imperial British East Africa Company background, it is unsurprising that the Colonial Medical Service initially continued the narrow Imperial British East Africa Company policy of providing healthcare exclusively for Europeans and their families in support of the burgeoning British infrastructure. The earliest Colonial MOs, to use the words of Michael Worboys, 'followed trade and the flag'.[36] This policy gradually widened to include the care of Africans working for Europeans and then to Africans in urban centres in general. It was not until after World War One that concerted policies were initiated to tackle the healthcare of African communities more generally.[37]

During this early period doctors provided a predominantly clinical service. Much less money was spent on preventive medicine or on investigation into epidemic or pandemic disease. Research and sanitary expeditions from metropolitan institutions concentrated accordingly upon economically important colonial towns and ports.[38] Consequently there was very little interest in healthcare in rural areas except in crisis situations when disease could affect the stability of the colonial regime, particularly through diminishing the productivity of its workforce. When wider campaigns were undertaken, such as those against sleeping sickness in Uganda (1901–14) or plague outbreaks in Kenya (intermittently between 1902 and 1913), they were crafted chiefly as responses to crisis, rather than the implementation of longer-term medical plans.

This type of medical administration largely occurred because, during the early years, the priority was the creation of an infrastructure. The first most important stage was the building of the Uganda railway, soon followed by the building of roads, the establishment of residential areas and the introduction of a telegraph and postal system.[39] Within the realm of medicine, hospitals, staff housing and early dispensaries all needed to be established, with early MOs often participating in their design and construction. A few early hospitals, such as the CMS Hospital at Mengo (1897), had been established by the missions, but in general it was a government concern to provide for and oversee the establishment of medical facilities.[40] Characteristically, European hospitals were usually founded before native ones and as a rule remained better equipped and serviced. During the first decade of British rule European hospitals were established at Mombasa, Entebbe and Nairobi.[41] In the earliest years the only stations with dispensaries in the entire region were the coastal townships of Mombassa, Malindi and Lamu (all trading centres of the Imperial British East Africa Company). The first native hospital was in Fort Hall, although others soon followed at Kisumu and Mombasa.[42]

When Tanzania became a British mandated territory in 1919 roads, government buildings and a telegraph system had already been established under German rule.[43] The first PMO, John Davey, could happily state that the British had 'inherited from the Germans some medical buildings which compare favourably with any in Tropical Africa.'[44] Hospitals, notably those at Tabora, Ocean Road and Sewa Haji, were already in existence. There was a relatively well-stocked laboratory, founded in 1897, where Robert Koch (1843–1910) had researched malaria, and a rudimentary public health programme in the form of a smallpox vaccination campaign and a health office.[45]

Over time the territories naturally developed their own medical agendas in line with local priorities. Each country was home to different indigenous peoples with their own cultures and customs; the geographical and economic features of each area were dramatically different. In Kenya the British presence seemed quite secure by the 1920s. The British government had backed schemes to encourage settlement through land grants in the country and, although plague outbursts were frequent and it suffered from endemic malaria, health risks were comparatively manageable. Indeed, the Kenyan highlands, were presented as an ideal location for British life, offering a land of opportunity for aspiring settlers.[46] In contrast, Uganda lacked widespread European settlement, and avoided the settler issues of Kenya. Uganda was, rather, characterised by a strong missionary presence that later formed into a nucleus of officials around Makerere. The establishment of tertiary education in the region arguably dominated all other considerations in the colony. A major shaper of health policy in Uganda was the hugely devastating sleeping sickness epidemic that occurred around the Northern shores of Lake Victoria between 1899 and 1905, killing around 250,000 people.[47] Following this devastating epidemic sleeping sickness controls continued to dominate the imperial agenda in Uganda throughout the colonial period.[48] Tanzania, where the European population was significantly reduced after the German defeat, had the smallest white community of the three countries under consideration. Moreover, the European inhabitants had less of a sense of permanence than their Kenyan and Ugandan counterparts precisely because it was a mandated territory rather than a direct British Colony with all the accoutrements of permanent rule. When Tanzania came under British control an eclectic mix of officers were drawn from all over the Empire and it took several years for the new medical administration to gel.[49] As a large mandated territory with considerably more isolated stations and widely dispersed officers the European community was more scattered than in Kenya or Uganda.

Despite regional differences, however, colonial life in British East Africa was established upon roughly similar lines and it is still possible to talk about the three countries as a united group. In 1924, several years after Tanzania joined the Empire, plans were revived to implement closer union between the three major

East African territories. Although these plans never came to fruition, parliamentary discussion over official closer union — strenuously supported by the Governor of Kenya, Sir Edward Grigg (1925–30) — continued until 1931.[50] The idea was attractive since Kenya, Tanzania and Uganda shared borders with Lake Victoria at their geographical centre. Mombassa acted as a port of entry to the whole region, and the Uganda railway served as a vital link for commerce and politics. After 1922 trade and interchange between these three countries was facilitated through the introduction of a common currency (the East African Shilling) in the region. By 1949 all three regions were further united under a joint High Commission that oversaw common services such as communications, posts and telegraphs and research.[51]

The organisation of medical provision in Kenya, Uganda and Tanzania developed along similar lines. The early years were characterised in Kenya and Uganda by the rather *ad hoc* establishment of the medical administration, concentrating particularly on carving out a presence in urban centres and providing healthcare mainly to the European officialdom. After the mandate had been awarded to the British to rule Tanzania (1919), serious reappraisal began. From the early 1920s moves were made to broaden medical care and to streamline the administrative channels through which it was managed. [52] The health of indigenous African communities moved further up the colonial agenda; colonial medical services were extended to rural areas, and schemes were initiated to train Africans as medical support staff. Bureaucracies were rationalized with more emphasis on the decentralisation of medical administration. Some responsibilities for public health and basic clinical medicine were delegated to native authorities, distancing central government from the minutiae of everyday affairs. Theoretically, this freed the headquarters from cumbersome routine bureaucracies and allowed them time to concentrate on the development of medical policies.[53] During this period both documentation and nomenclature of medical job titles were standardised for the first time and administrative procedures were reassessed. [54]

The impetus for this radical overhaul after World War One can be best understood as part of the prevailing political mood. In the 1920s colonial governments in East Africa began to reflect upon their relationship to the people they governed, and to draw up statements of the ideal considerations and responsibilities of a colonial government.[55] Although still self-serving and overbearingly colonial, with few concessions to local governance, a marked change in the rhetoric of colonialism was evident. East African colonial governments moved away from top-heavy European administration and began to favour systems of indirect rule as devised and practised by Sir Frederick Lugard (1858–1945) while High Commissioner in Nigeria (1900–07). This became the favoured model of British colonial governance, distinct from the French and Portuguese system of *administration directe* that aimed for the complete assimilation of colonial dependencies with the government systems of the ruling country.[56] As a means of implementing indirect rule within East Africa, the political administrations of Kenya, Uganda and Tanzania were divided up into regional blocks formally under the charge of British district administrators working in coordination with officially appointed native authorities. Demarcations of areas assigned to local control were made according to assumptions (subsequently found to be misinformed) that tribal affiliations were geographically fixed. Even the Kingdom of Buganda in Uganda Protectorate, which had traditionally had a 'special' relationship with its British masters, became assimilated into this idealised model of indirect governance after World War One. [57] Tanzania presented in some ways the most difficult case. German rule had divided Tanzania (Deutsches Ost Afrika) into administrative divisions called *akidas*, but rather than use these existing district divisions as the template for their own version of indirect rule, the British (reflecting a nationalistic, anti-German agenda) sought to reorganise local government in ways supposedly reflective of earlier 'natural' tribal boundaries. The result paid no heed to government systems that local people had become accustomed to under German rule and imposed new tribal delineations that took no account of a rapidly emergent complex series of Tanzanian identities.[58]

The organisation of medical services after 1920 followed the pattern of the political reorganisation of district administration. The increased reliance indirect rule put upon native authorities was reflected within the medical sphere, with Native Authority Ordinances stipulating their responsibilities for the supervision, regulation and funding of health in each locality. This was partially a pragmatic response since the ever expanding European populations of the three countries demanded an effectively organised health infrastructure, but it was also a reaction to the increased scrutiny colonial medical departments underwent after the First World War to provide healthcare facilities to Africans.

Although health emergencies and long-term priorities differed between the three territories, similarities in the general trajectory of medical development can be easily discerned. The East African region presented a comprehensive administrative unit: the same British government body ran the Colonial Service throughout Empire and the structures of all medical departments were broadly uniform. All Service positions were filled through the same recruitment procedure and there is evidence that, even during the early period, the colonies were regarded in official mentality as existing in uniform regional blocks. [59] Even before the official moves towards closer unification, when arranging transfers could be administratively awkward, officers were often moved, especially between contiguous colonies. The importance of the career as a binding agent was something that official pronouncements increasingly emphasised, especially after the recommendations of the Warren Fisher Committee. In July 1930 the Secretary of State, Lord Passfield (1859–1931) acknowledged that the government could not 'help the diversities of climate and local conditions' but declared that the government would do as much as it could to foster homogeneity under the umbrella of the Colonial Service.[60]

The colonial medical career unified individuals more than it divided them. This book will describe how this unification went beyond the institutional and will illustrate how Colonial MOs enrolled in a lifestyle that tacitly and explicitly embraced common attitudes and behaviours. This analysis acknowledges the way Empire was culturally understood at the time. However crudely generalised the assumption may seem today, before World War Two Empire was popularly and officially seen as a single entity, or at the very least a series of regional blocks (East Africa, West Africa, the Far East). The Empire was a manifestation of British rule and British pride rather than a series of different countries with individual characters, both from the perspective of the people taking part in the imperial adventure and the British public they left at home.

The Colonial Service and Colonial Identity

There has been relatively little written on the Colonial Service and virtually nothing specifically on the Colonial Medical Service.[61] When studies have considered the government medical cadres specifically they have typically touched upon their wider imperial mission, with little or no consideration of their constitution and character.[62] This is surprising as the Colonial Medical Service, after the Colonial Administrative Service, was the second largest recruiter of men to the Colonial Service. While Harrison and Crawford have specifically profiled the cohort of the Indian Medical Service (IMS), there is a conspicuous silence over their counterparts in Africa.[63]

Of direct relevance to this study are the works of Ann Beck, who between 1962 and 1981 contributed the largest academic analysis of the medical administration of Kenya, Tanzania and Uganda during the colonial period in two monographs and several journal articles.[64] Writing shortly after colonialism had crumbled in the region, Beck's historical examination described a linear trajectory of gradual medical improvements towards the eventual achievement of a mainly propitious medical situation in British East Africa.[65] The doctors she described were largely depicted (when described at all) as having chosen to work in Africa through genuine altruism or missionary-type zeal and there was little examination of the broader factors that may have informed their decisions and moulded their subsequent attitudes.[66] Although a useful starting point for British medical policy in East Africa, Beck's aims are rather different those presented by this study. This research concentrates upon the Medical Service personnel themselves, the sorts of experiences they had and the cultural standards they embodied.

Through highlighting questions of culture in colonial history, this book necessarily relies on a familiar post-colonial literature that explores whether group identities were created by the peculiarities of the colonial situation, or whether they were primarily replications of familiar, traditional cultures back home.[67] Eric Hobsbawn and Terence Ranger have argued for a nuanced understanding of colonial identity, one that borrows from the home context as well as inventing traditions to fit the new one.[68] The imperial subject, dislocated from a familiar home milieu, imported to his new social, cultural, political and economic space communal presumptions and expectations that were adapted to the specificities of the colonial context. These were ritualised in turn through collective behaviour that both confirmed and extended group loyalties while simultaneously differentiating them from other groups, particularly indigenous ones. Furthermore, as Ranger has argued, colonial neo-traditional behaviour in Africa not only helped to define European relationships with the colonised, but was actively used by some African peoples to capitalise on the colonial situation for their own ends.[69] Traditions were invented by all sectors of colonial society as a means of confirming and extending collective identities.

These arguments, and others, stress how the political peculiarities of Empire brought about the development of widely dispersed micro-communities, all with joined allegiance to the British crown and core (albeit remoulded) British values.[70] At the same time, other important works have placed more emphasis on ubiquitous images of exoticism and difference in the creation of imperial identities.[71] From this perspective, conceptions of colonial identity have relied heavily upon prevailing public enthusiasm for exotic images, particularly in travelling writing, colonial literature and journalism.[72] The Colonial Office utilised precisely these popular associations to stimulate recruitment to Empire careers (see Chapters 2 and 3). In important ways the popular paradigms of colonialism can be seen as self-fulfilling prophesies of what the colonial identity constituted during different times. The Colonial Office recruited a type; that type had certain common expectations (because they were selected using the same criteria) that in turn informed the wider colonial communities of which they were a part. Accordingly, the shared identities of Colonial MOs could be seen as intimately tied to popular conceptions of public servants and the colonial lifestyle they were expected to lead.[73] Furthermore, as Felix Driver has argued, the European in Africa attained great popular status because of the growing significance accorded to colonially-acquired expertise and knowledge attained through fieldwork and first-hand observation. These associations lent important cultural value to research in the exotic locations of Empire, notably for the furthering of modern metropolitan (in Driver's case, geographical; in this case, medical) knowledge.[74]

Complementing studies that rationalise and contextualise the reasons for, and constitution of, colonial identity, are detailed descriptions of colonial communities themselves. These are usually presented as a hybrid of exaggerated Britishness and specifically colonial exoticism. Some accounts have scrutinized the Colonial Office mindset in the moulding of London-based policies or the shared perspectives of Colonial Office employees.[75] Other historians such as Alex McKay and Henrika Kuklick have analysed specifically the careers of public servants, emphasising the influential factors of time and place in the development of close-knit colonial cadres.[76]

Another important contribution that emphasises the importance of local context over external factors is that of Dane Kennedy. Kennedy has presented a subtle picture of the 'conformity of values and unanimity of purpose' espoused by the people that made up Kenyan and Rhodesian settler societies.[77] The cultural communities that Kennedy described were the natural outcome of the negotiation of ideas between the colony and the metropolis. These were not only influenced by broader political obligations and theories of imperialism, but were also created locally in response to proximately gathered opinions and evidence. Rather than ideas being pure replicas, or exaggerations, of Britishness, home-grown values were often bent and even drastically distorted to present a homogenous colonial identity: an identity, moreover, that was articulated defensively precisely because it was associated with a demographic and racial minority.[78]

One of the pleasures of Kennedy's work is the way it presents medical discourses — notably those about climate — as revealing of the preoccupations and anxieties of settler society in general.[79] Somatic and psychological models of tropical health presented ideas that were anachronistic in the home setting (e.g.

acclimatization theories), but unified people behind a justifiable orthodoxy in the colonial one. This constituted what Kennedy termed a 'common culture'; one that was locally derived and which superseded other broader differences within colonial society. [80]

While Kennedy has argued for the endurance of nineteenth-century ideas of acclimatisation in the colonial context, other authors have argued that medical and scientific modernity (particularly the wonders of tropical medical) were used to define colonial communities and those they ruled. Several important works present imperial medicine as defining itself through modern 'rationality' and 'objectivity' as opposed to the superstition that was thought to dominate the 'primitive', non-scientific, indigenous cultures. Megan Vaughan has examined the way western medicine influenced images of the African. She has concluded that one important non-variable, in an otherwise constantly shifting cultural and political landscape, was the over-riding idea of 'difference' that ultimately defined European-African encounters. The African was reduced to a pathological specimen, a creature of disease and dirt.[81] Interestingly, Vaughan also looked at popular images of European doctors in Africa, particularly the way the image of the hero-doctor further demarcated the relationship between British and African people.[82]

These academic debates, and others, have sought to rationalise how a colonial identity could be created. The principal question is whether these common defining features were chiefly a means of self-definition or rather a means of defining the uncivilised 'other'. Were the specific medical manifestations of colonialism as much about the sustainment of old traditions as the celebration of new ones? Were new values inculcated as much to replicate home as they were to define a new location? To what extent did allegiance to colonial identities discipline the actions of individual subjects? These and similar questions provide a basis for a fresh evaluation of colonial medical identities. Seemingly ambiguous strands can be drawn together to form a balanced understanding of apparently conflicting determinants. Considerations of tradition and modernity, self-definition and the definition of others, reveal the group's strengths as well as weaknesses. As many historians have pointed out, the creation of colonial medical identities allowed the legitimisation of whiteness in historically non-white places.[83] At the same time, identities were subtle local negotiations between colonised and coloniser: far more complex than just an imposition of arbitrary values from above.[84]

Adding to this rich intellectual tradition of secondary analyses are images derived from the sources themselves. Memoirs, diaries, even obituaries, relate familiar experiences from which ideas of shared collective perception and self-identity can be gleaned. Accounts of African careers show surprisingly uniform notions of colonial life in general and the colonial medical endeavour specifically. Such ideas were self-perpetuating. Narratives were written in such a way as to fulfil prescriptive expectations of what being a good colonial entailed.[85] This was not merely mythmaking; certain motifs were repeatedly drawn upon because they were precisely what a reading public would want to hear. Particular images were so intimately associated with colonial life that they were regarded as imperative to the construction of an interesting account. Of course, not all colonial accounts consciously followed a script, but most emphasised certain aspects over others and used metaphors evoking an imagined idea of Africa.[86] This concept was as much about the realities of geography as about the identity that the British were creating for themselves in Africa. Moreover, the shared themes of colonial careers were vividly realistic descriptions of communal experiences that were central to creating certain attitudes. Colonial doctors wrote about similar things because they experienced similar things and because they came from shared backgrounds. Furthermore, the career became imbued with nostalgic overtones, especially after the collapse of the British African Empire during the 1960s.[87]

This book considers what type of candidate entered the Colonial Medical Service, suggests their motives and examines their subsequent experiences. While the trends and tables present an accurate profile of colonial medical personnel, other claims, especially surrounding the ways doctors looked at their work and career, are more impressionistic. In describing group motivations and identities there is always the danger of clouding the subtleties and idiosyncrasies of individual incentives, opinions and sometimes facts in misleading generalities. The findings presented within these following pages should therefore not be taken as definitively representative of unanimous and collective opinion, but rather to reflect one cultural historical aspect of a wider story. Regrettably, but typically, most available information comes from the elites who left evidence in the form of memoirs or had obituaries written of them. Some of the longest-serving officers left almost no historical traces: often nothing more than a name, departmental position and sometimes date of appointment within the *Colonial Office Lists*. These doctors, who represented the regular public face of health care, would have served thousands of people but left no memoirs.

A potential pitfall of a study of this type is that it examines the work and roles of a group who can, without much difficulty, be retrospectively identified as embodying the racist ideologies and presumptions typical of the colonial era. The modern-day postcolonial spirit naturally influences approaches within history and prevailing attitudes often emphasise the Service's negative, oppressive, or at the very least, exclusionary, aspects. The ideal balance is a challenging one to achieve: to make fair assessment of the work of those that went abroad in the service of Empire without condoning colonialism and all its attendant baggage. This study attempts to represent a body of professionals and makes no judgments over whether their attitudes, opinions and preconceptions were intrinsically 'right' or 'wrong'. Rather, it considers this historical culture in the same light as anthropological studies treat their subjects.

Chapter 2: Recruitment into the Colonial Medical Service

We want good men, but not Oslers or Treves.[1]

This chapter describes the bureaucratic recruitment processes to the Colonial Service in general and the Colonial Medical Service specifically. Its purpose is to explain the administrative context of this first stage of the colonial medical experience by revealing the processes that applicants had to undergo and the terms under which they were employed. This description will provide a framework for subsequent discussion of the reasons for joining the Service (Chapters 4 and 5), the 'reality' of colonial medical experience (Chapters 6 and 7) and the shared experiences, inherent in the Medical Service identity (Chapters 8 and 9).

An analysis of recruitment helps to situate the significance of choosing the appropriate colonial servant. It was extremely important to select the proper candidate, as these personnel were the direct representatives of the British Government in the localities — the man on the spot (and it was normally a man) had to epitomise the values of the ruling country whilst also getting on with valuable work for the Empire. In the first section, the relative status of the Colonial Service as a professional choice is described. It focuses upon the way interested people could obtain information about possible vacancies and on how the Colonial Office managed the recruitment process. General application and selection systems and criteria were routinely applied to all branches of the Colonial Service, so it is important to understand this common context to grasp the fundamental tenets of medical recruitment. The way medical recruitment specifically differed from this broad model is analysed in more detail in the second section. Lastly, this chapter then goes on to explain the rules and regulations under which the Colonial Medical Service doctors were employed in East Africa. This will help to frame subsequent consideration of the career's (perceived and real) advantages and disadvantages. This encompasses the official constraints on practice that doctors in the field needed to negotiate both individually and collectively.

Recruitment into the Colonial Service

The Colonial Service benefited and suffered from its prestigious connection with other Government Services. On one hand, its reputation was inextricably bound to the high-status perceptions of the Foreign Service, the Home Office Service and the Indian Civil Service as worthy and highly respected career choices for young graduates. On the other hand, it was commonly regarded, particularly until the 1930s, as a somewhat poor relation. Much of this bad press was because it was a comparatively new public service lacking a centralised bureaucracy. Before 1905, when the responsibility for many Colonial territories was moved from the Foreign Office to the Colonial Office, the Colonial Empire's staff were decentralised and non-uniform; in the candid words of one medical observer it was, administratively speaking, 'in a muddle'.[2]

Added to these organisational problems was the small size of the Service. Recruitment opportunities were fairly rare and, when vacancies did occur they were considered poorly paid. Furthermore, selection was conducted by interview, with its associations with patronage and informal influence, rather than through the competitive examinations instituted for entry into the Indian or Home Services. This made the Colonial Services relatively unattractive to first-rate candidates fresh out of university. Without overplaying this point — the career still held many prestigious nuances through its association with the government and politics — the image of a 'small and haphazard' Service, especially during the first twenty-five years of the twentieth century; was pervasive enough to cause governmental concern.[3]

A markedly defined hierarchy of eminence existed among public service careers abroad. The most elite services included the Sudan Political Service and the Indian Civil Service and the man in charge of Colonial Service recruitment, (later Sir) Ralph Furse, spent most of his professional energies in nurturing a similar *corps d'élite* in the Colonial Service.[4] Furse's Colonial Office career spanned more than three decades (1910–48) and he was indubitably the single most important figure in terms of raising the profile of, and organising, Colonial Service recruitment. He was himself a patronage appointment — his own job interview had only lasted ten minutes — a stalwart Tory who had attended public school and then read classics for a third-class degree at Oxford.[5] In many ways his values represented the most traditional and the conservative elements of society and can be seen to be both the symptom and the cause of the prevailing Colonial Service ethos.[6] His most notable achievement was the Warren Fisher Committee (1930) which was called for by the then Secretary of State Leo Amery '[l]argely as a result of Furse's representations' at the end of the 1920s.[7] This important Committee examined the question of Colonial Service recruitment in detail with an aim of streamlining and centralising the previously cumbersome procedures. It marked the beginning of bureaucratic modernisation within Colonial Service recruitment; unifying the various branches into vocational groups, with standardised conditions of service and more opportunities for inter-territorial transfers. The hope was that the Service would acquire a more international and unified ethos. As a direct result of the Committee appointments were overseen by a central Appointments Board, which was part of a newly established Personnel Division. Furse handled recruitment and training, and Charles Jeffries (1896–1972) was in charge of conditions of service and promotions.[8]

Before these reforms the system of recruitment was based on patronage — a selection system that had been in existence since the beginning of the Colonial Service in the 1830s. Candidates were selected through a system of 'introductions', usually by a friend or relative who was known to the Colonial Office; any candidate who was then deemed suitable was subsequently 'invited' to apply for a position.[9] By the inter-war period, however, when Colonial Service recruitment problems necessitated widening the recruitment base to encourage more middle-class candidates, patronage became recast as increasingly old fashioned, unfair and untenable. By the 1920s, a warning against any attempt to exert personal influence over any part of the selection procedure was routinely published in the official recruitment literature, advising that any evidence of a candidate interfering with a selection decision may 'seriously prejudice his chances of success.'[10] Although Colonial Office rhetoric increasingly distanced itself from patronage the system was not formally abolished until the implementation of the recommendations of the Warren Fisher Committee. Despite attempts by Furse to minimise his department's associations with patronage, the Committee felt obliged to conclude that up until that point the system of Colonial Service recruitment had been 'at any rate in theory, a system of patronage.'[11] It is easy to extend this argument even further. Furse himself reminisced that Colonial Service recruitment was run primarily through a system of 'personal contacts' throughout his tenure, which ended in 1948.[12] Furse actively controlled the markets in which the Service career was promoted and placed official liaison officers in favoured universities. He organised visits to suitable (i.e. public and sometimes top grammar) schools to stimulate recruitment, rather than push towards entirely open and meritocratic selection processes for all, regardless of educational background or social standing.

In accordance with this tradition, the Colonial Service rarely advertised positions; indeed it was thought that to do so would cheapen its appearance. The Service relied on its reputation and on an informal network of recommendations and hearsay, to stimulate interest.[13] There were several ways, however, that interested people could obtain information about the Colonial Service. During the early years of the twentieth century, the annually published *Colonial Office List* was an obvious first port of call. As well as including detailed historical and statistical information on each of the territories to allow prospective candidates to get a feel for the job, it published related parliamentary papers and information about major, historical and current, colonial developments. Each volume included a copy of the most recent colonial regulations (also obtainable as a separate publication) as well as a section offering information to prospective candidates called 'Information as to Colonial Appointments'.

A prospective applicant could apply for further information from the Colonial Office, who issued a series of slim pamphlets, outlining extended guidelines for appointment.[14] Many of the original versions of this literature are extremely rare and difficult to locate, but there is evidence that this modest marketing exercise was in existence as early as the last decade of the nineteenth century.[15] Interestingly, the titles of these pamphlets reveal that, even during the first few years of the twentieth century when Britain was still coming to grips with her newly acquired territories, there was a sense of the Colonial Empire staff being managed in broad vocational and regional groupings. Geographically, the colonially administered Empire was seen as being divided into (in the loosely accepted order of superiority) the Eastern, West African, East African, West Indian and Western Pacific Services.[16]

The colonial personnel of each territory were funded internally from that government's funds; recommendations over staffing needs were therefore usually made from within each colony. Governors would fill out a vacancy request form and through this would inform the Secretary of State of the staffing needs of their country.[17] In the early formative years, Governors would often recommend the establishment of new positions as well as requesting candidates for current ones. After Colonial Service unification frequently revised staffing schedules were created that listed the names of all staff positions in each dependency. Staffing needs were, technically at least, tied to the filling and refilling of these core positions.[18] In principle, the Secretary of State had to approve all appointments, except those at the very lowest end of the Colonial Service where candidates were recruited locally and were hired on salaries of less than one hundred pounds a year.[19] In practice most lower (i.e. almost exclusively non-European) appointments made by the Governor were merely rubber-stamped by the Secretary of State. In exceptional instances, especially in times of severe staff shortages, local European candidates could be appointed on a temporary basis by the Governor of the Colony or Protectorate. These temporary appointments were, however, then to be subsequently applied for via the usual application form and confirmed centrally by the Secretary of State for 'fuller investigation than may be possible to the Governor' before the position could be made permanent.[20] Europeans were seldom appointed in this way: it was considered more desirable that local applicants return to the United Kingdom and apply through the normal procedures instituted in London.[21]

Selections to the Colonial Administrative Service and to Services where professional qualifications were required (such as the Medical, Legal, Accounting or Scientific Services) were made through application and then interview through the Colonial Office in London. For posts in Ceylon, Hong Kong, the Straits Settlements and the Federated Malay Straits, cadetships offering on-the-job training for civil administrative posts within the colonies were available to young British subjects.[22]

Applicants not wishing to apply through one of the cadetship schemes — including all administrative and medical appointments — had to submit an application form (P1), obtainable from the Colonial Office, outlining their career history and qualifications as well as their preferences for colonial employment.[23] They also had to submit six copies of testimonials covering all stages of their educational and professional career as well as names of at least two referees who could vouch for their 'character and capacity'.[24] At this stage the Colonial Office would often make 'further enquiries' as well as obtaining references.[25] If assessed as suitable, candidates were called for an interview, usually conducted by one of the Assistant Private Secretaries (later, a member of the recruitment department), but sometimes, in the case of specialist appointments, by regularly meeting panels of relevant subject experts.[26] On successfully passing this stage of the application procedure, the candidate's name was then put onto the colonial vacancy list, along with the class of employment for which they were thought suitable. The Colonial Office was at pains to stress, however, that 'no definite prospect whatever can be held out' that a place on this list would lead to the offer of a colonial posting.[27] Candidates were instead encouraged to pursue other employment in the knowledge that, were they fortunate enough to be offered a post, the Colonial Office would contact them and allow time for them to work out their notice. This system which could not guarantee a position even after selection by interview further damaged the career's reputation, in that it failed to hook good candidates before they were offered alternative employment elsewhere.

In the period before 1930 the entire application process was overseen by the Assistant Private Secretaries (Appointments), of which there were two after 1910. They were directly responsible to the Secretary of State and, theoretically if not actually, presented all recommendations for selection to him.[28] After 1930 this same recruitment procedure was overseen by the Director of Recruitment (Colonial Service), who chaired the monthly meetings of the Colonial Service Appointments Board.[29] It was during this period, that stronger links were forged with the British Universities as part of Furse's project to improve the profile of the Colonial Service career among graduates.[30] One practical result was the reduction in 1925 of the minimum entry age for all candidates destined for tropical Africa from twenty two to twenty one and a half; a small change which meant that graduates could start their colonial career straight, or very soon, after finishing university.[31] Another change introduced later in the 1930s was the imposition of definite deadlines upon the application procedure for many branches of the Service, thereby aligning start dates with the university calendar. Vacancies for the Colonial Administrative Service, for example, were to be applied for between 1st January and 30th April, with selections usually made after the academic year had ended in July or August. It was hoped that the opportunity of securing a career almost immediately after graduation would encourage applications.[32] From an early date, Furse encouraged the active involvement of university-based appointments committees in putting forward suitable candidates. This was part of a promotional programme for the Colonial Service throughout the universities, particularly Furse's approved universities: Oxford, Cambridge and London.[33] By 1936 appointments committees based at these universities were formally stipulated as the most useful first port of call for graduates, even before they contacted the Director of Recruitment.[34]

Although candidates from the Dominions were theoretically eligible to take up Colonial Service positions, feelers were put out during the 1920s to make the career path more widely advertised and accessible to them. Previously, these potential entrants had to conduct their applications long-distance and could have been interviewed only if they had happened to be in England or had travelled there especially.[35] Naturally, physical distance combined with an ever-growing sense of independence from the mother country meant that applications from this group were rare, not least because of the difficulty of quickly obtaining information. To improve things Furse appointed contacts within universities in the Dominions. These liaison officers promoted the career and put forward suitable candidates to a central Appointments Board rather than having to send them to London. The first of these was set up in Canada in 1922 (operational in 1923). Others soon followed in Australia and New Zealand. Notably (and perhaps reflecting a concern to keep Colonial Service management fundamentally British), all recommendations of the Appointments Boards were still formally subject to the approval of the Secretary of State in London.[36]

Gradually, formal courses were established to give special training for those selected for colonial appointments, usually to be attended before the official start of the contract. Specific tropical medical training was given for Colonial MOs from 1899, a decade before a specialised training course was offered for entrants to the Colonial Administrative Service.[37] Specialised courses and scholarship schemes were later set up for some other services; schemes initiated by Furse as part of his effort to revive the profile and value of entrance to the Colonial Service. [38]

Entry Criteria

Certain restrictions upon entrance into the Colonial Service were enforced routinely. First and foremost candidates had to be naturalised British citizens, providing proof of their status through submitting their birth certificate (or a certified copy) early on in the application procedure.[39] Exceptionally, some lower-level vacancies were filled locally, by non-British candidates. MO positions in the West Indies, or some administrative positions in Malta, were open to non-Europeans, but the candidates had to have received all or part of their education in Britain.

The minimum age limit for most posts was 22.[40] A university degree was virtually essential.[41] After World War One, it became obligatory for all applicants to have served, providing they were of suitable age, in the war effort, as it was not thought appropriate that someone who had not been able to serve their country in a military capacity should do so in a civil one.[42] Although there was never an explicit ban on appointing women to the Colonial Service, most appointments throughout the period were of men. Women were increasingly considered as potential applicants as time progressed, but they were generally limited to fields considered specific to their gender, such as education, secretarial work, nursing and child health. In the early years the Colonial Office specified the undesirability of appointing married men to the Colonial Service. This was modified in 1920 to a statement that although married candidates had to obtain special permission from the Secretary of State if they wished to take their wife with them, particularly on a posting to tropical Africa, which was considered unsuitable for women.[43]

Candidates could express a preference on place of posting, but the Colonial Office reserved the right to appoint people as staffing needs required. Some places were naturally considered more desirable than others. West Africa presented perhaps the most mixed bag. On one hand, the governance systems and bureaucratic structures were more established and organised because of the longer

British presence in the region, yet on the other, it was the most dangerous place to go in terms of health. Because of this reputation, appointees in West Africa received a higher rate of pay than colleagues in the East of the continent. West African appointments also enjoyed many 'special privileges in respect of leave, absence and pension…on account of the unhealthiness of the climate'.[44] Once an officer had undertaken a posting in West Africa, it was made clear that a transfer was unlikely: Later editions of the 'Information as to Colonial Appointments' stipulated that 'no applications for transfer can be entertained until an officer has served for five years in West Africa.'[45]

In summary, the Colonial Service clearly experienced prestige problems in the period leading up to the First World War. In an attempt to amend this, Furse improved communications with the leading universities and created contacts in the Dominions to make the career more accessible to a broader range of people. Specialised training courses were also initiated in an attempt to foster institutional identity early on and to provide skills relevant to the tropical world.

Throughout the period the Colonial Service remained true to its meritocratic principles: a tenured career path for gentlemen, to be entered at a junior level with fixed steps towards promotion. Although prominent outsiders were sometimes appointed to the most prestigious positions, it was more common for officers to work their way up the Colonial Service career ladder.[46] Most strikingly, even after the setting up of the Colonial Service Appointments Board on the recommendation of the Warren Fisher Committee, many of the core mechanisms of application and appointment remained virtually unchanged. The most conspicuous shift was one of emphasis. Before 1930, discourses about the Colonial Service were very regional in their descriptions of the separate and individual public services; after the Warren Fisher Committee (and in accordance with its intention) stress was placed upon unifying factors rather than on any differences. This in turn had positive effects on the status of the career in the popular imagination. By 1939 the Colonial Service was presented as a single, integrated entity offering an attractive opportunity to work within one of its many unified branches in a stable, flexible, varied and rewarding career.

Recruitment into the Colonial Medical Service

Medical appointments were outlined in detail within Colonial Office memoranda produced for potential candidates and available upon request from the Assistant Private Secretary (Appointments), later the Director of Recruitment. Most relevant in terms of East African recruitment were *Miscellaneous No. 99: Medical Appointments in the Colonies (except West Africa)*; and *African (East) No.1103, Regulations for the East African Medical Service*. These were usually revised and updated annually, but less frequently during the 1930s. After 1930 all colonial memoranda were heavily revised and a new, simpler numbering system was introduced to reflect the clearer-cut, modern systems of the new Appointment's Branch. *Miscellaneous No.99*, for example, reappeared in 1931 as *Colonial Service Recruitment No.3A* [Later 3]. A fundamental format which was retained after Medical Service unification in 1934.

The Colonial Medical Service was promoted each September, in the educational number of the *BMJ*. This consisted of an article explaining opportunities for, and types of, employment. In accordance with the Colonial Office preference not to advertise, it was only during times of recruitment shortage, as in the late 1930s, that further advertisements were placed in the *BMJ* and *Lancet*.[47]

From the mid-1920s, further interest in the Medical Service as a career was stimulated through promotional visits by Colonial Office employees to British medical schools, especially through contacts with the Deans, but also through lectures to medical students.[48] One tactic was to invite officers to return to their former medical schools to give short lectures on their colonial experiences.[49] The practice of 'direct communication' with the medical schools was considered so successful, that in 1931 it was suggested that liaison officers be permanently appointed (as at Oxford and Cambridge Universities).[50]

From the beginning of the century until 1930 official publications emphasised the separate territorial medical staffs as distinct groups with their own rules and regulations. Accordingly, official Colonial Office literature stressed that transfers between the geographical areas were usually only offered at senior levels. Two exceptions were the West African Medical Service and the medical staff of the Straits Settlements and the Malay States. Both these had been traditionally presented as single, self-contained, Services with a higher level of regional integration that offered more systematic promotion schemes, regularised pay scales and opportunities for inter-territorial transfer within the group.[51] The West African Medical Service, established as a single service in 1902, particularly was upheld, even in the earliest days of its existence, as the model Medical Service. 'A properly organized entity' that the other medical services could benefit from emulating.[52] Even though the East African Medical Service was not formally run as one regional service until 1921, it had long been regarded in the colonial administrative mentality as a single entity. Early Colonial Service staff lists, for example, listed the Eastern African areas together as one unit, and officers saw themselves in terms of this regional identity.[53]

Just as there was a hierarchy within the colonial civil services, there was one within the medical services, which, despite the necessary professional qualifications of their candidates, fell some way behind the prestigious civil services in terms of status. Heather Bell has persuasively argued for the pre-eminence of the Sudan Medical Service as the one offering the best terms and conditions of employment at the beginning of the twentieth century, as well as benefiting from its associations with its famously elite sister Service, the Sudan Political Service.[54] The Indian Medical Service came a close second, and although its reputation waned from the end of the nineteenth century, it had a long and distinguished history. It was difficult to get into, boasted several famous medical researchers, and enjoyed close ties with the prestigious Indian Civil Service.[55] The West African Medical Service was probably the next most prestigious. Despite the unhealthiness of the West African climate the West African Medical Service was a model of professional organisation with a relatively attractive remuneration package. The East African Medical Service lagged behind as a fourth-class option.[56] The attraction of the Colonial Service career from the perspective of applicants will be discussed in Chapters 4 and 5. It is worth reiterating, however, that once an applicant had decided to apply for a Colonial Service position, rather than an Indian or Sudanese position (both which required taking a further examination), no guarantee could be given as to which region the applicant would be appointed. Applications for all territories were dealt with centrally and positions were filled as they became available.

It is difficult to assess how hard it was to get into the Colonial Medical Service, not least because the comparative numbers of enquiries, interviews and resulting appointments are unknown.[57] There was certainly a perception that it was a good thing to try for if all other attempts to get work in Britain had failed, but recruitment uptake naturally varied depending on colonial staffing needs. Figures surviving for the five-year period 1924–29, suggest, 'approximately 1 out of every 4 men, whose applications receive definite consideration, gets an appointment'.[58] A 1931 report stated: 'In the last year or two the fact that the large majority of MOs who make application are eventually appointed is an indication that there is now a general impression that the Service requires only well qualified and experienced officers'.[59] This period was a boom period for both general Colonial Service and Colonial Medical Service recruitment, so it is hard to assess how this compares with depressed periods of staffing, when presumably it was easier to be appointed.

The general pattern of recruitment to the Colonial Medical Service followed that of the Colonial Service (outlined above). The candidate had to fill out a slightly different application form, a P1 (Med), rather than the standard P1. This contained additional questions about medical experience, details of prizes and distinctions, contributions to the medical literature, and a history of the candidate's clinical appointments. It was also explicitly stipulated that one of the testimonials to be supplied should be from the Dean of the medical school at which the candidate was educated.[60]

Submission of colonial medical applications were originally called for in April of each year, but by the early 1900s this policy changed and it was decided that colonial appointments could be applied for at any time of the year and filled as circumstances required. [61] After the appointment of Sir Thomas Stanton as the first Chief Medical Adviser to the Colonial Office in 1926, suitable applications were vetted by his office, as well as being assessed through interview by the Colonial Medical Appointments Committee which met twice monthly.[62]

The criteria for eligibility changed very little throughout the period. In the very early years it was specified that medical candidates should be 'between the ages of 23 and 30 (25 and 32 in the case of West African appointments)',[63] a rule that was later extended by increasing the upper limit for all Medical Service positions to thirty-five.[64] Later entry requirements were simply framed as 'under 35 years of age' although 'definite preference' was given to applicants under thirty.[65] In East Africa there was a scheme whereby older, more experienced, candidates could apply to the Colonial Medical Service. These appointments were made for a fixed period of thirty months residential service and were paid at £700 per annum; [66] they were offered only on a temporary basis and without any pension rights.[67] This scheme under which several MOs were employed, appears to have been abolished by 1930.[68] The average age of entry into the Colonial

Medical Service in East Africa from 1893–1939 was 30 years, quite young considering the figure is inflated by the higher ages of officers who entered the career on a temporary basis in their forties. As with the Colonial Service in general, another unwavering criterion was nationality: applicants to the Medical Service were ineligible unless they provided proof of British citizenship.[69] For some services, including the West African Medical Service, they had furthermore to be of European parentage on both sides. Although this specification was not formally stated for the East African Medical Service until 1925, the policy was effectively already in operation.[70] It was always tacitly understood that Colonial Office officials were to refuse non-European candidates, although, in the interests of keeping the policy discrete they were 'not to base their non-selection on racial grounds if candidates ask why they have not been selected'.[71] The application form requested not only the candidate's birthplace and nationality, but also that of both parents. This information was plainly important, as the applicant's referees were specifically asked to confirm (to the best of their knowledge) the nationality of not only the applicant but of their father too.[72]

Ideally, and in contrast to the Colonial Administrative Service, the Medical Service did not want candidates fresh out of university. It was preferable that candidates should have gained a couple of years' practical experience as house physicians or house surgeons.[73] This was justified in terms of the particularly trying experiences young doctors might meet in the colonies where: 'a quite junior officer may often be placed in the position of having to deal with serious emergencies on his own responsibility, without the opportunity of consultation'.[74] By the 1930s more mature candidates with special skills were being actively sought: those who had public health experience or 'special knowledge of anaesthetics, radiology, surgery, medicine, ophthalmology, gynaecology and midwifery, diseases of the ear, nose, and throat, venereal diseases, etc.'.[75]

As far as basic medical qualifications went, applicants were required to have passed their qualifying exams in both medicine and surgery.[76] This ordinarily meant the joint bachelor's degree awarded from a British university, or the double qualification (the conjoint) of the English, Irish or Scottish professional corporations.[77] Initially it was not specified that all candidates were to be registered in the United Kingdom under the terms of the 1858 Medical Act, so theoretically British subjects who had obtained their medical qualifications overseas, could apply. When the unified Colonial Medical Service was officially created in 1934, however, these rules tightened. It was decided that all new entrants must possess a British qualification, although those already in the Medical Service without qualifications registered in the United Kingdom would not be penalised.[78] No provision had been made for British or foreign subjects who had obtained medical qualifications abroad until the [Medical Act] Amending Act of 1886, but reciprocity with all the larger Colonies (now Dominions) was established by 1902.[79]

Finally, the medical positions were mostly available to men. This partly reflected the gender ratio output of medical schools, but also the perception that Africa, in particular, was largely unsuitable for women, especially for extended periods of time. In East Africa 'Lady' or 'Woman Medical Officer' was a specific job title requiring specific skills deemed appropriate for a woman to undertake.

There were occasions, especially in the first thirty years of the period, when women were turned away from MO positions, not because they were under-qualified or unsuitable, but simply because the one post available to women was filled.[80] Such vacancies as were available to female MOs were usually confined to West Africa and Malaya and normally specified experience in child welfare work.[81]

In accordance with broader Colonial Office policy, taking wives to tropical climates such as East Africa was discouraged, although it was allowed with the express permission of the Secretary of State. In the very early years it was stipulated that 'preference will be given to unmarried candidates',[82] but as this rule was later relaxed, to the point were it was expected that officers proceeding to East Africa could 'usually take their wives with them on first appointment'.[83]

Interviews were held at the Colonial Office, usually, but not always, conducted by a specialist sub-committee.[84] Colonial medical experiences varied: one eventual Principal Medical Officer (PMO) of Tanzania, John Owen Shircore, recalled a very unhurried, although formal interview, in the early 1900s: 'Those were the days when candidates for such posts were expected to attend for interview in morning dress with top hat; the pace was appropriately more leisurely.'[85]

This formality, typical of the establishment, was reiterated in an unpublished memoir by Peter Clearkin (Sierra Leone, Kenya, and Uganda). He described his colonial medical interview in 1913:

[I was] conducted to a waiting room with half a dozen other applicants. Only one appeared to be a provincial like myself, the others, a superior class with a superior accent were dressed in the orthodox professional outfit of the day to wit, morning coat, striped trousers and appropriate accessories, plainly Londoners and very self-assured. They rather daunted me and I felt like slipping away from such an array of talent and elegance. However, I maintained a brave front emphasizing, if it were possible, my provincialness, attired as I was in a rough tweed suit and brogue shoes more suitable for the moors of Yorkshire and Durham than the pavements of Whitehall. My qualms were not diminished by conversation with my fellow provincial. He asked if it was the first time I had appeared before the selection Board. When he heard that it was and that I had been qualified less than a year he said I hadn't a hope but would be told to return when I had more experience; he, himself, had appeared before them twice without success but was hopeful this time.[86]

Clearkin goes on to describe the questions asked by the 'assortment of elderly bearded gentlemen' that constituted the interview panel: '[a] few enquiries were made about my amusements, hobbies, games etc.' although he makes no mention of any questions relating to medical competence.[87]

Once all the criteria had been met and an interview conducted there were still two further stages to be overcome before an appointment was confirmed: the candidate had to pass an examination in tropical medicine; and had to successfully undergo a physical examination. In accordance with the long held belief that diseases of tropical places required special medical expertise a qualification in tropical medicine was a crucial requirement for the Colonial Medical Service. One of the principal aims of the London School of Tropical Medicine (later the London School of Hygiene and Tropical Medicine (LSHTM)) was to provide a specialist education for MOs proceeding to the tropical world.[88] Even during the year of its opening, 1899, the 'Information as to Colonial Appointments' published in the *Colonial Office List* predicted that 'all [Medical Service] candidates will eventually be required to undergo a course of training there after selection, and prior to taking up appointments'.[89] As the School became established, the Diploma course it offered became a 'required' qualification for all MOs taking up positions in Africa.[90] Although it was recognised (especially in times of staff shortages) that officers would sometimes have to proceed without attending the necessary course, permission to do this could only to be obtained under the special directions of the Secretary of State. If granted, the MOs concerned were required to take the course during their first leave in the United Kingdom.[91]

As the discipline of tropical medicine grew, it became possible to take the diploma course in several universities.[92] By 1939 three options were available: a five month course (The Diploma in Tropical Medicine and Hygiene) at the London School of Hygiene and Tropical Medicine, examined by the conjoint board of the Royal College of Physicians and Royal College of Physicians in London; two ten week courses (The Diploma in Tropical Medicine and the Diploma in Tropical Hygiene) offered by the Liverpool School of Tropical Medicine; and the eleven and ten week long 'primary' and 'secondary courses leading to a Diploma in Tropical Medicine and Hygiene run by Edinburgh University.[93] Between 1904 and 1933 the University of Cambridge also ran a diploma course.[94]

Provided that the attendees passed the final examinations within the allotted time, took up their appointment as instructed, and did not resign within three years of assuming their post, the costs of attending these courses and sitting the examinations was borne by the colony to which the recruit was assigned.[95] The course attendee was also eligible for a board and lodging allowance which, during the 1920s was £3 a week, with an additional training allowance of five shillings.[96] This figure was raised after unification to £25 a month and continued to be paid after the diploma course finished until the day before embarkation (when the officer would be eligible to receive half of his regular salary until the day of arrival at the port of destination).[97]

The final hurdle the candidate had to overcome was the medical examination. This was a routine requirement from the start and was conducted by one of the consulting physicians to the Colonial Office. Between 1898 and 1919 this was Patrick Manson himself.[98] Later, when applications were allowed from candidates residing in a colony or dominion, it was performed by a MO appointed locally.[99]

The official guidelines under which Colonial MOs were recruited changed very little between the beginning of the twentieth century and the commencement of World War Two. MOs had to be young, Caucasian, physically fit, doubly qualified, have had a couple of years' hospital experience, and have taken the Diploma in Tropical Medicine (later the Diploma in Tropical Medicine and Hygiene). What is more, this close vetting upon entry, more frequently than not, entrenched in the officious language of both firm and particular regulatory requests was to be the start of a career filled (often to officers' annoyance) with a mass of bureaucratic requirements.

Terms and Conditions of Colonial Medical Employment

Once a place became available on the Secretary of State's list of colonial vacancies an offer of employment was sent out to the successful applicant. This letter revealed the place where the officer would be posted and informed him when and where he should attend the course of instruction in tropical medicine and hygiene.[100] All officers, once employed by the Colonial Office, were subject to three tiers of rules and regulations: first the general *Regulations of His Majesty's Colonial Service*, which was updated yearly and covered all the various services in all the colonial territories; second the 'Laws, Regulations and General Orders' of the dependency in which they were to serve; and third any special terms or conditions particular to each individual's appointment.[101] Together with the appointment letter, each selected candidate was also given a pamphlet outlining the particular terms on which they would be employed in the region to which they had been posted.[102]

MOs for East Africa were initially employed for a two-year probationary period (three years in West Africa). Subject to satisfactory performance (which for most of the period included passing local Kiswahili examinations as well attaining the Diploma or Certificate in Tropical Medicine and Hygiene), appointments were made permanent.[103] In the East African countries probationary service, once effectively passed, was counted as pensionable.

Pay was a constant bone of contention. It was a central issue in the BMA's arguments with the Colonial Office over terms and conditions for medical staff in the 1920s.[104] When the first MOs were appointed in Kenya and Uganda the starting salary was £400, with the Principal Medical Officer drawing a salary of £650.[105] By 1939 the starting salary for MOs in East Africa had risen to £600 per annum, an unchanging figure since the beginning of the 1920s.[106] Even after unification and the accompanying standardisations, East African MOs received the lowest starting salary, £60 less than the yearly rate offered to new medical recruits to the West African territories, and £100 less than those starting work in Malaya.[107] Although yearly salaries and allowances were given in pounds sterling, up until March 1922, salaries in East Africa were paid in local florins, at a fixed exchange rate of 10 florins to the pound.[108] This was eventually changed in all three territories to payment in East African shillings, issued at a fixed rate of twenty shillings to the pound.[109]

The financial depression of the 1930s did not help matters. Many of the colonies were so short of funds that they imposed temporary levies on salaries in the early 1930s, leave moratoria, suspension of local allowances and compulsory retirement.[110] In response to these financial difficulties, and to the negative publicity colonial salaries received in the medical press, later editions of Colonial Office memoranda concerning the terms of employment of Colonial MOs stressed the advantages of the *overall* remuneration package. Although the salary rate might not have seemed particularly competitive on first impression 'the actual value of an appointment is considerably greater than is indicated by the salary alone'.[111] Prospective employees were reminded to take into consideration the pensionable nature of the position; whether income tax was payable; accommodation and other local allowances; and the provision of free sea passages.[112]

Salaries rose yearly in fixed increments with 'efficiency bars' set within each scale. These 'efficiency bars' were fixed points within the capped salary scale beyond which an officer could not progress unless he had fulfilled certain requirements. In the very early years passing an efficiency bar could mean simply satisfying the Director of Medical Service's requirements for satisfactory service. It was later stipulated that this should normally involve improvement of their professional knowledge through taking a special course of study. In 1921, for example, a new MO's pay started at £600, and rose in annual increments of £25 to the top end of the salary scale for that level of appointment, which was £900. This meant that it could take a doctor, provided they passed their efficiency bars (set at £700 and £800), 12 years to reach the top end of their pay-scale.[113] Promotion gained this way was rightly portrayed as being very slow.

Although starting-rate pay for MOs was the same in 1934 as it had been in 1920, after the unification of the medical services in 1934, and accordance with the goal of standardisation, a single efficiency bar was set within that pay-scale at £840. Types of study acceptable for passing this bar were specified as a further degree, a specialist medical or surgical qualification, or 'a recognized diploma or degree in public health, sanitary science, or State medicine'. These requirements reflected the growing emphasis within the Colonial Medical Service, from the 1930s onwards, towards specialised personnel.[114]

A few positions were available at a slightly higher starting rate. New recruits possessing the Diploma in Public Health (DPH) were often recruited as Medical Officers of Health (MOH) and received £50 to £100 per annum above the standard salary, (though the supplement was non-pensionable).[115] Some positions also had a 'duty allowance'; an extra, non-pensionable, emolument paid to officers who took on extra duties, usually but not always, on a temporary basis.[116]

During the early years officers were given an outfit allowance in advance of their first trip, to help them to purchase clothes and equipment necessary for the tropical climate. This was abolished in the early 1920s, but newly appointed officers were frequently offered an advance of a month's pay to cover any initial settlement expenses.[117] A final (temporary) allowance was the war bonus, which was introduced for officers serving in Africa during the First World War in order to compensate them financially for the extra professional burdens imposed by the war.

With these financial allowances and supplements, doctors in East Africa did perhaps not fare particularly badly. All three countries in this study were among those where no income tax was payable by European residents, and, unlike in West Africa, MOs were allowed quarters free of rent for themselves and their families. [118] They were also given free first-class passage to the country in which they were to serve on first appointment and subsequently whenever they went on leave. At first there was some debate as to whether the fares of accompanying wives and children should be paid for. By the 1920s it had been decided that newly appointed officers would receive half the cost of these extra passages, and by the 1930s wives and children were paid for at the full rate, so long as they followed the Officer within twelve months of his appointment.[119] In 1935 the Colonial Office thought better of its generosity, stating only that a married officer posted to East Africa '*may* be granted an allowance towards the cost of his family's passages'.[120]

Each tour of duty was followed by leave, offered on full salary. For the East African territories the recommended tour of service was officially between twenty and thirty months long.[121] The officer was then entitled to five days leave for every month served, so that an officer having finished a thirty month tour of duty could expect to receive 150 days (approximately five months) leave.[122] These terms were tightened up around 1925. While the length of the tour of service remained the same, leave entitlement on full pay was reduced to two and a half or three and a half days per month's residential service depending on the district in which the officer served.[123] Sick leave was available, up to a maximum of six months full pay, with the option of a six months extension on half-pay for officers who would 'ultimately be fit to return to East Africa'.[124]

Before the Warren Fisher Committee, pensions were granted to officers who had served in the Colonial Service for twenty years or had reached the age of 50: whichever was sooner.[125] In the years before the recession of the 1930s, however, an officer could apply to continue his service past the official retirement age, subject of course to Government consent.[126] After 1934 a general arrangement was reached whereby pensions were calculated at the rate of 1/600th of the officer's salary and some allowances (such as the value of free living quarters) received for each month of service, irrespective of any transfers that may have occurred between territories. All officers were entitled to this pension after having completed ten years continuous service.[127] Any officer who wanted to retire earlier could do so on a gratuity, which was essentially a one-off payment taken in lieu of other pension rights. If an officer decided to take this option in East Africa he was entitled to a lump sum of £1,000 after nine years' service (of which a minimum of six years had to have been spent in residence) or £1,250 after twelve years (of which a minimum of eight had to have been spent in residence).[128] If an officer died in Service, his family received a sum equal to the gratuity to which he would have been entitled, depending on his length of service.[129] Officers also were obliged (even if unmarried) to contribute from their salaries to an insurance policy for widows and orphans in event of an officer's death. The details of this were famously complicated and were extensively overhauled and reviewed in 1936.[130]

The nature of the job necessarily required quite a large amount of travel. This was paid for as standard by the colonial government. By the 1930s, officers were encouraged to acquire their own cars or motorcycles to take them through their districts; although Government would not pay for the vehicles, petrol costs were reclaimable.[131]

The most controversial and hotly debated regulation centred on whether medical practitioners should be officially allowed to undertake private practice whilst also holding a government position. The general Colonial Office Regulations throughout this period expressly stated that Colonial Officers' pay was 'fixed on the assumption that his whole time is at the disposal of the Government [and therefore he] is prohibited from engaging in trade, or employing himself in any commercial or agricultural undertaking' or to 'undertake any private agency in any matter connected with the exercise of his public duties'.[132] In fact, private practice was never explicitly banned in any of the regulations issued by the Colonial Office specifically dealing with doctors. The Colonial Office realised the potential backlash if an avenue allowing officers to more money and increase their social standing was closed. Throughout the period a debate occurred at home and abroad over what was enviously considered by many non-medical colonial servants to be a substantial perk. Disquiet over the issue focused upon three main areas. First, the conduct of private practice presented an invariable clash of interests, not least in terms of time spent attending to government matters. Secondly, there was a worry that doctors would charge for services (perhaps even using Government medicines) which under the colonial government's system could also be obtained free of charge and effectively creating a two-tier level of service. Last, concerns were voiced that doctors were simply making too much money in this way, and in so doing distorting the aims and objectives of the Colonial Medical Service career, which Government did not want associated with lucrative private practice. During the interwar years it became obvious that it would be impossible to prohibit private practice entirely. All the high administrative posts as well as laboratory and sanitary appointments, were expressly prohibited from practising, but the rank and file MOs were allowed to undertake practice so long as it did not 'interfere with the faithful and efficient performance of their official duties' and on the express understanding that any abuse of the system would result in the privilege (and it *was* constantly stressed as a privilege) being withdrawn from the individual concerned.[133]

Supplementary fees could also be earned through undertaking other duties, such as conducting *post-mortem* examinations, acting as expert witness in local court cases or processing passport applications. To standardise the payments doctors could extract, fees charged for undertaking these extra duties were fixed throughout the Colonial Medical Service.[134] Medical care for all government officers was free, as it was for the families of all officers in the lower ranks of the Colonial Medical Service.[135]

The Colonial Medical Service system of promotion was based on meritorious service and senior appointments were usually made from within the Service. Promotions were put forward to the Secretary of State for approval by the head of each Medical Department through the local Governor. The assessment of an Officer's suitability would usually be conducted through annual confidential reports that the Director of Medical Services submitted for every member of staff working in his territory.[136] Although the official ethos barely changed throughout the period, it became specifically stressed after 1930 (probably in response to arguments put forward by the BMA that promotions could take years to attain) that all officers could theoretically be considered for promotion if they had 'rendered good service' regardless of whether they had reached the top of their salary scale. After unification, transfers became used even more frequently as a way to forward promotions. If no senior position was available in their current location, officers deserving of advancement were offered a higher position in another territory. Such transfers were consequently rare during the early years of an officer's career.[137] Jeffries outlined the situation in 1938:

[A Colonial MO] may expect an initial salary of £600, more or less. Provided that he is reasonably efficient in the performance of his duties, he may normally count on reaching, within from 13–15 years, a salary of £1,000, plus allowances and, in many cases, some private practice...even the average officer may legitimately aspire to reach at least the Senior MO grade, and there are reasonable chances of rising higher still.[138]

Essentially, the terms and conditions for MOs changed very little throughout the period. After the Warren Fisher Committee, certain precise criteria were introduced and other terms were expressed less ambiguously, but there was actually little material improvement in salary or leave entitlement. The unchanging nature of pay, leave, allowances and pension rights led to much disgruntlement among the medical personnel. These regulations, provided the framework under which officers were employed and largely prescribed and delineated their actions. What this actually meant for Colonial MOs in terms of daily practice and duties is discussed in Chapter 7.

*   *   *

Joining the Colonial Medical Service involved a set of procedures pre-arranged by the British Government. It naturally presented a much more bureaucratic process for medical graduates than they might expect to go through when opting for other medical careers. Not only were the rules and regulations of colonial medical employment dense and often location-specific to different parts of empire, but, as has been seen, the official selection criteria specified a certain type of profile. Some of these criteria were enshrined in terms of objective policy; such as the requirements to be of a certain age, ethnicity and educational calibre, but, as will be explored in the next chapter, it was also clear that there were other less publicly declared, but nevertheless ubiquitous, ideas upon which candidates were consistently and intimately judged.

Chapter 3: Subjective Selection and Recruitment Trends

> [S]uccess as a Medical Officer can only be achieved if his personality is such as to command the respect and trust of the native inhabitants of his Colony as well as the confidence of the local European community.[1]

Selection for service in the Colonial Medical Service was not based on rules alone. Official expressions of policy should be supplemented through an examination of the rather more subjective criteria of selection employed by the Colonial Office. Naturally, these criteria directly impacted upon the type of person who was chosen and are of central importance to later analysis of personnel profiles (Chapter 8). In many ways the ideal 'type' looked for by recruiters can be seen, unsurprisingly, to mirror the standards of the first Director of Recruitment, Ralph Furse, as well as the prevailing values of society at large. The first section of this chapter argues that long after the patronage system was officially abolished in 1930, an informal network still operated aimed at recruiting socially, ideologically and physically, the 'right' sort of officer. Next, medical recruitment changes throughout the period are examined and quantified, identifying periods of pressure as well as periods of relative ease. This analysis reveals that opportunities of entering the medical service were not constant throughout the period and that the Colonial Medical Service rose and fell in popularity; though not necessarily in accordance with other broader economic fluctuations, as might be expected.

Ralph Furse and the Subjective Side to the Selection Process

The question of having the appropriate 'character' to be a good colonial servant was central to its recruitment procedure. The decision to select candidates through personal interviews was predicated around this. Although much-criticised, periodic attempts to dispense with the interview as a central tool of selection, were uniformly rejected.[2] Advocates of an examined entry system felt that it would improve the public status of the Colonial Service since a better quality of candidate would be attracted by a competitive examination. From the start, however, the Colonial Office upheld the view that the particular exigencies of the tropical world presented sufficient reason to assess candidates more on their character than any ability to pass an examination, especially when many had just been through university or medical school. The career was one in which 'the variety of problems involved and the tact required are infinite, and hence it could hardly be made into a regular profession, with a rigid method of admission and promotion.'[3]

Admittedly recruitment standards to the Colonial Medical Service, unlike some of the other services, could be measured more objectively because of the candidates' professional qualifications. By implication, they relied less exclusively on the more nebulous concept of 'character' than appointments to the Colonial Administrative Service, for example. Nevertheless, collective notions of character had a very significant part to play. Every piece of information on the entrance procedure for the Colonial Service in general and the Colonial Medical Service in particular makes specific use of the word 'character' in its application information. Partly this is just the usual rhetoric of selection, but other evidence confirms that 'character' was indeed a clearly defined personal qualification that had received much official consideration. An early Private Secretary, Edward Marsh, described the interview process: although qualifications were naturally taken into account, it was necessary to take careful note of 'what we called the impression they made'.[4] Furse himself was particularly eloquent on the need to select the 'right sort' of person for a colonial position. As officers were required to 'represent the British Government personally' among the native races, he believed the 'qualities of character, personality, tact and address' were of the utmost importance, and ones that he felt could only be ascertained through personal interview.[5] The overhauled recruitment guidelines after Medical Service unification could not have been more explicit: although practical and academic experiences were very important, equal, if not more, importance was placed upon character.

The assessment of character was sometimes undertaken before formal interview. The desk diaries (spanning the years 1899–1915) of the Assistant Private Secretary (Appointments), reveal that a snap decision was usually made when personal callers came to the Colonial Office to enquire about potential employment. Someone deemed suitable was likely to leave with some promotional literature and an application form, while less suitable types were dismissed with a polite excuse, if not a flat refusal. Kirk-Greene has shown how the 'always subjective, often dismissive and frequently highly "politically incorrect" process' which candidates underwent changed little between 1899 and 1948.[6] The same sort of instant character assessment was certainly applied to medical enquiries, irrespective of the fact that doctors could be argued as being self-defining in terms of academic quality. Some of the comments about medical candidates in these early patronage diaries clearly refer to doctors who subsequently joined the East African Medical Service. William Owen-Pritchard (Kenya and Tanzania) was described as 'a very nice doctor'. An entry for Dr Lamborn may well refer to an early enquiry from William Lamborn (Tanzania), who although assessed as 'not a gentleman' was nevertheless 'extraordinarily cheerful & pleasing'. Anstruther Rendle, who went on to have a long colonial medical career (Uganda and Kenya) was judged, somewhat blandly, although by no means negatively, as a 'rather nice man' who 'would do well', unlike his (also medically qualified) brother who accompanied him and was written off in the same note as 'anaemic looking, much younger, rather colourless, [although] apparently inoffensive.' Two men who became heads of medical departments also had their preliminary interviews noted: John Owen Shircore (Tanzania) made a good impression being 'gentle & well-liking' and if the Dr Milne interviewed in early 1909 is Arthur Milne who headed the Medical Department in Kenya, then the impression that he was 'quite passable' was retrospectively an understatement.[7]

After application forms had been received — with a photograph appended to the back just to rule out any physical peculiarities or degenerate signs — the next stage was the personal interview.[8] Furse, characteristically vocal over the intrinsic importance of finding the right 'type of man'[9] described his interview technique as follows:

> We sat as far apart as we could so that a candidate who was being interviewed by one of us need not feel that he was being overheard by the others. At the same time we could often help each other by unobtrusively watching the other man's candidate from a different angle. Interviewing boards normally sit on one side of a table with their victim on the other. By so doing they often miss significant details. For instance, a man's face may not reveal that he is intensely nervous. But a twitching foot, or hands tightly clenched under the table, will tell you this, and you can make the necessary allowances or deductions, which are often important.[10]

Clearly, much rode on first impressions. Even as late as 1948 the confidential *Appointments Handbook* (made up of Furse's recommendations, compiled by his deputy) reminded interviewers that body language was all-important: 'You will have in mind the truism that weakness of various kinds may lurk in a flabby lip or in averted eyes, just as single mindedness and purpose are commonly reflected in a steady gaze and a firm set of mouth and jaw.'[11]

Ideas of good character were further explored through the P.7 form. This was the form letter and statement issued by the Colonial Office to be completed by the referees named on the application form. Among the statements for the referee to complete were questions as to whether the candidate was '(a) honest? (b) of strictly sober and temperate habits? (c) industrious? (d) of sound moral character [and] (e) of active bodily habits?'[12] It was not enough for Colonial Office staff to judge a good character independently; they also relied on others to divulge character faults they might have missed. The Colonial Office even had a secret list that rated the reliability of some referees over others.[13]

Ideas of the right type can be roughly divided for into six groups of traits, all of which were necessarily interconnected and inseparable within any overall assessment: social qualifications, athleticism, mental stability, ability to rule, morality and self-reliance.

*   *   *

The pervasive idea that 'the ethos of the ruling classes was the ethos of the Colonial Service' had a long history stemming from the elite nature of early patronage appointments. [14] This was largely true of all foreign Public Services, epitomised in the description of the Sudan as 'that country of blacks ruled by blues.'[15] The actual class composition of the Colonial Medical Service will be discussed in a later chapter; what is important here are the impressionistic ideals of the model entrant. There was a clear sense that the right sort of candidate upheld upper-middle class British values. Even if he had not necessarily been to a public school, many of the qualities traditionally associated with the British public school were deemed essential and selection was based upon what Robert Heussler called 'the traditional cult of the gentleman'.[16] These values included the characteristics of leadership, militarism, conservatism, sportsmanship or fairness, a strong sense of social propriety, manners and consciousness of British tradition.[17] In Furse's opinion 'public school training is of more importance than university training in producing the personality and character capable of handling the natives well.'[18] He made many attempts throughout his career to encourage candidates with this type of education.[19]

With the abolition of entry by patronage it would be natural to assume a reduction in emphasis within the Colonial Service on status and social qualifications. In some ways this did occur: non-Oxbridge universities, although still not largely represented, gradually became more visible; the middle-classes too, after entering universities that were progressively more accessible to them, were increasingly seeing Colonial Service as a viable career. It was still a job for the educated elite, but less founded on social connections than in the pre-war period. The associations did not disappear entirely and while Furse was in charge of recruitment his conservative ideas held considerable sway. As one colonial historian assessed the situation in 1945, 'the two way stations on the road to C[olonial] S[ervice] careers....were [still] the great British Public Schools and the two ancient universities of Oxford and Cambridge.'[20]

Ideals of breeding and gentility and were closely associated with broader upper-middle class prejudices over race, religion, gender and sartorial presentation. A strong, barely hidden, element of racism characterised Colonial Service recruitment. Advice on appointing an Indian doctor is illustrative: '[i]n dealing with Indian applicants our method so far had been to do all we can to avoid telling them openly that they are ineligible on racial grounds.' Rather brutally the Colonial Office allowed Indians to fill in all the application forms and then found 'some excuse or other' to turn them down.[21] The nationalist agenda extended beyond even racial concerns to the point where candidates from the Dominions were regarded as a second best option. If a decision had to made quickly, the British candidate was to be chosen over any foreign one every time.[22] White British men were considered by far the best choice, although it was known that this policy had to be conducted guardedly: 'whatever happens, it is most important that no indication should leak out that men are rejected for Colonial Services on account of colour.' The same minute went on to say:

The gist of the matter is that for various reasons, into which I need not go, it has been found unwise to appoint to positions in the public services of almost all the colonies, persons who from a knowledge of their antecedents, or from their personal appearance, might be suspected of having a mixture of non-European (I mean of course, coloured) blood.[23]

Similarly there was institutional discrimination on religious grounds. Although theoretically non-Christian beliefs were no bar to a colonial appointment, they did often play a part in character assessments, particularly earlier in the period. [24]

The requirement for physical fitness meant candidates would 'stand or fall by the medical examination'.[25] This assessment, was also required for entry into physically demanding jobs, such as the army, but the emphasis on athleticism is surprising for a sedentary profession such as medicine which did not typically require sporting prowess.[26] Being a colonial doctor, however, laid stress on this quality and nowhere more so than in the taxing climate of tropical Africa. The Medical Adviser could deny entry to those who were 'insufficiently developed physically', just as the Private Secretary could apply the same type of check on those who were not 'sufficiently developed from the point of view of character'.[27] This integral emphasis on sport and physical robustness was intimately connected (largely through the influence of public schools) with ideals of Empire. 'Without hard exercise men in hot countries rapidly lose their health and often mental serenity. The result is a loss of efficiency and, in some cases, a tragic disaster.'[28]

Closely associated with physical fitness were ideas of mental strength and stability. The form candidates had to complete and give to the consulting physician asked for a declaration of whether they had suffered from any nervous complaint as well as asking if there was a history of insanity in their family.[29] This question not only suggested that mental disease was hereditary, but also assumed that the stresses of residence in a tropical climate might bring out undesirable psychological traits, a view that was in accord with some medical recommendations:

> The best kind of man to go to the tropics is the good ordinary type of Britisher, with a clear head 'well screwed on', an even temper, not over intellectual; one who can take an interest in things around, not unduly introspective, not ever sighing for the flesh-pots of Piccadilly...The unsuitable man is he who is a victim of migraine, headaches, any hereditary mental taint, or epilepsy; who bears heat ill, or suffers from insomnia, or is neurotic in any way.[30]

This was in accord with longstanding associations between residence in the tropics and the deleterious mental and physical effects of the hot sun and climate.[31] This belief, stemming from the earliest days of tropical exploration persisted until the end of the period, although by the 1930s it was often expressed publicly in more diluted and culturally acceptable idioms. One danger claimed for tropical life was nervous exhaustion (sometimes termed tropical neurasthenia). It was chiefly on the basis of this enduring belief that those of weaker constitutions — namely women and children — were discouraged from spending extended periods of time in the tropics.[32] Since most Colonial Medical Service doctors served in Africa, they were considered particularly exposed to 'stresses that do not operate to the same extent in a temperate climate' which meant that selection techniques had to take this into consideration: '[t]he fundamental qualification for such an official is *mens sana in corpore sano* [a sound mind in a sound body]', read the promotional feature on the Colonial Service as a career in a late 1920s issue of the *Public Schools' Employment Bureau Bulletin*. [33] Repeatedly, 'the importance of avoiding nerves' was cited as an important factor in the selection of the right sort of candidate.[34] Even at the end of the period, a proposal from the Governor of Uganda, Philip Mitchell, suggested that the tour of duty for MOs there be reduced from thirty to fifteen months, because 'the climate of Uganda…has a deteriorating affect on mental efficiency.'[35] The Colonial Office still held, as late as 1939, that the East African climate was 'liable to produce nervous manifestations after lengthy residence.'[36]

James Mangan and James Walvin have examined in detail the emphasis on morality in relation to societal values during this period, especially the way this perceived asset permeated middle-class opinion.[37] The Colonial Service, too, laid explicit stress upon conventional moral values and specifically asked that candidates be sought who displayed good fibre.[38] The P.7 referees' form asked whether the candidate was 'a fit and proper person' to hold a 'responsible appointment in the Colonial Service', requesting information on any potential character deficits 'in connection with matrimonial affairs, temperament etc.'.[39] This assessment could also be made at interview: a scribbled note on a candidate expressed doubts over his 'moral character'.[40]

Another strong ideal was the ability to rule, to be a self-reliant and confident leader. This not only embodied public school leadership values, but additionally a certain tact and ability to respect native cultures and not offend native inhabitants.[41] The ideal choice of candidate was one who could 'command the confidence and respect of the native; for it would not be an exaggeration to say that we rule these great areas primarily through means of personal influence'.[42]

Furse was looking for candidates who would feel part of the Service and were likely to uphold the traditions of Empire. The most desirable candidate therefore held a single-minded commitment to his work, was ideally a bachelor and someone who 'takes up the Colonial Service as his career from the start'. The 'unsatisfactory candidate' would have 'made but an indifferent success of life elsewhere and comes to us *faute de mieux* at the age of 27 to 35.'[43] Indeed, one of the conclusions of the special departmental committee appointed to look into the Colonial Medical Service in 1920, which led to the unification of the East African Medical Service, was that the unification was desirable particularly when one appreciated the 'great esprit de corps' of the West African Medical Service.[44] It was believed that dedication to service needed to be inculcated while young, the aim being to produce leaders loyal to the ruling government and proud to participate in all the pomp and ceremony that displayed and reinforced the values of Empire.[45] This dedication could partly be fostered through giving preferential treatment to sons of officers who had already served in the Empire.[46] Even after the loss of India in 1947, it was still thought desirable that Colonial Service candidates embody some sense of the tradition of Empire; that 'the colonial Empire struck some chord in his mind even as a boy'. It was also felt that best candidates come from 'stock that has proved its worth, generation by generation in the professions or in the public service.'[47]

The good colonial servant believed in crown and country and therefore candidates of less certain political convictions were to be avoided. This went beyond considerations of race; it was an issue of national security. In 1925 Medical graduates from the Irish Free State, for example, were considered unsuitable for Colonial Service employment because their political loyalties could not be guaranteed. The opinion of Mr Flood, a member of the Colonial Medical and Sanitary Advisory Committee, was very definite: despite possessing a reasonable medical school at Trinity College Dublin, the service is better off without them [Irish Medical graduates]', not least because they came from a disloyal country, rendering them 'unsuited for any service under the crown.'[48] Concerns were similarly voiced that candidates from the Dominions lacked the prerequisite 'tradition of service to the state' and were therefore unlikely to be as committed to the imperialist enterprise as their home-grown contemporaries.[49] Even when Dominion candidates were considered suitable, it was noted that particular care should be taken on 'the question of personality'; presumably code for deficiency in allegiance.[50] Selection was therefore not solely associated with whiteness, but also with ideas of national loyalty. Even white settlers in Kenya complained that their peers from the home country were more likely to be offered a Colonial Service position than they themselves were.[51]

Officers were united not only in their common aims and goals, but also through a pride in their united government service. But while the need to feel part of a broader group was an essential characteristic, this was combined with the requirement for the individual to be self-reliant and independent. The tropical world was different and challenging; racially and culturally isolating for the Europeans who went there. It therefore needed a special type of person to cope with life on their own. An early reference sets the tone for the rest of the period: The ideal colonial MO 'must be a self-reliant man, and should early on in his career seek to exercise a clear and independent judgement. He must accustom himself to act alone, and to have the courage of his convictions, for he will seldom be able to summon prompt assistance from his brethren.'[52]

These assessments of character were entirely bound up with the pervasive mind-set of the ruling classes. It was natural, for example, for Furse to uphold the values of the social group to which he belonged and to respect the same common denominators subscribed to by Colonial Office colleagues.[53] Similarly, the predominant focus on ideals of manliness reflected the inherent gender values of the period. The dearth of women working in the Colonial Office meant that women's interests were rarely put forward and even when they were, the male dominated Colonial Office could summarily dismiss them as being irrelevant to the Services' staffing composition.[54] Particularly up until the inter-war period, one of the main tasks of Colonial MOs was to provide medical care for the European civil administration resident in the colonies, and as these were mostly single men, women doctors were seen as less relevant in the types of medical skills they could offer.

The heads of the medical departments working in the colonies reinforced many of these opinions on necessary character traits. When asked to assess the type of person he wanted in his Medical Department, William Kauntze (Director of Medical Services (DMS), Uganda) was unequivocal: '[g]et sturdy men; avoid temperaments. Highlanders and Irish give a lot of trouble.'[55] In a later letter Kauntze was even more specific:

> Professional qualifications are important, especially if they include additional ones in public health, but they are secondary to character so long as they indicate a reasonable standard of medical knowledge.

> From my experience here and elsewhere temperamental people (particularly with the Celtic temperament) suffer more from climatic strain and are consequently much more difficult to manage departmentally. The really well-educated man with interests outside as well as medicine, usually serves us better that one with a narrower education.[56]

Equally revealing are opinions voiced in the private correspondence of Mr Edward Cooke (who served on the interview committee for colonial medical appointments during World War One) to Furse. Character was so important that it could even surpass professional qualifications. The Colonial Medical Service did not need first-class doctors as much as needed 'good types', especially in times of recruitment shortfall:

> For general appointments, I do not think that we need to attract the very best men. Such men are more useful at home. In the colonies we want a good all-round general practitioner with a good physique and a sporting temperament. Higher attainments are not required, and an unfit man for appointment in so far as there is probably no less satisfactory officer than a man who is too good for his job.[57]

Colonial Medical Service recruiters had a very clearly defined idea of the 'type' of person they wanted staffing the British imperial possessions. This type, broadly speaking, supported (even if it was not socially part of) a traditional and conservative worldview customarily associated with the British upper classes. It also upheld and reinforced the manly values of Empire by recruiting (principally) men who were white-skinned, loyal, sporting, firm-minded strong leaders. Academic attainments became progressively more important as the period progressed, but were not valued nearly as strongly. Character was the guiding principle of recruitment.

Recruitment Trends

The overall trends of colonial medical recruitment shed light on overarching issues that faced both recruiters and recruited throughout the period before World War Two. During the early years of Britain's tropical Empire, the Colonial Office presented a discouraging message about an individual's chances of gaining an appointment. The 1899 *Information as to Colonial Appointments*, stated that unless the candidate was enrolled in one of the cadetship schemes or professionally qualified, there were 'scarcely' any openings.[58] By 1908 this rather negative tone had softened: there were 'few openings for candidates from this country except in tropical Africa'.[59] A cautious phrasing that was dropped altogether by the 1920s.

It is important to differentiate between number of applications made and the number of positions available: in the early period there were generally more applications than positions to fill. Analysis of a selection of Patronage desk diaries, although necessarily imperfect (interest in a specifically medical career would not necessarily have been noted), sheds some light on the popularity of the colonial medical career in relation to other services during the period before 1914. Although peaking in 1903 interest in medical positions was remarkably steady until just before the First World War started (Figure 3.1).

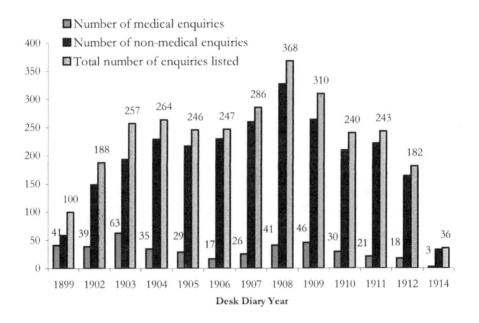

Figure 3.1: Appointment Enquiries for the Colonial Service, 1902–12, 1914[60]

No official records were kept of actual recruitment numbers in the years preceding 1913, but the 1899 Selborne Report counted a total of 447 MOs in the Service of Empire for 1895.[61] In 1912 there were 23 Colonial Medical Service doctors in Kenya and 25 in Uganda, so new openings for doctors in this region were not plentiful, not least because in the first decade of the century West Africa was perceived as having the most pressing need for medical staff. Some impression of vacancies is possible. In 1899, for example, it was stated that an average of fifteen medical appointments a year was to be expected.[62] By the end of World War One the medical establishments of the African colonies were beginning to grow and it was estimated that there would be 'over 50' vacancies for doctors in the Medical Service overall.[63] Nonetheless, even when vacancies did increase, recruitment sometimes remained depressed. One of the problems plaguing the medical services until the late 1920s was the failure of candidates to come forward. Private Secretary John Davidson summed up the dramatic reversal in trends: 'instead of a glut of candidates and few posts, there are many posts and no candidates.... A very keen imagination is not necessary to picture what the state of the candidates list will be directly peace comes.'[64]

The effects of World War One were felt for some time in the Medical Service as well as in the other branches. Furse felt that the war had created a 'stay at home' mentality in the post-war generation; families who had lost sons or fathers in action were perhaps keener than before to 'keep a boy at home'. Further, economic stringency meant that it was harder to send sons to university and more appealing to send them into business than in the pre-war years.[65] For the medical services the war caused a shortfall that took nearly a decade to recover, and this coupled with the growing opportunities for doctors within the UK, 'mainly owing to the expansion of various social services', meant that the starting salary offered looked even more unappealing than formerly.[66] In 1919 Furse admitted confidentially to the Secretary of State, Leo Amery, that for some time the appointments branch had found itself in such a position where they had had to 'take on several men since (and still have to) whom one would rather not see get a place.'[67]

The trouble seemed to lie in the poor popularity of the Service as a career rather than in any deficiency in the number of doctors *per se*. In July 1920 a minute on the issue recorded:

> The position as regards medical vacancies is that we have now about 100 vacancies in all, (mainly E Africa, W Africa and Malaya): we have had enquiries as a result of the last advertisement (in last weeks Lancet and BMJ) from about 25 medical men (British and apparently qualified) a few lady doctors...and a few non-British. I understand that, from previous experience, out of 25 enquiries, one cannot expect to obtain more than ten definite candidates, and this is scarcely sufficient to keep pace with the present wastage, apart from making up the arrears; and the position in E and W Africa, and Malaya can, I understand, justifiably be described as 'dangerous.[68]

By 1922 a low point had been reached resulting in retrenchments of existing staff, notably in Kenya.[69] Things had not improved by the mid-1920s and Furse later reflected how 'At the end of 1925 there were about 130 vacancies unfilled; suitable candidates were not forthcoming and the position was definitely unsatisfactory'.[70] One scheme proposed was to expand the recruitment base to the Dominions, initially in Canada, but later in Australia, New Zealand and South Africa. Canada was thought 'most likely to be of special use to us in supplying our very serious deficiency of doctors'; not only would it help the personnel shortage, but it was thought that the inclusion of Canadian doctors in the colonial medical staffs would advance relations with the self-governing Dominions in general. It was hoped that ties to England would be improved through Canadians 'taking a definite share of the "white man's burden"'.[71]

Unsurprisingly, this need to broaden the recruitment base for the colonial medical services did not extend to doctors of other races. Although some non-

European doctors were employed on the Mauritanian medical staff and that of the West Indies, they were effectively ineligible for most Colonial Service appointments, irrespective of their qualifications. With regard to East Africa, which contained a large Indian population, no formal declaration of this policy was inserted into the recruitment literature until 1925, but even in earlier times of severe recruitment shortage, it was considered preferable to have no MO rather than an Indian one.[72]

If the immediate post-World War One years were ones of slump and slow recovery, the years between 1925 and 1929 were 'marked by a large expansion of cadres and very high recruitment'.[73] Despite protracted arguments over terms and conditions of service between the BMA and the Chief Medical Adviser to the Colonial Office, Thomas Stanton, this period saw the most concerted effort to enhance the Medical Service's reputation through personal contacts with the Deans of London and provincial medical schools. The results were very positive; 'a steady stream of well qualified and experienced candidates was regularly forthcoming', and confidence was so high (albeit temporarily) that it was decided that it was no longer necessary to advertise within the medical journals.[74]

Medical recruitment was going well in 1930, but the situation deteriorated between 1931 and 1934, and although figures later improved, they did not return to the highs of the late 1920s. Although worrying, however, the sharp reduction in medical recruitment that occurred between 1930 and 1931 was less dramatic than was experienced in other branches of the Colonial Service, including the Administrative Service.[75] Indeed, the Medical Service attracted the most recruits in 1931 and was consistently, second only to the Administrative Service as the biggest overall recruiter up to 1939. Furse was quietly confident that, although recruitment to most branches of the Service were in a troubled state, the situation regarding medical recruitment was, contrastingly, 'satisfactory'.[76] Other figures produced by Furse show that career interest in the Colonial Service was increasing. By 1931 the Colonial Office received more enquiries and interviewed more (and better) candidates than ever before. In Furse's assessment, the profile and popularity of the Colonial Service had substantially improved even if there were very few positions available for successful candidates to fill.[77]

The anomaly of relatively sustained medical recruitment throughout the depression of the 1930s has not yet been analysed by historians. Furse put it down to the fact that doctors were drawn from 'ready made material' meaning that in times of economic stringency they could serve successfully in the Colonies without having further public money spent upon them, unlike Veterinary, Administrative or Forestry officers, for whom a specialised training course before departure was imperative.[78]

Most services in the 1930s lost staff through retrenchments. It was estimated as early as 1932 that approximately one thousand retrenchments had taken place in a year and a half, though the medical services had, once again, not been hit particularly hard.[79] The figures for the East African Medical Service bear this out: compared to other parts of Africa — particularly the Gold Coast — Kenya, Uganda and Tanzania did not suffer too severely.[80] Furse in typically loyal style even gave a positive spin to the problems faced during the early 1930s: 'however tragic and regrettable' retrenchment had the advantage of having 'relieved the Service of its weakest elements'.[81]

Towards the end of the 1930s, however, quiet optimism was replaced by mounting concern: medical applicants were simply not coming forward in anything like the numbers needed to sustain, let alone extend, the medical services in the Colonies. Unease was so great that in 1938 it was decided to set up a special committee to look into these problems. As the committee reported, since 1935, 'the number of [medical] applicants has been limited, so much so that it is seldom that there is more than one applicant for a particular post.' Furthermore, it was stressed that the standard of the applicants that did present themselves 'cannot be regarded as high.'[82] In order to understand and assess the phenomenon, the various heads of medical departments in the colonies were consulted and the opinions of the men in charge of recruitment to the military medical services and the Indian Medical Service were canvassed to see if they were also experiencing such trends. The results were worrying: although the Navy and Air Force medical services had noticed a decline in applicants, the Royal Army Medical Corps and the Indian Medical Service reported that recruitment, though not up to capacity, had, nevertheless, 'improved very much'.[83] The final report of this special committee located four problems at the root of the downward trend: first, the effects of the depression, which meant that many well qualified and suitable candidates had been turned away, resulting in the image of a Service difficult to get into (even for those with experience); second, that retrenchments had contributed to a sense of 'uneasiness' over the stability of the career; third, that competition from similar services had increased;[84] fourth the perception that wives or fiancées were not encouraged in the tropics (especially West Africa) had allegedly put off many young doctors, a point that was of increased importance in the 1930s when independent enquiries confirmed to the Colonial Office that doctors were marrying younger than ever previously.[85]

Among the suggestions put forward to improve the situation was the appointment of doctors immediately after qualification followed by experience in the hospitals of the colony to which they were posted (rather than sending them out to a district, as was normally done). It was hoped that this would enable the Colonial Office to select the best products of the medical schools, before they were lured away by the offer of a permanent hospital position. This idea was dismissed as being impracticable, not least because hospitals in the territories varied so considerably that they could not be guaranteed to have the personnel or facilities to train new staff. It was thought best to revive connections with the Deans of medical schools and to pursue a vigorous promotional campaign, revitalising the service's reputation and expunging any myths that may have resulted from the problems of the preceding years.

Yet, scarcely had these plans been formulated, when the outbreak of the Second World War brought a further destabilising knock to recruitment. Hurriedly, the Colonial Office put together a series of letters and articles for publication in *The Times* in an attempt to 'reassure any such candidate, who may be in doubt where his patriotic duty lies. He may feel absolutely confident that, in offering his services to the Colonial Office, he is acting in accordance with the

national interest.' It was stated that this admonishment applied with 'special force'
to the Colonial Medical Service:

> In the tropical countries of which the Colonial Empire so largely consists, the
> problems of public health are of basic importance. We simply cannot afford
> to fall back; nay more, we cannot afford not to go forward. The Colonial
> Office therefore must continue to recruit young doctors for appointments in
> the Colonial Medical Service, and it is earnestly to be hoped that suitable
> candidates will continue to come forward.[86]

The Colonial Medical Service clearly experienced different recruitment
tensions at different times. Although few vacancies arose before World War One,
demand for colonial doctors was high from 1914 until the mid 1920s.
Unfortunately, for various reasons, candidates did not come forward in anything
like the numbers needed effectively to supply the growing medical needs of
Empire after the war. An extensive recruitment drive in the late 1920s specifically
aimed at medical schools, together with improved relations with the British
Medical Association and the receding effects of the War, ushered in a period of
relative boom. Following this period of prosperity Colonial recruitment fell as the
effect of the worldwide financial depression made itself felt, but the Medical
Service did not suffer as badly as other Colonial Services. By 1935, just when
other branches were beginning to make a recovery, medical applications again
became worryingly low — a state of affairs that continued until after World War
Two.

*   *   *

If medical recruitment did not necessarily mirror recruitment peaks and troughs as
experience by the Colonial Administrative Service, it did hold many similarities to
its important sister Service in terms of the way recruits were selected. Perhaps this
emphasis was surprising as doctors made up an already self-selecting group in
terms of their pre-requisite medical qualifications. Appointments were not based
solely on academic and professional qualifications, but on a mixture of objective
and subjective criteria aimed at selecting the type of person who could operate
best under the perceived stresses of the tropical world. This careful selection
procedure, with its emphasis on personality, suggests that doctors working in the
colonies had a broader socio-political role to play than they necessarily would at
home. They needed to have the sorts of characteristics that could survive well in
the potentially isolated and alien environment; more importantly, they were
symbols of the ruling country and had to be assessed in terms of their potential to
uphold its values. For these reasons Furse insisted on interview as the central tool
of recruitment, and selection right up to the 1950s was based upon many of the
same central principles.

  If this is the picture from the side of Colonial officialdom, what of the
appointees themselves? Why, when terms and conditions of service were
considered to be relatively inflexible and uncompetitive, did doctors choose the

career over other professional alternatives available to them? That is the subject of the next two chapters.

Chapter 4: Identity and Experience I: Practical Reasons for Being a Doctor in East Africa

T]he Service offers an attractive career for the keen and well-qualified young officer. It is attractive professionally, financially and socially.[1]

The reasons why doctors chose to undertake public service careers in Africa were necessarily diverse. Yet, however multifarious individual motivations were in their different personal, and public, influences, certain common themes can be identified as informing the decisions of colonial doctors before World War Two. Some were economic (the attractions of regular pay and a future pension); some practical (it was, for the 'right sort', easy to get the job); some social (the respectability and prestige associated with the career); some professional (the chance to gain practical tropical medical experience); and all were culturally determined (the then fashionable allure of Empire). Although doctors in their reminiscences sometimes identified a single, dominant reason for their career choice, on closer scrutiny, they all contribute to a much broader world picture. In some ways the point is commonplace: doctors were influenced in their choices by the circumstances of the period in which they lived. It is still worthwhile, however, to explore the individual and group motivations that occurred on much more than just the level of conscious choice.[2]

The divisions between the main factors that influenced Colonial Service career choices discussed in this chapter and the next have been created for thematic order. They are inevitably false distinctions, as varying combinations of inter-related factors contributed to individual choices. What is more, the weight of each factor changed relative to other social economic and cultural influences of the time while the balance between factors was never static. In the earlier period, for example, the missionary connection, riding on the back of Livingstone's popularity, may have encouraged ideas of working in Africa, in the later period this was less persuasive and was replaced by growing professional individualism among doctors specifically and more general ideas of Empire building. The post-war generation of doctors had very different priorities from their pre-war equivalents and by the 1920s a new rhetoric of development began to replace former ideas of Empire building for exclusively European purposes. Although the period is chronologically short, it covers a time of great social flux.[3]

This chapter explores the various stimuli affecting colonial medical career choices, interweaving personal recollections of MOs with broader historical social and economic factors. As much of the evidence is autobiographical, compiled from personal papers, biographical descriptions in obituaries and other sources, it cannot be said to represent the unanimous opinion of all Colonial MOs. Naturally, only a small (generally elite) proportion of the 424 doctors identified left detailed accounts of their lives or had obituaries written about them. Moreover, the accounts were written from varying perspectives and with different motives, so that they are inevitably eclectic and non-standard. However, recurrent themes and shared standpoints can be easily identified and related back to arguments over subjective recruitment criteria presented in the previous chapter. Since individuals were specifically chosen by the Colonial Office for the way they were anticipated to contribute to the shared perspectives and common values of the group, they understandably demonstrated some unity of purpose. Such issues, and others discussed below, help piece together an informative perspective of how and why doctors perceived the career as they did.

The Economic Factor

Any decision over job choice necessarily took account of its economic viability. Although recruitment to the colonial medical career fluctuated before the Second World War, the highs and lows were related more to pressures on the medical profession at home than to any particularly persuasive financial appeal of the career itself. The colonial option did have certain features that made it desirable in many doctors' minds, but these were rarely cited as being purely (or even partly) economic. When it was difficult for doctors in the United Kingdom to find secure jobs a position in the Colonial Medical Service must have been relatively attractive — a regular salary, even if quite low, was better than none — but that is far from saying that the salary was in itself an attraction to colonial medical work. On the contrary, pay was mostly portrayed as uncompetitive, especially relative to the difficult local conditions and the level of expertise required. This section examines how the home economic situation in the pre and post-World War One period stimulated Colonial Medical Service recruitment in different ways and discusses the ambiguous influence of pay.

Medical historians who have researched the dynamics of medical employment in the Victorian and Edwardian periods have pointed out that professional market pressures at home were among the most significant forces acting upon doctors taking up an imperial posting. Douglas Haynes, building on work on the English medical profession by Anne Digby and Jeanne Peterson, strongly reinforced the idea that professional overcrowding at home after 1850 created a medical market that was increasingly competitive. By the 1880s and 1890s this had become acute enough to cause many doctors to look for alternative ways of making a living —

one of which was in the newly expanding Empire.[4] In the context of this increasingly competitive environment, the Colonial Medical career offered an attractive option for medical graduates in need of a stable assured salary. Furthermore, the growth in the medical market at home had brought certain other pressures. Doctors who had obtained domestic employment often found that they were not necessarily guaranteed the prosperity they may have expected from the profession. Increasingly, therefore, the Colonial Medical Service became seen as an alternative for practitioners faced with the difficult reality that 'passing an examination is one thing, finding a subsequent job is another.'[5] Anne Digby has examined these conflicting tensions in detail. On one hand, the medical profession at the end of the nineteenth century had established itself as a viable and interesting career, but on the other it was very crowded and did not necessarily bring large financial rewards. Despite doctors' claims to gentility and social prestige, the reality of medical life, Digby persuasively concluded, was that, for most practitioners, it was rather difficult to 'make a medical living' in Great Britain.[6] Even Samuel Squire Sprigge, who tended to minimise the importance of medical overcrowding in his assessment of the problems medicine faced in 1905, acknowledged the competition for practices and patients and admitted that the 'grievances of the general practitioner are very substantial.'[7]

The pressure on medical jobs was particularly acute for Welsh, Scottish and Irish doctors. Their problems were often compounded by their comparative lack of access to the prerequisite capital or connections enjoyed by their wealthier English colleagues. Doctors qualified in England were more highly regarded by potential employers, even though those trained in Scotland, Ireland or the provinces held qualifications of equal professional status. Until the Great War, a certain amount of snobbishness afforded priority to English candidates who had a qualification from the Royal College of Surgeons or the Royal College of Physicians of England.[8] The difficulty in obtaining post qualification employment in Britain — allied to the rising output of doctors from provincial medical schools — goes some way towards explaining the existence of a large Celtic contingent within the Colonial Medical Service.

Although almost uniformly characterised as comparatively poorly paid, a Service career offered relative professional independence within the stable framework of an organised civil service with prospects for promotion and advancement as well as reasonable pension rights. These attractions could have been particularly important to the less well-off middle classes who were increasingly going through medical schools, but who did not have the capital to establish themselves in private practice. Hugh Trowell, for example, admitted that as a 'scholarship boy with no private means' his options for a medical career in 1929 were seriously curtailed, as he could neither afford to go into private practice nor work in hospital.[9] This prioritisation of the domestic economy as a factor driving medical career decision-making can be also sustained for the post-war period.

Although the medical profession continued to grow after the war, vacancies were created in the home profession through war fatalities and the growth of opportunities for doctors within the public and military services as well as within the increasingly competitive worlds of business and commerce. Although the growth of the medical profession continued to be publicised in the medical press, the pressures on the home market were reduced and doctors subsequently were more easily accommodated within the United Kingdom. Applications to the Colonial Medical Service went down correspondingly.[10] The increased presence of women in the medical job market, particularly after the First World War, made little difference to Colonial Medical Service recruitment, because of the inherent bias towards accepting men which continued until the end of the period.[11]

Similarly, the major downturn in medical service recruitment that occurred after 1935 can be interpreted as having been chiefly led by the market forces at home. During the depression of the 1930s it again became more difficult for doctors to find work in the domestic market, but when times became better, and employment chances for doctors at home improved, recruitment to the Empire Services dropped off.[12] Economic issues were insufficient to account for the ups and downs of recruitment alone and there were occasions, such as those experienced in the late 1920s, when Medical Service recruitment was high while the home market was also buoyant.[13] But, while there is no exact correlation, as a general rule periods of increased interest in the Colonial Medical Service can be said to have happened at times of professional pressure on doctors at home.

Of course, more personal issues also influenced choice. A sensible candidate to any profession would make a thorough assessment of the overall future economic prospects. The backdrop of fluctuating supply and demand at home would clearly play a part, but for most people the daily economic influences on choice boiled down to a question of how much they were to be paid. It is perhaps a testament to just how bad conditions were elsewhere, and how good perks of the career were perceived to be, that despite the enduring perception of poor pay, applications to the Service far outstripped available positions before World War One and during the second half of the 1920s. Not all officers thought that the starting salaries were inadequate. Arthur Boase in 1924 thought that £600 a year 'seemed like a lot of money' but in general, the salary was thought to be uncompetitive, given the dangers, stresses and expertise integral to the job. [14]

Compared to what newly qualified doctors could expect to receive as a houseman, however, salaries were a significant improvement. [15] Peter Clearkin, who came from a large Irish Catholic family with limited financial means, recalled that he had to choose his post-qualification hospital residency carefully because some simply did not pay enough for him to survive without parental help. After only four months as a houseman financial considerations forced him to move to private practice and it was only after it became clear that this did not suit him either that he decided to apply for the Colonial Medical Service in 1913. Although Clearkin complained that the Colonial Medical Service pay 'could not by any stretch of the imagination be called generous', the salary he would have received from the Colonial Service was still considerably more than the £125 per annum that he had received as a young assistant in private practice a few months prior. [16]

Farnworth Anderson similarly recollected a frugal state of affairs during his period as a houseman in the early 1920s:

All we could hope for was two or three guineas occasionally for assisting one's chief with an operation on a private patient in a nursing home. One's chief came in three or four times a week....The rest of the time you had to look after the patients and to supervise the work of the dressers on the firm, write to patients to come in to hospital, see return out patients, and of course to assist in any operations. Occasionally I was allowed to do an operation if my chief was feeling indulgent and satisfied with my capabilities.[17]

Although colonial salaries were better than those that doctors could generally expect to receive immediately after qualification, it should be remembered that the Colonial Medical Service preferred to recruit doctors who had already had a couple of years' hospital experience. Some officers did manage to join straight after qualification, but most considered the career only after having completed a hospital residency. It is only through comparison with typical post-residency salaries that colonial medical pay could be viewed as low.

During the period under consideration, the starting salary for Colonial MOs was only once raised. Between the beginnings of the Colonial Medical Service in East Africa and April 1920, a new MO could expect to receive £400 or, after 1910, £500 per annum, compared to a share in a private practice in Great Britain in 1909 that paid £1,000 per annum.[18] The situation clearly caused grievances amongst the officers; in 1918 East African colonial doctors Henderson, Massey and Small complained to the British Medical Association (BMA) that the starting salaries in the East African Medical Service had not increased since the turn of the century.[19] And even when the rate of colonial pay was finally updated to £600 per annum (the rate at which it remained until the end of the period), it was not long before this too was perceived as out of keeping with inflation and analogous salary rates in other medical jobs.[20] A comparison put forward by the Director of Medical and Sanitary Services (DMSS), Sierra Leone, JCS McDouall in 1931 is indicative. To support his argument that the low colonial salary was at the heart of recruitment problems, McDouall included several job advertisements for public medical appointments that he had found in the *BMJ*. These showed that the position of Assistant School Medical Officer and Medical Officer of Health in the County Borough of Blackburn was offered a starting salary of £600 p.a.; a job at the County Bacteriological Laboratory in Staffordshire started at £700 p.a. and Deputy Medical Officer of Health and Assistant School Medical Officer for Caernarvonshire County Council also offered a starting salary of £700 p.a.[21] Plainly, colonial salaries were uncompetitive compared with other positions opening up for British doctors.

The vocal complaints about colonial salaries made to the BMA peaked in 1920 and forced the Colonial Office to put some public effort into justifying the pay scales through a series of organised talks to medical schools.[22] Andrew Balfour, in a enthusiastic address calling medical students to consider Colonial Service opportunities, had to admit that salaries could be described only as 'fairly satisfactory' (something, he playfully commented, Scotsmen — such as he was addressing — would find particularly hard to swallow).[23] Several years later the apologetic tone remained; Charles Jeffries in his book on the Colonial Service was at great pains to justify the salary that MOs could expect to receive. Potential candidates were reminded that the post included considerable and generous benefits, such as free or subsidised housing, healthcare and passages as well as a non-contributory pension provision. The overall package meant that the 'real wages of an appointment are very substantially more than the salary would suggest.'[24] By 1939 the Assistant Medical Adviser to the Colonial Office was confident that the career choice offered a 'comfortable', although not luxurious, living for the officer and his dependents.[25] The other perks, not least the reduced local costs, meant that officers could hope to live 'in a style that he could not hope to maintain in this country.'[26]

Doctors joined the Colonial Service not only because there were few other alternatives available to them; indeed, some newly-qualified doctors were attracted to the career over alternative options for gainful employment. Examples from both the early and later periods show that the poor salary did not necessarily deter people. Arthur Bagshawe was said to have shunned an offer from his uncle to join him in his large private practice in Sussex, in favour of deciding his own path and taking a job in the Colonial Medical Service.[27] Arthur Williams similarly caused his father 'sad disappointment' when he also made such a decision in the early 1930s and refused to join the large family practice in Northumberland.[28]

Different economic dynamics affected recruitment patterns in different periods. Whereas attractive salaries might persuade doctors to stay at home, especially in times of domestic economic difficulty, this was not always the case. Despite the language of justification and explanation that characterised official commentaries on the issue, the career clearly offered opportunities that were more substantial than those represented by the salary rates. To see why doctors went to East Africa, these other factors should be given due assessment.

Practical Considerations and the Social Factor

There were other practical reasons why doctors may have chosen the Colonial Service career route: first in accordance with Colonial Office assurances, the overall remuneration *package*, gave opportunity for financial security, if not prosperity; second, the career was comparatively easy to get into and was quite well advertised in a respected forum (the *BMJ*) especially compared to other Colonial Service careers that were mostly completely unadvertised throughout the period; third, the need for a medical qualification made it intrinsically more meritocratic in that it was open to a larger portion of the middle classes than, for example, the Colonial Administrative Service (which still looked primarily to Oxbridge and the public schools as markers of suitability); last, the Colonial Medical Service offered a respectable governmental career that had enough prestigious associations to confer some social respectability, even if it did not have the equivalent status of the Indian or Sudan Medical Services.

A posting in East Africa was particularly attractive because the region was regarded as climatically healthier than West Africa.[29] This not only made the East African Medical Service more directly appealing, but meant that it was more feasible for young doctors to take their wives and families with them on a first posting. Although these factors were in some ways unexceptional, they all contributed to the attractiveness of the colonial medical career.

The cost of living in the colonies was substantially less than at home, for a start, officers did not have to pay income tax in East Africa and the job provided free living quarters, paid passage, financial provision for widows and orphans, a non-contributory pension scheme and the opportunity to supplement pay, if it was desired, through private practice. Most important, especially during difficult economic periods at home, was the promise of regular monthly pay, with annual increments and fixed steps to promotion. '[C]ertainty' emphasised one Colonial Medical Service selector, rather than any other incentives (including 'extra emoluments') was what 'the majority of candidates expect to find in the government service.'[30] To some the idea of a fixed tenure, once they had completed probation, was a real draw to the career as it gave them the option to remain in the Service for the rest of their working lives.[31] On the other hand, although the perceived stability was attractive, it was sufficiently flexible for doctors to leave the career if it did not agree with them or their families. In fact, it is difficult not to see some relationship between the average length of service for doctors in East Africa, which was eleven years, and the fact that ten years was the minimum length of service needed to qualify for a gratuity upon discharge.

Another practical consideration for potential entrants was that an appointment into the Colonial Medical Service was relatively easy to secure when compared to the highly competitive entrance examinations that both the Army and the Indian Medical Service required.[32] Both of these examinations were followed by mandatory six-month instruction course — much longer than that which was required to achieve the Diploma of Tropical Medicine and Hygiene needed by Colonial Medical Service entrants after 1899.[33] This reason for entering the Service is not mentioned in memoirs or obituaries, but this is not surprising as it would be unusual for any candidate to admit 'ease of entry' as a reason for choosing a career, not least because it would portray the individual as being unambitious (or worse, aware of their intellectual limitations) and would imply a lower status to the career. Although there is no explicit evidence for this factor it is likely to have been at least a subconscious motivation in some cases. After the demanding examinations that doctors needed to pass in order to qualify, the prospect of another test would be very unappealing. The fact that Furse admitted that the Medical Service was not always staffed by the most outstanding candidates gives further weight to ease of entry as a factor.[34]

Despite Andrew Balfour's bitter complaint in 1924 of 'lamentable ignorance' among medical graduates about the possibility of a government career in Empire, it was relatively easy to hear about the career as a young medical graduate.[35] Not only had there been a concerted campaign since the mid 1920s to promote the career in lectures to medical schools, it was one of the few Colonial Service careers that regularly advertised and several doctors mentioned that an advertisement in the BMJ prompted their application.[36] Also, as the period progressed it became increasingly easier to obtain detailed information on the tropical world. As well as popularising Africa more generally in the public imagination, this allowed young men to judge whether a tropical career would suit them. Throughout the period prospective candidates could obtain information on the life, climate and living expenses of the colonies from an ever-expanding literature of handbooks and travel advice manuals, some published by the Colonial Office itself.[37]

East Africa held specific appeal because it seemed a relatively healthy option, especially when compared to West Africa. Of course, the difference was only relative. Clare Wiggins related the story of his entrance interview (c.1900) when he was told in response to an enquiry over pension terms: '[p]ension, *pension*, Good Heavens, boy, no one lives to draw a pension!'[38] But East Africa was certainly seen as safer. Arthur Williams turned down an offer of a posting in Nigeria because of its reputation as 'white man's grave' before taking one to Uganda, which he thought a rather safer option.[39] Hugh Trowell too declared that he had been quite put off by the 'rather grim stories about West Africa' and had therefore quite consciously decided that he would wait for a posting in East Africa, especially as he hoped to have a family with his wife there.[40]

The prospects of a healthy environment for Europeans must have been particularly persuasive to doctors, a group with a professional interest in debates surrounding matters of health. In the earlier part of the period discussions over the suitability of Europeans to long-term residency in the tropical world frequently featured in the medical press. Medical orthodoxy emphasised the fundamental inability of Europeans to acclimatise as one of the strongest obstacles to settlement, but doctors such as Luigi Sambon challenged these notions.[41] The old views became replaced by a new faith in (tropical) medical science, particularly in the benefits of public health measures that allowed Europeans successfully to survive in hot and unwholesome places. Gradually the image of Africa as 'white man's grave' gave way to cautious optimism: the tropics needed to be managed through special precautions and routine, but this management was quite possible. Some of the negative health images — particularly an enduring view that women and children were not suited to long term residence — remained throughout the period, but perceived risks receded in the public and medical imagination from 1900 onwards.[42] Colonial Office publications actively promoted the climatic advantages of the Eastern regions. with descriptions of the Kenyan highlands tending to stress familiarity rather than unusualness.[43] For Africa in general Europeans needed to take 'elementary precautions' (and trips back to the United Kingdom), but this was far removed from earlier ideas that questioned the suitability of Europeans for any lengthy periods of residency in the tropics at all.[44] Indeed colonisation was presented in some forums as a way to further the boundaries of medical science by making areas more habitable.[45]

Closely associated with this promotion of the climate of East Africa as especially favourable, relative to the majority of the Continent, were the considerations doctors had for their wives and families. Many doctors mentioned that the East African Service appealed to them particularly because it meant that they could take their wives with them. Arthur Cole took the Colonial Service option over his preferred career in the Sudan Medical Service principally for this reason. Robert Hennessey made a similar point. Similarly, Arthur Williams preferred a Colonial Service career to becoming a missionary in 1931 because he thought that the latter would not allow him to have a wife.[46]

To add to these considerations was the appeal of a government position as a marker of social respectability. As the period progressed and public pride in the British Empire rose, the colonial career gained kudos and a more favourable reputation. This was something that Furse had been keen to nurture. He articulated this quite conscious goal:

> Above all, the prestige of the Colonial Service must be raised in the eyes of potential candidates, and of their parents and advisers. The Service must be 'put on the map', and a woefully ignorant public made to appreciate the scope and variety of its achievements, and to realize that it offered one of the most interesting and spiritually rewarding careers open to the cream of the country's youth.[47]

Furse must have felt satisfied at the end of his career in 1948 that all branches of the Colonial Service had grown in size and repute. Yet his vision was an essentially conservative one, based on the rank and behaviour of the ruling classes and the retention of essentially feudal ideas of ownership and management. In holding these ideas, he naturally turned his back on the modern ideals of egalitarianism, and gender and racial equality that emerged in the 1930s.

If a medical training was (as one East African MO called it) a route to a 'rational choice of career' which conferred respectability upon its members as a learned and established profession, its public status was heightened even further through the explicit and implicit associations that a governmental position held with the standards and attitudes of the ruling classes.[48] Furthermore, in the colonies, where health was at a premium, being a doctor was a particularly high profile community position, perhaps even more so than in Britain. Taking up a Colonial Service career meant that an increasing number of middle class medical graduates could expect to share some of the social privileges they might otherwise not have had opportunity to experience at home:[49]

> [A]n officer of the Colonial Service can enjoy in many ways a higher standard of living than would be possible on a similar salary in this country. He can command much more in the way of personal service though the service may not be the most efficient. He has a definite rank and social position and does not, outside his office, become merely one of the crowd.[50]

One closely related argument that has been put forward — by David Cannadine — was that the Colonial Service career held appeal precisely because many class elements of the colonial lifestyle echoed the values of a bygone era of British landed society; one that was, furthermore, becoming increasingly untenable at home owing to the effects of urban growth, industrialisation and commercialisation.[51]

A survey of the evidence supports this idea. Much of the colonial promotional literature stressed the way Eastern Africa particularly could offer conditions suitable for those with conservative, landowning, rural overlord ideals that were no longer acceptable back home.[52] One Colonial Service doctor recalled his 'early horror of the peri-urban industrial housing sprawl' he encountered on his train journeys to and from medical school, as being one of his leading incentives to practice medicine in Africa rather than in his home context.[53] In the same way, contemporary concerns, particularly present in Kenya, over the issue of 'poor whites' entering the country seemed to further reflect a desire to preserve, if not a real ruling elite, certainly one that espoused its values.[54]

Aside from social prestige, a job in the Colonial Medical Service offered other unique social benefits. In the colonies an MO was a member of a small and exclusive ruling elite, who could expect to have servants and other accoutrements of his newly acquired status.[55] The lifestyle was said to offer a 'much freer existence', than that which existed in the home country, not least because the Colonial Service was mostly staffed with young people.[56] Perhaps even more persuasively, the life was presented as fun. Colonial communities, although scattered, could usually converge at a central social club that typically held dances and other collective events. Thus, it was recommended that those travelling to East Africa should bring formal evening wear to wear at the club in Mombassa.[57]

Even the smallest station boasts a club where people gather in the evenings for a game of lawn tennis and a drink at sundown. In the larger stations, there are, of course, greater facilities for recreation, including polo and golf. There is also some measure of social life, and officers' wives live active and happy lives.[58]

First and foremost it was a place attractive to outdoor types and it was warned that 'anyone whose interests lie in the direction of art, music or literature, may expect to find his opportunities for such pursuits restricted.' [59] Not only, said Lord Cranworth, were there abundant opportunities to hunt 'some of the finest game animals in the world' but 'bird-shooting is almost everywhere good' and fishing was 'generally obtainable'. Group sports were frequently played: Cranworth seemed to think that prospective inhabitants would be hard pushed to find themselves so far away from a station that they would have to miss out on lawn tennis or 'the occasional game of cricket'.[60] Furthermore, it was even declared that '...the general standard of play in games is considerably higher than that found at home', apparently because sports had a natural place within the 'routine of living' for Colonial Officers.[61] Harrison has acknowledged this emphasis on the attractions of the sporting life in his work on the Indian Medical Service. Most famously Ronald Ross's initial choice of posting to India seemed to have been closely connected to his desire for adventure: '[i]t was only late in his Indian career that Ross acquired an interest in scientific research and in public health. The recreational activities which attracted him to the Indian Medical Service also loom large in the diaries of other Medical Officers stationed in India; often to the exclusion of any detailed description of medical practice.'[62]

It is debatable whether these images accurately reflected the realities of tropical colonial life, which must have regularly been isolating, alien and characterised by the lack of home comforts. However, the perception of colonial life projected within these positive images *did* clearly influence doctors' choices. Arthur Williams turned down an initial job offer in the West African Medical Service in Nigeria because he felt that (as well as being more deadly) the place offered fewer opportunities for big-game hunting.[63] Philip William Hutton reminisced that he had been attracted to Uganda, not only because the medical school there offered opportunities to teach, but also because of the sport, especially sailing, offered by the close proximity of Lake Victoria.[64] John Buchanan was attracted by the sporting life too; as he had enjoyed a successful rugby career in Scotland and wanted to keep up his interests.[65]

The East African based colonial career therefore offered several attractions that doctors may have taken into account when making their career choices. These practical considerations included the overall employment package, the accessibility of the career, the comparative healthiness of the places to which they would be posted, the ability to take families with them, and the way the career also seemed to promise new recruits increased social standing and a dramatically improved lifestyle. With these advantages, it is hard to imagine why anyone should have wanted to stay at home. The way doctors heard about these perceived advantages, through either word-of-mouth or family connections, also played a crucial part in awakening this interest.

Connections

As discussed in the preceding chapter, although recruitment based on patronage was officially abolished after 1930, many of its fundamental tenets informed the actions and decisions of the Appointments Department well into the late 1940s. Personal recommendations, whether through a medical school Dean, a university liaison officer or a friend or relative who was already in the career (or a similar one), were vitally important both in terms of Colonial Office officials hearing about good candidates and the applicants themselves hearing about the Service. Furse's policy of promoting the Colonial Service to medical graduates by the use of promotional talks by ex (or current) officers and Colonial Office officials would, it was hoped, attract the right sort of candidates.[66] This time-honoured idea of leading by example was similar to that traditionally employed within the hierarchical discipline and duty structures of public schools. The usefulness of close personal connections was acknowledged at the time. Medical school Deans recommended, for example, that talks by former medical students were better received than those given by people less intimately connected with the establishment.[67] The system did indeed seem to produce good results; by the 1930s Furse was satisfied that 'the appointment of officers who were holding good public appointments in institutions has in many cases been found to lead to applications from their successors or colleagues.'[68] Not only were these publicity methods felt to be useful indicators of individual suitability; they were actively nurtured as an effective way of keeping up continuity and loyalty (the idea of a sense of tradition) to the Service.

There is no doubt as to the importance of personal influences upon MOs' career choices. Even if this factor was not as strong as that of economics and Empire enthusiasm, the officers themselves frequently mentioned it. The attractions of the career were publicised through medical families, personal or familial Colonial associations and information passed on about the Service career from friends and colleagues.

The importance of precedent, particularly as a guide to career choices in medical families during the nineteenth century, has recently been examined by historians.[69] Crowther and Dupree have persuasively downplayed the importance of family succession in determining medical careers. Although they acknowledge the importance of having a medical parent as a potential guiding light into future career decisions, they prefer to emphasise networks of influence and patronage formed at medical school, as loose group markers and identifiers which usually persisted into later life.[70] These findings are borne out by the findings of this study (Chapter 9): doctors related particularly strongly to colonial colleagues who had been to the same university or medical school as themselves. A sense of group belonging was overlaid and extended by the particularities of the colonial setting. These felt connected through common purposes and expectations; what Dane Kennedy has labelled the 'islands of white' of the colonial sphere.[71]

Many Colonial MOs came from medical families.[72] Arthur Williams recalled how he had had an interest in life overseas but felt a 'filial duty' to take over his father's country medical practice; the Colonial Medical Service seemed to offer a way to reconcile both urges, especially as he confessed 'an uneasy feeling of professional incompatibility' with his father and did not want to follow exactly the same career path as he had done.[73] Perhaps even more pertinent is the large number of MOs who had connections with Africa, or other colonial territories, through their families. Perhaps the most striking example is Philip Edmund Clinton Manson-Bahr, who joined the Colonial Medical Service in Tanzania in 1939: his famous grandfather was Patrick Manson and his father, Philip Manson-Bahr. As one obituarist pointed out, 'this milieu exerted a significant influence on his future career.'[74]

The importance of these factors with regard to recruitment into the Indian Medical Service has also been acknowledged. Not only were a substantial proportion of recruits from medical families, but from colonial medical families, particularly those with Indian connections.[75] The relative newness of the East African Medical Service meant that it was unlikely, at least until the end of the period, that East African doctors had parents in the same service (the Indian Medical Service had been in existence in some form since the 1600s), but many had relatives with medical missionary or governmental medical service backgrounds. Arthur Morley's father had been a medical missionary in China;[76] Arthur Cole referred to the 'considerable overseas tradition in his family' as having influenced his decision to take up a colonial medical career. His grandfather and father had both been medical missionaries, in India and China respectively, and his wife's parents had served in Nyasaland in the early expeditionary days.[77] Alfred Mackie was born in Antigua in the West Indies where his father was a Colonial MO.[78] Arthur Boase's father worked in the Medical Service of British Guiana, and accordingly felt that the Colonial Medical Service seem 'the natural thing' to do after he had qualified.[79] Some were sons of Indian Medical Service officers: John Shircore's father had been a captain, as were the fathers of Herbert Duke and Raymond Price.[80]

It seems reasonable to attribute Ernest Cook's initial decision to join his famous uncles (Albert and John Cook) at Mengo in Uganda to family influences and expectations. Rather than remain a missionary, Cook transferred to the Colonial Service after 1926 (until 1936).[81] Farnworth Anderson decided to go to Kenya partly because his second brother had gone there before him and had 'loved it'.[82] Similarly, Albert Owen was attracted to his Colonial Service career through the experiences of his elder brother Hugh, in Uganda.[83] Brothers James and Percival Ross both took up medical careers in Kenya. Although little is known about Robert and Victor van Someren, or the two Twinings they qualified around the same time from the same institutions and were probably related.[84]

Many MOs came from non-medical colonial backgrounds: William Kauntze descended from a famous Doctor of divinity, William Carey, 'the well-known Oriental scholar, who had been one of the earliest missionaries in India'. Dowdeswell and Ansorge were both born in Bengal; Dawson Milne was born in Kingston, Jamaica; Robert Moffat, Mary Turton and Colin Carothers all came from South African backgrounds; John Buchanan was born to an early colonial family in Nyasaland; and Philip Hutton was born to colonists in India.[85]

Many officers joined the Colonial Service because they had been influenced by positive accounts of colonial life from relatives or friends. Charles Wilcocks sold his private practice and joined the Colonial Medical Service because of the enthusiastic reports of a friend in the Service.[86] Arthur Cole recalled the positive influences of his brother-in-law who was a member of the Nigerian Medical Service.[87] Raymond Barrett described how he was influenced in his future career while employed as an assistant in what he described as a 'working class practice'; one of his bosses had previously worked for the Medical Service in Kenya and was an 'ardent advocate' of the advantages of the colonial medical life.[88] Similarly, Hugh Calwell decided on an overseas public service career after being impressed by a lecture by Sir John Megaw, then Director of the Indian Medical Service, while still at medical school in Belfast. He changed his focus from India to Africa, however, after meeting Peter Clearkin who told him about his life in the Colonial Medical Service in Tanzania.[89] Similarly, John Gilks remembered that the appointment in 1912 of Arthur Williams, had resulted from their discussions in London sometime before.[90]

Informal networks of professional influence should therefore be seen as crucial to Colonial Medical recruitment, although these often operated in an uncontrived way between friends and family members without any explicit promotional purpose. Nevertheless, these interactions were a crucial factor in underpinning group belonging and unity among Colonial Medical Service members.

Despite the importance of these practical factors, however, was the ubiquitous, perhaps less tangible, allure of Empire. Job prospects in the UK, salary perks of a colonial position with all the concomitant increased social standing, as well as the positive experiences of family and friends, would have shaped people's choices, but these assessments alone were unlikely to have sustained interest. Also imbued throughout the decision-making process were the extremely powerful, positive ideological associations of an Empire career.

Chapter 5: Identity and Experience II: Ideological Reasons for being a Doctor in East Africa

> One wonders why so many medical men chose tropical Africa when they could have lived an easier life in a temperate climate and under less burdensome conditions.[1]

Discursive representations of Empire before 1939 both created and sustained a number of powerful images that situated careers based in the outposts of Empire closely together with issues of national importance. Religion, adventure and professional heroism all had their parts to play in stimulating interest in the Colonial Service and helped to justify the less than satisfactory pay and dislocation from family and familiar society. To be actively working as a member of the Colonial Service, particularly at a time when criticisms of the imperial project were relatively rare, immediately conferred upon participants a certain amount of valour that might not have been achieved with such immediacy within the home context. For doctors, particularly, the intrinsically philanthropic nature of the work meant that it was intimately associated with positive ideas of Christian morality as well as being dynamically connected with a new, potentially life-threatening, medical specialism, that of tropical medicine. It is these close associations with religion and (both professional and non-professional) adventure that formed the basis of many of the ideological factors that influenced doctors choices when deciding to work overseas for the Colonial Service.

The Religious Factor

Reading through the reminiscences and obituaries of ex-Colonial MOs, the numerous references to Christianity are striking.[2] Firm and explicit Christian beliefs were intrinsic to popular middle and upper-middle class religious expectations typical of the period. A desire to continue a Christian tradition confirmed and extended a historically-based convention that related many of the ideals of masculinity, including those needed for an African adventure, with Christian principles.[3] It is reasonable, therefore, to link some individuals' decisions to join the Colonial Medical Service to the religious connections specifically forged between medicine and the tropics through the work of medical missionaries. Missionaries had for a long time shouldered the burden of responsibility for medical care in the continent. Some medical graduates found Africa attractive precisely because it provided an opportunity to combine their professional preferences with these enduring images of Christian good works. In the context of Empire, a Christian identity further demarcated European communities from the uncivilised 'other' and was one of the key markers, especially in the early period, of civilised, rational and moral life of the white ruling communities. In choosing to become Colonial Medical Service doctors, rather than missionaries, some young graduates were engaging with these influential images of the Christian in Africa while pragmatically choosing a higher paying, more sociable and less religiously rigorous alternative to the missionary life.

Much of the fashionable literature that would have been read by potential candidates associated Empire with Christian values.[4] Many popular books and magazines portrayed the imperial adventure in Christian terms. Although by the end of the Edwardian period much of the unconcealed Christianity in these texts became increasingly overtaken by a more jingoistic rhetoric, many of the core Christian values remained.[5] The popular Boy Scout movement too, although never overtly Christian (indeed, keen to distance itself from being too much so), had a tone that was 'certainly moralistic' and typical of the nineteenth-century ideals that linked good moral fibre with imperial adventure.[6]

Many MOs were the children of clerics or missionaries.[7] It was a tradition moreover, of which some officers were self-consciously proud. Dawson Milne, who wrote a short history of the East African Medical Service, was keen to stress the Christian legacy. He presented the Colonial MOs he worked with in a direct line of succession from David Livingstone himself. The first government PMO, Robert Moffat, was, he reminded his medical department colleagues, the grandson of Livingstone's father-in-law and it was felt proper that MOs would be aware and proud of this tradition stemming from its brave medical missionary beginnings.[8] Moffat himself was said to have chosen a government career over a private one precisely because it gave him the opportunity 'to do good work'.[9]

Personal recollections provide a revealing insight into doctors' motivations. One of the earliest medical men to join the Colonial Medical Service in Uganda in 1895, William Ansorge, did so after being rejected by the Church Missionary Society.[10] Arthur Williams remembered how his image of Africa had been specifically influenced through its strong connections with the missionary movements and the Christian literature of his youth that had stressed associations between religion and Africa. His faith was so strong that he even considered giving up medicine at Cambridge for a career in the church, but persevered and eventually became a candidate for the Universities' Mission to Central Africa (UMCA). The Colonial Service seemed like a good alternative only when he discovered that missionary life with the UMCA would not allow him to marry.[11]

William Kauntze similarly chose medicine only as 'an after-thought in that it would prepare him for missionary work'; the tropical medicine certificate course additionally activating his interest.[12] During his time as a Colonial MO he continued his active religious involvement and enjoyed many years as a churchwarden to All Saint's Cathedral, Nairobi.[13]

Hugh Trowell, whose religious faith was so strong that he was ordained an Anglican minister after he retired from service, succinctly summed up the missionary/adventurer associations that coloured his pre-application image of Africa. He described his decision to be a doctor in Africa as having been driven by a 'mixture of idealism, a background of Christian belief, and a desire for adventure'.[14] His involvement with the Student Christian Movement while studying medicine had aroused his interest in a colonial career, as it highlighted the Colonial Service as a means of tying his medical education to his humanitarian beliefs without becoming a missionary — the group was 'not quite certain how much they wanted to convert people'; rather they wanted to help create an infrastructure in Africa.[15] Trowell was not alone in adopting a religious career after resigning from the Colonial Medical Service. A small, but significant minority took a similar path demonstrating how close the link could be between governmental medical works and missionary ideals. [16]

There was mutual suspicion between missionaries and government officials, particularly after 1914, but the boundaries between the two groups were not as rigid as has sometimes been argued. [17] The Colonial Medical Service temporarily employed missionaries with relevant experience during times of particular personnel shortages. Thus Charles Edwards, who had been a missionary in Kenya since the mid 1890s, served, according to the *Colonial Office List* of 1911, for a year as a temporary MO. Also Robert Stones, who had worked for the Church Missionary Society in Africa since 1911, spent a year on secondment to the Colonial Medical Service (Tanzania).[18]

Associated with this Christian motivation was a less explicitly religious humanitarian motive. This subtle change in emphasis was particularly evident after World War One, when the direction of colonial rhetoric turned to caring for African communities, rather than just the Europeans stationed there. Humanitarian issues began to feature in the promotional literature as a motivation for joining the Service: 'In few other branches of human activity can the work so surely be its own reward.'[19] Doctors became increasingly self-conscious about the part played in the improvement of public health conditions and health education for those in less fortunate positions than themselves. Some members of the Colonial Medical Service were motivated to work in Africa by work they had already undertaken in underprivileged areas of Britain. Raymond Barrett remembered that part of the career's attraction (aside from the enthusiastic press it had received from his boss) was the humanitarian side to the work. 'My experience of general practice in a rather insalubrious neighbourhood certainly influenced my decision', he recalled.[20]

Not everyone who became a government doctor in Africa did so solely to help those less fortunate than themselves, but these were notable factors within career selection. Associations between Africa and Christian missions were long established in the public mentality and it is striking how many Officers recalled some religious connection in making their choice. Furse himself was aware that the Colonial Service offered a new secular opportunity to take on some jobs that had formerly been associated principally with religion. He outlined how the career was a suitable choice for 'the idealist who wanted to serve his fellow men, the sort of man who, for example, would probably have gone into the Church 50 or 60 years ago.'[21] As will be discussed in the following section, the fashionable allure of Empire manifested itself in many other ways, but the association between Africa and good Christian works was an important part of the complicated tapestry of cultural appeal that held sway over people's choices.

The Adventure Factor

Public enthusiasm for Empire was at its peak in this period. In opting for an Empire career young doctors were taking part in something that held very distinct connotations of national pride, adventure and exoticism. Furthermore, while most people in Britain only experienced Empire at a distance, whether through the books and magazines they read, the music hall songs they knew, the imperial exhibitions they attended, the statues and memorials in public parks and (later) the cinema films they watched, active involvement immediately conferred extra status, perhaps even a degree of valour, upon actual participants. [22] This section briefly traces some of the most ubiquitous motifs and their roots in popular conceptions of Empire. It then analyses the evidence that doctors quite self-consciously entered into the colonial career because it seemed to present adventure, excitement and difference.

The appeal of an African adventure had deep roots in the literary-romantic Empire-building enthusiasm illustrated by the immense popularity of travel writers and adventurers such as David Livingstone (1813-73), Richard Burton (1821-90), John Hanning Speke (1827-64) and Mary Kingsley (1862-1900).[23] Livingstone in particular forged links between adventure, medicine and religiosity — his monograph; *Missionary Travels* sold 70,000 copies in the first few months after its publication in 1857.[24] As Driver has argued, this fashion both caused and extended enduring popular representations of the explorer and traveller and 'helped to produce an image of Africa as a field for European endeavour, and the myths which surround them — above all the image of Livingstone as a humanitarian pioneer — provided a potent means of justifying subsequent imperial adventures'.[25] These early associations, which Driver pinpoints as having peaked in 1890 with the publication of Henry Morton Stanley's *In Darkest Africa*, were subsequently extended further and altered through the new enthusiasm for British Empire, especially after World War One when Britain's presence in Africa solidified. [26] Many novels produced as part of this tradition are still popular today such as Joseph Conrad's, *Heart of Darkness* (1899); JH Paterson's, *The Man Eaters of Tsavo*, (1907); Somerset Maugham's, *The Explorer* (1908); Karen Blixen's, *Out of Africa* (1937), indicating how deeply these ideas permeated society.[27]

Much work has been done on the type of rhetoric used to describe the colonial experience in fictional and non-fictional mediums.[28] But Empire touched people in many ways beyond the written word; it was promoted through schools, pageants, exhibitions, biscuit tins and Liberty's department store.[29] Clearly young men applying for work abroad were attracted to Empire careers as part of this wider tradition. Images of a strange land full of exotic creatures and people had great appeal, and Africa in particular became a place onto which people could project their fantasies. The game was bigger, the skies wider and the people were more different.

Magazines such as the hugely popular *Boys Own Paper*, *The Magnet* or *Gem* promoted the imperial life of adventure.[30] These publications, and others, reinforced prevalent ideas of masculinity and heroism; only the strong and intrepid, it was thought, could survive in such a difficult and alien place. What Stanley described as the prerequisites of 'pure manliness' rather than 'vain fancies' represented solid, enduring, character credentials that changed remarkably little between the 1880s and 1939.[31] They were, moreover, exactly what the Colonial Office was looking for in its selection of candidates.

When a local boy got a Colonial Service job it was treated as the beginning of an adventure.[32] This was not necessarily empty rhetoric. Many of the claims made for Africa were true; it was unfamiliar, it was unhealthy and especially, before the advent of air travel, a journey to the tropics was long, expensive and arduous. Preparatory rituals included going to the tropical outfitters — Waugh's *Scoop* offers an entertaining parody of the paraphernalia that was deemed necessary for an African journey — or the buying of special equipment.[33] One needs only to look at the advertisements within the flyleaves of a 1930s edition of the Royal Geographical Society's *Hints to Travellers* to sense the excitement over the sort of equipment required by the attentive traveller.[34]

Some of these popular associations actually served to damage the reputation of the Colonial Medical Service, particularly as career destination for serious researchers or specialists. The medical school staffs' reaction to Hugh Trowell's career choice in 1929, for example, aptly illustrates the reverse side of the positive images of adventure:

> When it came out in [St.] Thomas's [Hospital] that I was going, I was even given a bit of a lecture, by my immediate superior, the honorary physician. You couldn't do any good work, any good medical work, out there. You probably would take to whisky too much, and black women even more. I said I was getting married, so he shut up about that. But the feeling was very much against going abroad in any Colonial Medical Service. They were said to attract—not exactly the scum, but the people who wanted adventure, some shooting, big game. You would probably remain a bachelor most of the time. Then he said it was such a waste. I'd done reasonably well at Thomas's.[35]

In general, however, Colonial Service promoters used the rhetoric of adventure advantageously and for their own ends. Professional opportunities for doctors in Africa opened up by the rise of tropical medicine presented a fresh field in which to shine, with the added romance of brave, selfless individuals having to endure the hardships of an unhealthy and uncivilised place. Doctors could fashion themselves relatively quickly as experts in Africa, in a way that would have needed a lifelong research career or a high-ranking hospital consultancy to achieve at home. The market for health manual and travel advice books was enormous.[36]

Furthermore, pursuing a war on parasites and pathogens projected a heroic image for the folks back home; a parallel to the ever-present big-game hunting images of Africa played out at a microscopic level. Andrew Balfour himself explicitly used a very similar analogy; the tropical world offered, he told his audience, 'a happy hunting ground for both the sportsman and the tropical pathologist'.[37] The new field of tropical medicine was presented most dramatically by stressing the most grotesquely diseases, such as elephantiasis, or by making repeated reference to the gulf between African and European health practices. There was, of course, a medical reality behind this rhetoric. Despite and because of the reputation tropical (particularly West) Africa had as a 'white man's grave', it offered a particularly attention-grabbing environment in which European healthcare workers could practise.[38]

The successful Colonial MO needed to be of 'infinite resource and sagacity'.[39] But as Alex McKay has pointed out, it was the lure of the different 'with all that symbolised' that government service candidates wanted: '[t]hey did not seek the familiar'.[40] In fact, group similarities and common denominators were positively stressed (above discord and divergence which certainly also existed) to demarcate the boundaries between the home country and the colony, and the colonisers and the colonised (see Chapter 9). The colonial career offered scope and opportunities that were accepted — even positively welcomed — because the work and opportunities provided were 'often on a far more challenging scale than in Britain.'[41] The Colonial Office realised how potent these images of difference were and used them frequently in their promotional language: students at St Thomas's were told as late as 1939 that the career would especially appeal to the medical graduate 'who desires to break away from the traditional practice of medicine in this country'.[42] Furse reminisced similarly on the Colonial Service's need for adventurous types:

> The chief attractions of the Colonial Service to the type of man we needed were, and remain, spiritual: the challenge to adventure, the urge to prove himself in the face of hardship and risk to health, of loneliness often and not infrequently danger; the chance of dedicating himself to the service of his fellow men, and of responsibility at an early age on a scale which life at home could scarcely ever offer; the pride of belonging to a great service devoted to a mighty and beneficent task; the novelty of life in unfamiliar scenes and strange conditions.[43]

The romantic imagery of contrast between the modern world and the tropical world was used time and time again to encourage careers in the Colonial Medical Service. Emotive language stressed the 'interest and beauty of the setting in which the Colonial Medical Officer is often privileged to work'.[44] The student audience of Balfour's 1924 address, was led into the lecture through highly romanticised language; they were asked to imagine taking a tour in a plane 'from the capricious weather and the gloomy skies of the north into balmier regions with a bright, strong sun above, and a vivid blue sea below, and…a long coast-line, bordered by a ribbon of snowy surf.'[45]

One of the reasons why New Zealand candidates were predicted to be relatively uninterested in pursuing a Colonial Service career was because it was felt that this adventure ideal would not have as much influence on those who already enjoyed those elements within their own home cultures. Given that many candidates interviewed for the Colonial Service said that they applied through a desire to lead 'an out-door life', the Colonial Office worried that 'New Zealanders have plenty of that supplied on the spot'.[46] Oddly, an attempt to stimulate interest among Australians, did not credit the Australian landscape with presenting the same opportunities and reverted to the more conventional motifs of persuasion: 'a man in these services is able to enjoy a greater variety of life than his contemporary in Australia….Taking it all round it is a grand life — hard at times, but none the worse for that — and a young man who is fortunate enough to enter one of these fine services has before him a life of usefulness and interest.'[47]

Even when negative elements were mentioned, these seemed to revel in the potential hardships opened by the colonial career: This was part of the package and one, it was emphasised, that should be embraced. The Secretary of State, Lord Lloyd reminded a group of young Colonial Service recruits what their decision entailed in 1940:

> You are not going to have a soft job. You will indeed have plenty of hard work and not too many of the comforts of life, and quite possibly no lack of danger, but I know that you would not have it otherwise….In what other task can you have so much power so early? You can at the age of twenty-five be the father of your people: you can drive the road, bridge the river, and water the desert; you can be the arm of justice and the hand of mercy to millions.[48]

The potential to suffer in Africa conferred bravery and status on the participants and emphasized once again just how distant and different Africa was.[49] People did not go to have an easy option; on the contrary they went to have a different, possibly harder option. The difficulties in fact served to bind the group together with common experiences and further set them apart from those who stayed at home.

Some saw the career as a stepping-stone to permanent settlement in Africa.[50] Others saw it as a means of extending amateur interests in anthropology, exploration, sport or natural history. Undoubtedly, the career offered tangibly exciting prospects; indeed there were few non-military positions for doctors that could offer comparable opportunities. This is far from saying that the colonial life could always pay back all the dividends of excitement it promised. Many MOs were bored with the job at times, or found facilities basic and trying. Negative images, though, are much harder to find than positive ones. This is partly because those who enjoyed the career were plainly more likely to want to write about it. Also, pragmatically, exotic images of adventure could sell. Books written about the colonial experience were expected to be enlivened with drama and local colour; this did not necessarily reflect each individual's opinions or the reality of life.[51]

Many adventurous depictions of service in Africa were images created by the officers themselves. Often they came from their own attitudes and so should be seen as largely self-descriptive. Even if the key-players in the medical services came from 'ordinary' middle-class backgrounds, the Colonial Service held connotations allowing people, if not to transcend their background, then at least to magnify their role in the new social setting. Normal contexts of work and leisure became intertwined and their comparative status and respect was inflated. The adventurous associations of their new life took them out of the mundane setting of Britain. As one of the earliest MOs in East Africa admitted, there was 'an indescribable fascination in African travel and adventure, which draws one again and again to the Dark Continent' despite the fact that many people had died there.[52] The theme is a common one; Farnworth Anderson recalled that he had become interested in East Africa through his Grandfather's large library of travel books about the region. Further interest was stimulated through several visits, while still a house surgeon, to the Great Empire exhibition at Wembley in 1924: 'Every Dominion and all of the Colonies had their own pavilion, and I often used to go and learn about them all. It certainly looked in those days as if the British Empire was a stable institution, destined to last forever.'[53] James Hunter had a self-confessed enthusiasm for African travel literature life reinforced when he and his fiancée saw in the late 1930s 'a colour film of Uganda, *The Pearl of Africa*, at the Empire Exhibition in Glasgow'.[54] Arthur Williams also admitted that literature on Africa helped mould his early impressions as a young man.[55] Robert Hennessey romantically described how he was attracted, not only by the exotic diseases he would professionally encounter, but by the landscape in which he would find them.[56]

Images of adventure were potent, widespread and clearly influential. Even famous names, confident in their tropical reputation, admitted that they had originally been drawn to their careers by the adventure and difference it had presented. Patrick Manson justified his decision to take up employment in China because of his 'adventurous spirit'.[57] Aldo Castellani saw his decision to volunteer for the Royal Society Sleeping Sickness Expedition in Uganda as part of a tradition, in which 'every young man craved adventure'.[58] Adventure tied together colonial communities through shared risks (Chapter 9). Of course adventure was not necessarily sufficient reason alone for the choice of job. Doctors' daily duties also provided opportunities for field observation of tropical diseases, helped the very poorest communities, and set them apart as practitioners who were not afraid to 'get their hands dirty' in conditions which were peculiarly both far below and far above those they could ever experience professionally in the United Kingdom.

The Professional Factor

The professional opportunities offered to doctors through a Colonial Medical Service career were exceptional. First, doctors could expect to have relative professional independence, often being in charge of large districts with very little outside interference. Second, the job appealed to doctors who hoped for variety in their professional lives. The colonial doctor, at least in the early years of his career, had to be very much an 'all rounder'. Colonial medical duties usually meant that individuals had to man clinics or hospitals, perform surgery, complete all the pre-requisite administration, and take up local opportunities to observe tropical diseases that were relatively unstudied and unfamiliar. And third, while the interest in being a generalist no doubt appealed to some, evidence from both the Colonial Office and the colonial doctors indicate that it was also specifically the idea of being a tropical medical practitioner, if not an expert, that appealed to the majority. A career in the Colonial Medical Service played upon a certain amount of idealism in the minds of young medical recruits. It combined many of the powerful external values of the time (Empire, adventure, exploration) with professional opportunities of making new and necessary discoveries (within parasitology, zoology, helminthology, entomology and bacteriology) and with personal attributes that were valued highly in the early part of the twentieth century (independence, ingenuity, innovation and initiative).

The Colonial Office itself pushed the idea that the Medical Service offered an independent (even if hard) professional existence. The Assistant Medical Adviser to the Colonial Office, AGH Smart, emphasised that, although there would be a support network of subsidiary medical staff to assist doctors, at the end of the day what an officer 'makes of his Hospital and District will largely depend on himself'.[59] Charles Jeffries made a virtue out of the 'hands-on' nature of the career; Colonial MOs, he stressed, would

> ...deal not so much with paper problems as with men and women; he will be entrusted with responsibility, and will be able, according to his position in the Service, to reach decisions for himself, to take practical action on his decisions, and to see the results of his work.[60]

This emphasis on doctors defining the boundaries and focus of their jobs was linked closely to notions of leadership, independence, resourcefulness and sound mind stressed by the Colonial Office interviewers. Ideas of job self-definition also fitted in with the meritocratic values of the Colonial Service. Although all officers started at the bottom of the career ladder as generalists, they could subsequently specialise, especially after the 1930s when doctors were encouraged to take further specialist or postgraduate qualifications while on leave.[61] The Colonial Office was very keen to publicise the 'almost unlimited scope for work and investigation' afforded by the colonial medical career. Because life was '[l]ived more in the open a man has every chance to exercise personality, to show administrative flair and to indicate any special professional bias or aptitude he may possess.'[62]

As can be seen from some of the Officers' subsequent careers, there was a thin line between an amateur interest in natural history and a professional interest in medical zoology, particularly medical entomology. Many budding medical entomologists inclined towards work in East Africa because of the wide-ranging problems associated with sleeping sickness and malaria in the region. The Colonial Medical Service career could combine an outdoor life and interest in natural history with practical medical knowledge gained at medical school; the abundance of wildlife in East Africa presented ample opportunities to learn more about the natural world. For example the obituarist of Fairfax Bell wrote '[h]is great interest in natural history was probably a deciding factor in leading him to work in the

Colonial Service'.[63] Similarly, Geoffrey Hale Carpenter, who 'exemplified a peculiar British product, the doctor naturalist who allowed what was at first a hobby to become the pivot of his career', was influenced in his initial career choice through the abundance of opportunities for expanding his amateur interests in natural history in a more professional capacity. [64] After hearing a lecture on insect-borne diseases as a young student, he 'decided forthwith that the field was for him.'[65]

Other keen naturalists included Arthur Bagshawe, Enrico Bayon, William Lamborn, and Aubrey Hodges.[66] Some officers, of course, took natural historical interests in distinctly non-medical directions. Rather than study parasites or disease vectors, they concentrated on birdlife and big game. Foster's blunt historical assessment of William Ansorge, as one whose 'contribution to medicine in Uganda was nil' is supported by Ansorge's own description of his experiences in East Africa. [67] His book makes no reference to medicine, but concentrates on describing his explorations from the east to the west coast and the subsequent categorisation of his zoological findings.[68] For others, interests in the broader zoological aspects of natural history developed later in their lives, as a direct consequence of living in Africa. Ralph Brockman, John Shircore and Clare Wiggins were all remembered as great enthusiasts for natural historical pursuits.[69]

Closely associated with these proclivities for natural history was the self-conscious decision to be part of the relatively new specialism, tropical medicine. A career in Africa opened up new avenues for medical investigation. By 1931 Furse could analyse this appeal to doctors in the second of his progress reports for the Appointments Department.

> Experience has shown that Medical Officers enter the Service for two main reasons: (1) the attraction of work in backward countries as compared with that of a general practitioner or of an officer in one of the Fighting Services; (2) the desire to take up some special branch of medicine and surgery.

> Financial considerations prevent the average young practitioner, who has gained his experience by means of resident or other appointments on the staff of Institutions, from specialising on his own account. It is known that the Colonial Service offers unique opportunities for practice in general medicine and surgery and that every encouragement is given to an Officer to pursue any specialist work in which he may be interested.[70]

In the early years of the twentieth century with the growth of bacteriology and parasitology, a new medical optimism concerning the tropical world developed. Even though mortality statistics were still higher for those serving in the tropics than at home, they were no longer so drastic that a career in Africa meant an unacceptably high chance of premature death. Doctors furthermore were an essential component of schemes to manage Africa through health work, not least as the colonies presented 'opportunity for pioneer work in virgin or only partially explored fields.'[71]

Furthermore, although medical facilities were meagre, this was offset by the abundance of resources (specimens, cases), for doctors to establish, and perhaps later also expand, their position in the tropical medical field. A career *in situ* gave doctors greater authority to speak of the effects of particular diseases through first-hand observations, and to have a practical sense of the environment and the daily health problems of African life. The African job's associations with tropical medicine therefore offered a situation whereby a medical man could have a realistic chance of making a name for himself.[72] Significantly, many of the most important tropical medical discoveries had been made by doctors resident in the colonies, rather than by research scientists in the home country; for example, Manson in China, Castellani in Uganda, Ross in India. By the first decade of the twentieth century these successes must have held some sway on ambitious young men's choices.

A tropical medical career created an opportunity to add prestige to a fledgling administration (and to the nation back home) by playing an active part in the field. These issues were afforded even more national importance because of the cutting edge status of tropical medicine among professional medical researchers during the period.

The way doctors defined themselves in terms of this research science culture is briefly addressed in Chapter 9; what is important here is that the Service actively promoted these opportunities as a reason to join. When Furse described the reason why Canadian medical graduates should feel especially drawn to the career, one of the reasons he offered was that it afforded 'rich opportunities for research in fields otherwise inaccessible to them'.[73] Interestingly, the well-publicised lack of facilities in Africa was presented less of a hindrance than a challenge. As Andrew Balfour pointed out, Laveran, Manson and Bruce all worked in peripheral locations without modern laboratory facilities. The portable microscope rather than the laboratory was the most powerful tool of the tropical specialism: 'it and its appurtenances constitute a laboratory in themselves.'[74]

Officers confirmed the official tone. Many Colonial MOs listed 'good therapeutic prospects' offered by tropical medicine as one of the chief attractions of the job.[75] To Robert Hennessey, a talk from a West African Medical Officer, led him to decide, 'there seemed to be good opportunities in a variety of fields.'[76] Although he had expressed a preference for a posting in West Africa or Malaya, he was offered Uganda, which he concluded would be suitable, not least because '[t]ropical [d]iseases were in ample supply'.[77] The new tropical field of scientific endeavour with so many causes and effects to be uncovered and documented created far more chances (and adventurous challenges) for medical men to make a mark on the field.[78] By being transported far from the perceived mundanities of urban life, the right sort of man, enjoyed research opportunities, which although hindered by lack of facilities and rough conditions, were not only more numerous, but more urgent and pressing than the old-world diseases back home in England. To add further glory, they were intertwined with the successful establishment of Empire and, as the period progressed, with broader welfare policies concerned with the health and wellbeing of millions of indigenous peoples.

These professional attractions clearly influenced the decisions of doctors deciding upon their future careers. The Colonial Medical Service offered a job that was relatively independent and unrestricted, while simultaneously having an infrastructure that encouraged people to gain extra qualifications and specialise should they so desire. The career paradoxically had professional appeal to both decided and undecided graduates. On one hand the chance to do a 'bit of everything' could have been attractive to young graduates who were not yet sure which branch of medicine they wanted to pursue. On the other hand, the Service had definite attractions for the more focused student especially for those specifically interested in tropical medicine.[79]

*   *   *

This chapter, and the one preceding it, has surveyed the main factors that influenced doctors career choices; of course there were exceptions to this pattern. Most doctors would have applied because of a combination of attractions, and equally some may have applied for reasons not touched upon at all. This second point is particularly relevant to doctors who found themselves in colonial medical careers after other professional experiences had taken them to Africa. Some doctors joined the Colonial Medical Service after a period in the army, frequently having had their appetite whetted through a period of service in the Royal Army Medical Corps (RAMC) in Africa, or through their experiences as military doctors during the Boer War.[80] Similarly, some joined governmental service after being commissioned to go to East Africa on separately organised scientific reconnaissance exercises, particularly those sent to Uganda under the auspices of the Royal Society (e.g. Muriel Robertson and Herbert Duke). Another group that deserves mention were those who went to Africa as private practitioners and only subsequently sidestepped into a Colonial Service career.[81] Although the one notable exception is Walter Macdonald, who unusually walked the other way and had left government service to become a private practitioner.[82]

Doctors occasionally started Colonial Service careers in other unusual circumstances, but early career exposure to Africa was the most common stimulus to finding other permanent work there. For these doctors the Colonial Medical Service offered an opportunity to continue working in a place they enjoyed, and in which they had already made social, and often emotional, connections.

Relatively few doctors specified their reasons for joining the Colonial Medical Service, and even if the sample were doubled, interpretive problems would still exist. Although general themes can be identified directly and others pieced together through evidence presented by other historical studies, personal circumstances are invariably characterised by internal contradictions and a lack of definition. People rarely relate to their own lives in compartmentalised categories. Robert Hennessey's memoir best captures the problems of capturing this type of history:

It would be pleasant to be able to say that my arrival in the African medical field was the result of careful planning, to achieve a long-cherished ambition. Nothing could be further from the truth. There was no fixed star in my firmament; practical considerations led to deviations; my interests were apt to vary; and fortuitous happenings had unexpected effects.[83]

Yet, although no perfect explanations emerge, there are enough similarities to allow insight into some common motives and rationales. Doctors as a collective group were, after all, subject to similar professional influences and market pressures; the young recruits all existed communally in a time that held established conceptions of acceptable cultural values and expectations, and the Colonial Office's terms and conditions of Service offered a tangible check list against which officers could individually assess job prospects. Although priorities changed throughout the period and were liable to dissimilar interpretations by different individuals, a valid general assessment is possible.

Many of the reasons for joining the Colonial Service were closely connected to the selection criteria used by the Service. For example, the Colonial Office quite naturally preferred candidates who were enthusiastic about the ideal of Empire. As the period progressed the Colonial career became more popular. This gradual upward trend was not always reflected numerically in recruitment figures, which in turn were subject to separate economic and social factors. By 1931, however, the *BMJ* felt able to describe the Colonial Medical Service as ranking 'among the premier Services of the Empire'[84] and by the end of Word War Two, the Colonial Service, from the European perspective at least, was seen generally as a 'respected and sought after Crown career'.[85] Furthermore, it had increased its sense of common identity, one that still is evident among retired colonial officers today.[86] Although this sense of group belonging clearly grew out of shared practical experiences and common institutional purposes, it can also be related back to the circumstances in which doctors first chose the career above other options available to them. The expectations held in the home country shaped their professional perspectives to an important degree once they had begun medical work in East Africa. This was a chain of events that would colour what MOs deemed to be acceptable and unacceptable in their jobs, how they perceived themselves both individually and as a cadre and, later, even their memories.

Chapter 6: The Organisation of the Colonial Medical Service in East Africa

> You have no idea how primitive Africa is. You'll never do any good medical work. You'll take to whisky and black women.... Damn it man, it's such a waste of your talent.... All you will do in East Africa is shoot game, have a bit of an adventure.[1]

Whereas the preceding chapters dealt with the bureaucratic processes and issues raised in *becoming* a Colonial MO, this chapter and the others that follow examine some of the experiences of *being* a MO once appointed to British East Africa. Although several academic works have considered the medical history of the region, there has been little systematic description of the organisation of colonial medical administration or the collective experiences of government doctors in the field.[2] Most general Colonial Service histories have concentrated on policies rather than people, with no assessment of distinctively Medical Service experiences and nothing about them in the East African context.[3]

In an attempt to amend this omission, this chapter reconstructs some of the key elements of the colonial medical encounter. As no single official job description existed for the various ranks within the Medical Service, and no single organisational model provided an immutable template for all methods of colonial medical administration, this argument has been pieced together from a large evidential base. The resulting picture, therefore, describes the general situation at the expense of exploring the subtleties of individual experiences, which naturally differed depending on time, place and personality.

The first section describes the organisation of the Colonial Medical Service. Unsurprisingly, the discrete identities of the three colonies meant that each had their own particular focus or medical interest that encouraged certain types of medical organisation over others. Uganda was characterised by a strong missionary presence and had a relatively rapidly emerging schedule to educate Africans as healthcare workers; Kenya had a powerful and vocal white settler community with which to contend; and Tanzania a very different set of concerns resulting from its former German rule and relatively small British settler population. Although individual medical policies were affected by these differences, the general personnel organisation of the Colonial Medical Service followed the same basic pattern in all three places, perhaps natural enough as the Colonial Office in Britain governed them all. This section outlines departmental structures and the main job titles as well as broadly describing the official duties assigned to them. It describes the MOs' practices rather than the policies they followed, although there was some overlap in these two areas.

The second section goes on to outline the common denominators within the practical organisation of medical care and its administration in the three countries. The way healthcare was physically and demographically distributed is described, particularly highlighting the use of the dispensary system and medical safaris as a means of extending western medicine to the rural areas. The changing focus of medicine is traced, especially the growing status afforded to public health issues after 1919. This growing interest extended official duties in practical terms as well as broadening theoretical expectations of the role colonial medical departments were expected to fulfil.

Although there were clearly local differences, the structure of the Colonial Service created many similarities. In terms of bureaucratic organisation, the departments followed the structural model typical of medical departments throughout the British Empire. This administrative structure was heavily based on the organisation of the West African Medical Service (unified in 1902), which itself had been modelled on an earlier administrative prototypes used in the organisation of the Indian Medical Service.[4] In the early formative years, the medical departments of Kenya and Uganda were established on equivalent bureaucratic principles before they merged between 1903–08.[5] When British administration was established in Tanzania it also modelled itself on the Kenyan and Ugandan precedent.[6] Regional proximity and shared British rule meant that, especially after improved transport systems were completed, Medical Department heads would meet together and confer over policies and priorities, working towards coordination wherever practicable.[7] Building on these common roots, this chapter emphasises similarities above differences, to situate the character of the East African Medical Service together with the way it was structured and focused.

Official Structures and Policies

Described in the simplest terms, the medical bureaucracies were run in a conservative and hierarchical manner.[8] Officers were expected to work themselves into a position of pre-eminence and, until they had done so, to obey their superiors and to afford fellow officers respect fitting their rank.[9] This typical 'white-collar' method of bureaucratic organisation was similar to the quasi-militaristic ethos traditionally promoted at British public schools and was favoured within most public service cultures by at the time.[10] Four core grades of officer made up the colonial medical personnel during most of this period: the head of department, the deputy head, the senior officials and the rank-and-file MOs.[11] Supporting this contingent of medically qualified British staff, were European laboratory assistants, clerical assistants and nursing staff. There also existed a large network of non-European subsidiary staff, made up principally of Indians and (by the end of the period) Africans who worked as hospital assistants, compounders, sub-assistant surgeons, dispensers and laboratory assistants.[12]

Two points illustrate the bureaucratic philosophy of the Service and define the professional culture of which all officers were a part. First, the higher up an officer was in the Colonial Medical Service the less clinical and more administrative their job became. Indeed, some officers commented that they would prefer to be passed over for promotion than take on the onerous paperwork expected of the senior ranks.[13] Second, the Service prided itself on its meritocratic culture; all officers essentially received the same on-the-job training and rose up the ranks over time. The higher positions were filled through promotion of those who had 'rendered good service',[14] although occasionally they were staffed via transfers from the medical departments of other British territories or (rarely) through the establishment of special senior consultant positions.[15] This provided a very structured career path for Service entrants, although in smaller territories with few senior positions the possibility of promotion was dispiritingly remote, especially before unification in 1934.

As the medical departments grew job titles correspondingly became more varied, reflecting increasing bureaucracy and specialization. During the early years there were only two possible positions within the Medical Departments of Kenya and Uganda: those of PMO and MO.[16] By 1939 there were twelve different medical positions within the Kenya Medical Department, eleven in Tanzania and ten in Uganda.[17] The new job titles, while remaining structured around the four core positions, reflected the creation of specialised posts and a desire to establish a broader spread of senior positions. The aim was to make the administration less overtly top down and autocratic and increase prospects for promotion. Certain new senior positions accommodated changing health priorities, for example Principal Sanitation Officer (PSO) established in Kenya in 1913, Sleeping Sickness Officer, established in Tanzania in 1926 and Principal of Mulago Medical School, established in Uganda in 1928.[18]

The period before 1920 was one of establishment and consolidation of the colonial medical administration. During this time the medical departments sought to define and regulate the duties associated with each medical rank, as well as establishing procedures and setting up physical infrastructures, such as hospitals and dispensaries. By the late 1920s as Britain's position in Eastern Africa solidified, the medical departmental organisation became more complex. Departments were divided up into distinct branches and divisions as new regulations for the East African Medical Service were introduced.[19] Later, the centralising reforms of the 1934 unification encouraged a simpler and more standardised structure.[20]

From the time of the formal unification of the East African Medical Service in 1921 moves were being made to encourage homogeneity. Large-scale changes in nomenclature of the job titles were instituted in 1925 and 1934 not only to reflect more up-to-date ideas of departmental orientation, but also to contribute to the desired goal of an increasingly standardised service.[21] It was only in 1925 that the first formal guidelines were published briefly describing, the structure of the Medical Departments and the duties attached to each main position.[22]

The Four Core Positions

Headship of the Medical Department (PMO, DMSS, DMS)

The head of the Medical Department was directly answerable to the Governor. The post changed very little in its remit throughout the period, although by 1939 the head was responsible for a larger body of medical personnel servicing a much wider section of the population. Initially in all three dependencies as the head was called Principal Medical Officer (PMO). In 1925 Kenya and Uganda changed the title to Director of Medical and Sanitary Services (DMSS) and in Tanzania it was changed to Director of Medical Services (DMS).[23] At unification of the medical services in 1934 the title DMS was adopted in all three territories.[24]

The departmental headship was the highest-paid medical position in the dependency. The post carried ultimate responsibility for the 'administration and control of all Government medical and sanitary establishments and the distribution of their personnel'.[25] It was an exclusively organisational and management position, although a PMO might go out of his way to keep a hand in with the more practical aspects of medicine.[26] Despite the fact that the head of the Medical Department rarely, if ever, needed to practice medicine as part of his professional commitments, he was always a qualified doctor, usually one who had started off as MO and worked his way up through the Service.[27] The PMO customarily had a seat on the colonial government's executive and legislative councils and was closely involved in the overall governance and legislature of the colony, particularly issues related to public health legislation.[28] The PMO was also a prominent member of many urban administrative boards, especially those with medical interests.[29]

Additional to this political role, the PMO was accountable for the overall management of the Colonial Medical Service and the general regulation of medicine within the territory, such as the registration of private, commercial and governmental medical practitioners), the issuing of licences to Indian Sub-Assistant surgeons, and the allocation of medical expenditure and revenues.[30] In the earlier period, the PMO, often worked closely with the Public Works Department in organising new buildings and facilities for medical provision.[31] The PMO sanctioned all local Colonial Service appointments and assumed responsibility for all MOs once they had arrived in the colony. As the head of all personnel, the PMO granted leave, stipulated the posting and duties of doctors, enforced discipline. He arbitrated in professional disputes and investigated any complaints brought by non-governmental parties over the provision or quality of official medicine within the territory.[32] The PMO was responsible for the submission of departmental reports requested by central government in London; he had to submit the medical figures and estimates via the annual Blue Books as well as prepare the Annual Medical and Sanitary Report covering all aspects of medical administration within the colony. Theoretically (although it was often impracticable), the PMO was expected to undertake with his deputy periodic tours of their area to gain a 'proper appreciation of the medical problems of the country.'[33]

Deputy Headship of the Medical Department (DPMO, DDMSS, DDMS, DDSS, DDLS)

It was in 1902 (in Uganda) that first mention was made of the existence of a deputy position.[34] From that time onwards, with the exception of a short period in Kenya (1909–13 when the position was temporarily abolished), at least one deputy, but sometimes several, acted as second-in-command to the head of each Medical Department.[35] The position underwent many changes in both its nomenclature and designated responsibilities; changes that were directly reflective of the way the Medical Department was structured at various times.[36] From the mid 1920s to the mid 1930s, the favoured method of organising the medical departments in the East African territories was to separate them into medical, sanitary and laboratory branches. A director headed each branch with a title usually indicating their particular area of responsibility: Deputy Director of Medical Services (DDMS); Deputy Director of Sanitary Services (DDSS) and Deputy Director of Laboratory Services (DDLS).[37] After unification in 1934 this system was abolished and gradually it became normal for a single deputyship with the title Deputy Director of Medical Services (DDMS) to exist within each territory's medical hierarchy.[38] To compensate for lost posts, an assistantship (Assistant Director of Medical Services, ADMS) was additionally created at an intermediary level between the rank of deputy PMO and that of SMO.[39]

The DPMO directly supported the head of the Medical Department. A purely administrative position, it was the route by which the most ambitious officers could eventually rise to the directorship. The DPMO acted as the first in command during times when the PMO was away from office and assisted generally in all duties carried out by the head of department. Deputies who headed the separate branches of the colonial medical establishment, naturally had extended responsibilities. The DDMS supervised and organised the MOs as well as overseeing the running of hospitals and dispensaries; the DDSS was responsible for the organisation and duties of the sanitary support staff, often working in close association with the Public Works Department in the building of new hospitals and the hygienic planning of cities and public buildings; the DDLS was responsible for the management of the bacteriologists, pathologists, laboratory assistants, chemical analysts and microscopists. In accordance with this division of labour, it was expected that deputies would compile the section of the annual medical and sanitary report relevant to their realm of responsibility.

Senior Medical Officer (SMO)

The first SMO in British East Africa was appointed in Uganda in February 1904. The holder, Robert Moffat, had stepped down from his position as head of the Medical Departments of Kenya and Uganda because he felt that the joint directorship was not only excessively 'unwieldy' but also that its administrative focus had distanced him too greatly from his original professional interests.[40]

The number of SMOs in office at any one time varied. In the period before 1920, they usually made up around 5 per cent of the entire medically-qualified workforce and in the later period, they constituted between 10 per cent and 14 per cent of the medical department.[41] Unlike the higher positions, the grade of SMO remained a constant feature of all three medical departments from its institution to the end of the period and beyond. SMOs' responsibilities were mostly divided regionally. They managed several medical districts, undertaking a combination of administrative and clinical duties. While they carried a heavy burden of administrative responsibility, supervising a large geographical area, SMOs were also expected to offer practical assistance on difficult clinical cases and to participate in, as well as manage, local medical initiatives. The SMO had to prepare regional medical reports and report back to the head of department on any particularly interesting provincial developments as well as making suggestions for improvements. They were also required to undertake regular supervisory tours checking out and reporting on all aspects of district medical work. Depending on the geographical area of responsibility, an SMO was often in charge of a particular hospital or medical programme; if there was no SMO the nearest MO often carried out these duties.

Medical Officer (MO, DMO, MOH, HO)

Most colonial medical workers were MOs, sometimes known in rural postings as District Medical Officers (DMOs). These doctors constituted the main colonial medical infrastructure and undertook the bulk of the medical work in the colonial Empire. Most appointments involved taking charge of a (sometimes extensive) medical district within which officers usually attended to the local hospital, oversaw sanitation and provided basic medical and surgical care to the community. Unlike their equivalents in Britain, the MOs' job required considerable management skills. Not only did the government doctor have to care for a large number of patients, they also had to supervise and train the Indian and, later, African support staff who were responsible for much of the day-to-day medical work in the regions.[42]

Supplementary duties of a MO included medico-legal work such as acting as police surgeon, undertaking the duties of expert witness and attending executions.[43] They were also expected to conduct post mortems, issue death certificates, and examine and report on the health of government officials about to proceed on leave (or those who had been invalided). [44] Additionally, they could be called upon to examine locally appointed candidates for government service.[45] Particularly in the period before World War One, local government doctors often had to set up (sometimes from scratch) their own facilities in the areas to which they were posted. This became less frequent as the medical infrastructure became more established, but plenty of early evidence points to doctors' close involvement with house building, hospital planning, local staff training and the setting up of rural dispensaries.[46]

The character of a MO's job predictably varied depending upon whether they were located in an urban or rural posting; over time it also became further extended and formalised through different types of colonial legislation. In municipal postings MOs were sometimes expected to participate in many of the local government structures, for example the town planning boards, the central boards of health and the boards of medical registration. The legal remit of an

MO's duties was defined by laws passed to regulate infectious diseases and public health and by disease-specific legislation with regard to sleeping sickness, plague, malaria, venereal disease etc. The earliest public health responsibilities of MOs were set out in very specific and localised regulations (such as the 1899 East Africa Plague Regulations), and gradually this type of legislation became the model through which the policing and custodial role of the MO became extended and further enunciated.[47] The first general Public Health Ordinance was only passed in East Africa in 1913 (in Kenya). Many of the roles defined for MOs in this and later Public Health Ordinances —the issuing of health passes, the right to impose restrictions on the movements of natives, the enforced inspection of private business and dwelling houses, the power to demand cleaning and disinfection etc. — were simply more comprehensively articulated extensions of earlier Township Ordinances. Infectious Diseases Ordinances, passed in each territory and frequently amended throughout the period, provided Officers with the right to destroy or remove potentially infectious property, to prohibit the movements of possibly infected people and to order their removal to segregation camps. In accordance with the later implementation of a policy to govern East Africa through indirect rule, some of these responsibilities were gradually transferred to the native authorities.[48]

Public Health legislation fundamentally changed the remit of a MO's work.[49] The legislation, which was received with 'astonishment and incredulity' in many quarters, significantly 'modified' the views of all MOs.[50] Indeed, the public health role of the MO eventually became so important that it often took precedence over clinical duties. The officer who 'mastered the intricacies of the new Public Health Ordinance' reminisced one MO, 'became overnight a man with a future'.[51] This increased responsibility had, however, been long in the making. Although the job title of Health Officer (Later, MOH) was added to the personnel complement of Uganda and Kenya as early as 1904, the real kick-start to systematic interest in public health matters can dates to the visit of sanitary expert, Professor William Simpson to Kenya, Uganda and Zanzibar on the request of the British government in 1913.[52] After Simpson's damning report on sanitary conditions in British East Africa, MOHs possessing a Diploma in Public Health could be appointed on a slightly higher salary scale than regular MOs, usually to the larger urban centres or ports. In addition to their inspection and regulatory duties, Port Health Officers were responsible for enforcing quarantine regulations, inspecting in-coming vessels and issuing them with clean health certificates, where appropriate.[53]

The jobs of MOs and MOHs might be officially different, but the shortage of doctors and the close relationship between public health and general medical welfare was so intimate that most officers, irrespective of their title or possession of a Diploma in Public Health, performed both functions daily.[54] This enforced generalism was a regular feature of the colonial medical life: just as the difference between the duties of MOs and MOHs tended to be blurred, there was little official acknowledgement of the difference between surgical and medical positions.[55] Although surgical work was assigned to officers known to prefer such tasks wherever possible, most MOs were expected to perform basic surgery. The first specifically surgical job title was not introduced until 1920, when the position of Resident Surgical Officer (RSO) in the European Hospital, Nairobi was established. In the same year the part-time position of District Surgeon was set up in Kenya. This allowed some MOs to divide their time between settler farming and surgical work, and also helped increase staffing in remote areas that did 'not warrant the whole time services of a Medical Officer'.[56] The position of District Surgeon endured in Kenya, but other surgical job titles in East Africa were reserved for senior officials tied to hospitals.

Another role of the MO that expanded over time was that of the educator. As the first point of contact between the African people and the European medical services, the MO became cast more frequently as educator and public health advisor in accordance with the changing priorities of colonial administration. The pragmatic acknowledgment that MOs alone could not effectively manage the healthcare of such large populations led to a policy of placing nominal responsibility for health in the hands of the native populations themselves. Schemes were systematically introduced, from the 1920s, to educate Africans as auxiliary health workers.[57] In all three countries, the role of the MO went beyond formal tuition. He became increasingly used as a general mouthpiece through which matters of sanitary and epidemiological importance could be promoted. The role of the MO as health propagandist was increasingly enunciated, particularly under the influence of Drs Gilks and Paterson in Kenya and Owen in Tanzania.[58] As the head of the Uganda Medical Service formally pronounced in 1934, the MO 'must preach the laws of health in and out of season'.[59]

Although the multifarious role of the MO was stressed as being very hands-on, the amount of administration a MO had to undertake was quite considerable and the cause of many complaints (see Chapter 7). Duties included completing statistical returns, for their district, confidential reports on subordinate staff, stock-taking reports on medical supplies, an annual report on medical buildings and domestic medical quarters, as well as registers of pay, absence and ill health for all staff working in the district.[60] As annual medical funding from the colonial government was based on the demand for medical services, it was the task of the MO to supply detailed (and preferably large) patient figures — 'statistical obsession' which one MO cynically described as 'the ten-fold propaganda value of ten circumcisions as against the unitary significance of one hysterectomy.'[61] MOs, just like other civil servants, were required to have a certain level of administrative expertise and numerical proficiency. Indeed, by the 1930s administrative duties were so important that it was declared a 'first prerequisite' to promotion to the senior grades. Those officers who felt that their talents lay in other areas were recommended to consider specialist or teaching posts if they wanted to be considered for promotion.[62]

The ideal MO therefore espoused medical and surgical skill, management ability, educational interests, custodial duties and administrative proficiency. Personnel resources were never sufficient to allow for the luxury of exclusive specialisation before 1939. Even if the MO had ambitions, or even an official brief, to undertake specialist projects or detailed research on a particular medical phenomenon, these had to be fitted in with their core obligations. This makes it all the more remarkable that so many Colonial MOs contributed papers to East African and international research meetings. Aubrey Hodges' 1905 complaint, when appointed to head the sleeping sickness investigations in Uganda, 'more work for the same pay', is just an early example of problems that later MOs encountered when they found that they were required to organise specialist investigations around all the regular duties of a MO.[63] Although the priorities of MOs were subject to change and adaptation (for example, the need to establish medical facilities in the first decades of British administration were supplanted by other concerns once the infrastructure was set up), the 1920s were a crucial turning point. From this time onwards, the focus of medical care shifted demographically (from providing healthcare only for European officials to the entire population), geographically (from focusing principally on urban areas to opening up rural ones) and in its medical focus (from curative medicine to public health). Furthermore, these changes, once made, became fundamental tenets of the job description that were to endure well beyond World War Two.[64] To understand the context of these changes in the job responsibility it is necessary to describe the way medicine was administratively ordered by the British in the East African region.

The Organisation and Focus of Colonial Medicine

The way colonial medicine was organised within the period directly reflected changes in the focus of medical care and the expanding needs of the colonies. The practical organisation of the medical department, the role of its employees, and the policies it espoused were all interrelated facets of the different stages of establishment, development and, eventually, solidification of colonial medical administration in British East Africa. Broadly speaking, the history of colonial medical administration before 1939 can be divided into two distinct phases. The first stage (1893–1919) represented the period when the British presence in Kenya and Uganda was established. Government medical care during these formative years was organised principally for the benefit of the official European communities and, when offered to Africans, it was usually to those in European employment. The focus of medical administration tended to be one of health crisis management. Attempts to combat major epidemics had the aim of stabilising British rule, rather than contributing to the welfare of African communities. During the first years of civilian rule in Kenya and Uganda, the provision of curative medical services and the establishment of basic facilities took precedence over wider medical aims. In stark contrast the second stage (1920–39) marked a period of increased conviction that colonial rule in East Africa was to be around for some time. Medical departmental policies were significantly rethought in three major ways: first, there was a shift away from curative medicine towards preventive medicine; second, a complete overhaul of the medical administration was undertaken, moving towards a more decentralised system with responsibilities accorded to native authorities and provision made for rural African communities; and third, the first moves were made towards the official support of research medicine and the early development of specialisation. When Tanzania joined the British Empire the changes it underwent were more the result of these policy shifts than symptoms typical of the establishment of British rule.

As described in Chapter 1, the earliest incarnation of the Colonial Medical Service in Kenya and Uganda came directly out of the Imperial British East Africa Company. In 1895, when the company was officially disbanded, many Imperial British East Africa Company doctors transferred from company employment to government service and medical employees from the Uganda railway later joined them. In this period medical policies were first demarcated and procedures and job descriptions were defined.[65] The organisational model for the Colonial Medical Service in East Africa was broadly provided by the West African Medical Service, but medical administration in Kenya and Uganda did not, initially at least, have an equivalent organizational infrastructure on which to build. In 1928, former PMO of Kenya, Milne, described the difficulties staff faced, especially when everything had to be established from first principles.[66] Perhaps most cumbersome of all to the administration was the lack of delegation that the bureaucracy allowed for. With relatively few SMOs during the pre-war years, all MOs reported back through the same single hierarchical channel that meant that requests could take months to be dealt with. Although attempts were made to improve and coordinate the medical services, the fundamental problem of short staffing and the need to establish a basic infrastructure took precedence over all else before the end of World War One.[67]

A key change in Medical Department orientation was the movement towards preventive medicine. Although (as Beck argued) this chiefly got underway in the period after 1920, crucial inroads were also made into the issue before the war.[68] The importance of the early township ordinances leading to the first Public Health Ordinance in 1913 have already been mentioned; it is valuable also to acknowledge the changing of attitudes towards public health in non-legalistic ways. Most significantly, the metropolitan-based push for sanitary improvements in the colonies was met with approval by medical departmental staff in East Africa. Subsequent delays in implementing the suggestions were more to do with limited resources than any lack of will or concordance.[69] Furthermore, because priority had to be afforded to issues integral to the establishment of colonial rule, most early initiatives towards sanitary reform were almost exclusively limited to urban areas before 1919.

Since the beginning of the century, medical opinion was largely unified in its acknowledgment of the pivotal function public health issues had in the future of the colonies.[70] The government in London declared its support for the ideas and agreed the need to 'look to, and depend more on, prophylaxis than on cure' within the realms of colonial medicine.[71] These priorities were reflected relatively quickly within the colonial context. In 1904 the first post of Health Officer was instituted in Kenya, with Walter Macdonald as the first incumbent.[72] Soon after William Radford was made a MOH and became one of the first vocal campaigners for the East African public health cause. He frequently wrote to medical headquarters to express his dissatisfaction with the overburdened nature of his job and argued the need for concerted sanitary campaigns.[73] By 1910, Uganda had established a separate sanitary branch of its Medical Department and the medical secretariat in Nairobi was also agitating for change.[74]

This new phase of awareness of preventive issues within the British medical administration can really be dated to 1913 and William Simpson's (Public Health

Advisor to the British Government) visit to Kenya and Uganda. Simpson's recommendations were so important that they formed, *verbatim*, the basis of the subsequent Public Health Ordinance.[75] His recommendations included a call for the formation of a separate sanitary branch of the Medical Department in Kenya, where it had not yet been created, the re-organisation of urban areas, and the appointment and training of sanitary superintendents. Yet, although these proposals were embraced in principle, the systematic introduction of public health reforms was severely disrupted by the outbreak of the First World War, and change did not occur until the 1920s. From this time preventive campaigns were led by Gilks and Paterson in Kenya and by Shircore, who installed numerous sanitary superintendents for lower-level public health work in Tanzania.[76] In Uganda, the appointment of de Boer as DDMS in 1933 had a great influence on the development of public health awareness. De Boer was said to have converted 'not only the Medical Department but the entire Administration to the gospel of environmental health.'[77]

Increased bureaucracy of the Medical Department and new legislation underpinned this new public health focus. By the beginning of the First World War both Kenya and Uganda had split their medical administration into separate sanitary and medical branches as well as creating more senior positions within public health, such as Chief Sanitary Officer. When Tanzania joined the British Empire officially in 1919, it too reflected these developments by quickly setting up a Medical Department split into clinical, sanitary and laboratory branches. As well as the PMO and DPMO, a Senior Sanitary (later Sanitation) Officer was appointed together with a strong contingent of non-medically qualified European sanitary superintendents.[78]

To cement this new direction, more attention came to be focused upon the organisation of the Medical Service. The favoured system was one in which medical districts were overseen, whenever possible, by an SMO who 'directed and coordinated' the medical work of several districts within a single province.[79] Senior staff usually manned the most important stations with a few MOs, but in outlying areas MOs formed the basis of the local medical administration. Occasionally, a MO could be in charge of an entire district, especially in sparsely populated areas such as the remote Northern Frontier District of Kenya. More generally, the districts were divided up into smaller units, referred to as locations or stations.[80] In accordance with the policy of indirect rule, these stations were also meant to be loosely representative of tribal boundaries with the headman or chief of the relevant tribe acting as the principal spokesman for each station.[81] At each station sub-assistant surgeons, compounders and dressers assisted the resident MO.

The system of medical administration in operation from the 1920s was based upon close cooperation with the native authorities.[82] The MO was expected to meet regularly with local chiefs and elders and health information was disseminated and 'confidence was slowly gained'[83] through weekly meetings called, in Kenya and Uganda, *baraza*. John Carman reminisced that it was at these regular meetings that an MO would 'speak about anti-malarial measures, methods of preventing plague and sleeping sickness or matters concerning housing and general standards of living.'[84] This educational function was in existence before the administrative changes of the 1920s, but it was only after that time that the use of MOs as health propagandists was seen as central. It is difficult to gauge how successful these relationships with native authorities were. Hunter felt in Uganda that he had personally never had any difficulties and many others voiced the same opinions.[85]

As the MOs were based in the district stations with other British officials, rural health provision to outlying African communities was provided, from the 1920s onwards, by the introduction of dispensaries throughout British East Africa. The system had first been successfully tried in Uganda in the post war years and thereafter was applied to Kenya by Patrick Nunan (in 1920) and then Tanzania.[86] Dispensaries provided in and out patient facilities and were under the charge of an African resident assistant, although a European MO paid regular visits to oversee and provide supplies, as well as deal with any problematic cases. Interestingly, dispensaries were also seen as 'propaganda centres' for distributing public health advice.[87] Schemes for the development of the dispensary system, which really took off after 1926, were led in Uganda by Major Keane, in Tanzania by Shircore and Scott and by Gilks in Kenya.[88] Furthermore, 1920 was recognised as a turning point at the time; it was the year that Gilks took over the headship of the Medical Department of Kenya and plans were inaugurated to extend public health activities to, and establish hospitals in, the rural native reserves. It was also the year that the first plans were initiated in Kenya to make provision for the training of native Africans as subsidiary medical staff. [89]

Each station had at least one dispensary, but usually several, which in turn were connected with a larger district hospital (by the 1930s most administrative districts usually had a small hospital). Notwithstanding the popularity of the dispensary scheme, many of the plans to expand rural treatment centres were not implemented, and a formally organised official system of rural healthcare centres was not established until 1946.[90]

One of the ways MOs managed these dispensaries and surveyed their districts was through regular, often arduous, medical safaris.[91] Routine medical duties during such a safari included 'get[ting] round...dispensaries as often as possible, inspecting their work records, replenishing their stores, and possibly helping with or evacuating special cases.'[92] As well as overseeing the day-to-day healthcare of the residential population, DMOs often went on safari with a specific brief to investigate and quantify incidences of a disease.[93] These medical surveys were a frequent feature of duties right through the period, even before the large-scale establishment of dispensaries. They provided the means through which the central administration collected data on the medical profile of the country.

From the 1920s schemes to train Africans for lower grade medical work were a crucial part of the decentralisation policy and were crucial for the growth of the dispensary system.[94] These 'tribal dressers' were African healthcare workers who, with some basic training, were responsible for running the many rural dispensaries. The training of Africans did not really take off in Kenya until 1926, but the scheme was first organized in the 1920s in Uganda (under Major Keane) and Tanzania (under Davey and Shircore).[95] It was in Uganda that this project had the most success and Mulago became the centre of medical training for Africans, eventually, in 1964, to full (MB, ChB) degree level.[96]

This type of medical administration was not problem-free. It still largely relied upon local administrations reporting back to the centre so that initiatives were usually confined to local levels and it remained difficult to centralise policy or to implement country-wide initiatives.[97] Criticisms were still being made of the administration well into the 1930s, when it was felt that the medical services lacked coordination with disparate officers in outlying districts all reporting back at different rates and on different matters to a single authority. This, some argued, acted as a 'serious deterrent to organised progress' — particularly the implementation of wider reaching development initiatives.[98]

The first systematic encouragement of research and specialisation emerged towards the end of the period. MOs had actively engaged in research as part of their routine duties from early times, through collecting local disease data in medical safaris or through their own field investigations for postgraduate medical qualifications, but earmarked funding and facilities were conspicuously absent. As early as 1903 Sir Michael Foster, Secretary of the Royal Society, called upon the Secretary of State to support colonial medical research (especially into malaria and blackwater fever) financially and administratively.[99] A fundamental stumbling block to progress was the lack of even basic research facilities within the East African colonies. Even though the first bacteriologist, Philip Ross, was appointed to the East African Medical Service in 1903 (a specialist position that was paid at a higher rate than the other MOs), it was some time before laboratory services achieved equivalent status to the clinical or sanitary branches of colonial medicine.[100] In Kenya and Uganda laboratory facilities were first arranged as a separate division of the Medical Department in 1915.[101] In Tanzania, the British inherited relatively developed laboratory facilities set up by prominent researchers, such as Robert Koch and Friedrich Karl Kleine.[102] A separate laboratory division was therefore established in British Tanzania right from the start. Despite this promising precedent, research was simply not prominent enough on the British colonial medical agenda to allow for many concerted subsequent developments, especially given the disruptions of the war and later strains on colonial budgets during the depression of the 1930s. Research all too often suffered through lack of central funding and was only really given premium attention after 1945.

This did not mean that no earlier pressures for change existed. MOs themselves seemed keen to push for more colonially-based research facilities. Among improvements called for in 1919 by the departmental committee set up to consider the condition of the Colonial Medical Services under the chairmanship of Sir Walter Egerton, were study leave for MOs, the development of research services and an increased number of specialist appointments. From the 1920s research in the colonies became a topic of parliamentary debate.[103] In Kenya in 1924, doctors involved in research, many of whom were colonial medical staff, submitted a formal memorandum petitioning the chairman of a visiting Royal Commission for greater recognition of the problems facing research-orientated doctors. They complained that there was a 'very great lack of appreciation of such scientific work' and that the chronic inadequacy of staff, combined with the lack of centralised cooperation and unsuitable laboratory facilities, made it was very difficult to conduct any serious scientific research.[104] There were even early calls for the establishment of a Colonial Medical Research Service (which eventually became established in 1945).[105] Conferences on the Coordination of Medical Research, were held in the three territories in 1933 and 1936, but various other priorities always seemed to be more immediately pressing, such as the need for more medical manpower, better hospital facilities and increased funding for training programmes for Africans. The result was that the East African Bureau of Research in Medicine and Hygiene was not established until 1949 with former MO in Kenya, Kenneth Martin as its director. Beck identifies this organisation as marking the first serious movement towards state-sponsored medical research in East Africa.[106]

*   *   *

Changes in the organisation and focus of the medical departments were part of the developments occurring in the European administration all over British East Africa as it sought first to establish and then to consolidate its position. Between 1893 and 1919 medical administration developed with few formally developed central policies, personnel were mainly placed for European convenience and a single hierarchy ran all administration. Attempts had been made from 1913 onwards to broaden the remit of medical care, but these plans had to wait for the period of greater stability after the end of World War One to come to fruition. It was this next period that saw the most concerted moves towards change. In the medical sphere at least, decentralisation and application of the precepts of indirect rule were attempts to create an infrastructure to cope with more facets and levels of healthcare within such large geographical areas.[107]

One of the major reasons why concerted attempts to foster research and specialisation were made only after 1930 was the power of curative medicine. The high incidence of disease meant that primary health care priorities swallowed up the scarce resources. Although the importance of preventive medicine had grown dramatically — to the point where it was regarded as the area to which the MO should devote 'the major part of his attention' — the striking, often instantaneous, impact of curative medicine meant that it was seen as a principal means through which the 'confidence of the people must...be obtained'.[108]

Medical departments naturally had to react on a day-to-day basis to the most pressing health needs of the country. Special initiatives were put in place for particular health emergencies. The focus of colonial medical administration, however, grew over time to accommodate both the increased expectations of colonial medicine with the need for bureaucratic workability. Eventually the duties of MOs developed, they became broader and more standardised, while also adjusting to the need for specialisation by stratifying jobs and allocating the new ranks with special remits of responsibility. In turn, the gradually changing focus of the bureaucratic structures also affected in-field experiences.

Chapter 7: Experiences in the Field

> Awful shock when I saw the hospital, a filthy old German building, full of rats
> and dirt. Conditions almost indescribable. The place had heretofore been run
> by ... a typical babu. Sanitation in Songea almost non-existent. Operating
> theatre filthy; so started by ordering it to be scrubbed out and whitewashed.[1]

This chapter aims to provide a more personal understanding of Medical Service
lives. Based on official documents and personal reminiscence (memoirs, personal
papers, obituaries), which provide a wealth of evidence on the experiences of the
colonial career, this chapter gives an impression of the common colonial medical
experience and offers a synthesis of what, practically speaking, being a Colonial
MO in East Africa entailed for most officers.

First, the typical methods of induction into the Service are briefly described.
The overriding characteristics of the job likely to have been experienced by most
employees are also summarized. Naturally enough the job contained both
attractive and less attractive features; on one hand it offered officers a large degree
of independence and the ability to develop a broad skill base; on the other hand,
many MOs found things difficult owing to the rudimentary conditions and lack of
facilities. For some it was extremely pressured and even personally dangerous at
times. The examination of the less attractive features of the job presents evidence
of complaints over the problems inherent in the colonial medical career. Many
MOs were vocal in their discontent with general and local features of their
professional lives. Special mention is made of the arguments presented to the
Colonial Office by the BMA on behalf of Colonial doctors over the terms and
conditions of employment. Examination of frustrations and criticisms helps to
complete the picture of how medical colonial life was perceived by those who
participated within it.

The final section concentrates on women doctors of the cohort. In many
ways the experiences of this small group were identical to those of their male
contemporaries, but some important differences make them worthy of
consideration in their own right. Some medically qualified women came to East
Africa as colonial wives. Although never formally recognised on the colonial

payroll, they played a vital support role in the provision of routine medical services.

Life as a Colonial Doctor

Individual experiences differed, but a first posting to East Africa generally followed an established pattern. After appointment and successful completion of the Diploma in Tropical Medicine and Hygiene in the United Kingdom, new MOs were required to sail at the first available opportunity for Mombassa, or sometimes Dar Es Salaam, the ports of entry for the East Africa region.[2] Unless the officer was to be stationed at one of these ports, there then followed an extended overland trip to the capital city of the country of designation; after 1901 with the opening of the Uganda railway this would have been undertaken, at least partly, by train. Otherwise officers had to make the arduous journey overland usually with an entourage of native assistants with mules. After the 1920s things were made easier with the coming of motorcars to the region.

The first weeks of official work were commonly spent in a capital city, or at least significant urban centre; often in one of the major hospitals to give the officer a gentle introduction to the territory; near to more experienced staff. This initiation was as much social as professional, and it was during these early weeks that the new MO was introduced to colleagues and superiors within the Service and initiated into the codes and conduct of colonial behaviour.[3] After this urban orientation the MO was given wider responsibilities, sometimes allocated to a specific hospital in an urban location, or, more commonly, sent out to a particular district, often with a brief to conduct a regional medical survey. There were examples, particularly before 1914, where new recruits were sent out immediately to remote areas, but by the post war period this practice was extremely rare and avoided wherever possible.[4]

On a practical level, the newly arrived officer would be allocated a house (furnished by the Public Works Department), would typically acquire some form of transport, perhaps a bicycle or (in the later half of the period) a car, hire some local help (classically a cook and a house boy), start learning Swahili and perhaps supplement their supplies by a visit to the tropical outfitters.[5] With very little official initiation, other than a brief welcome meeting with a senior officer, professional life would formally begin.

Professional Independence

One of the most apparent features of the colonial medical experience was the amount of professional independence doctors were given. Staff-patient ratio 'bore no relationship to UK levels' and newly-arrived doctors were often responsible for large districts with dispersed populations.[6] In general, the exact definition of each individual's job and responsibilities was never officially articulated, beyond a very broad brief that usually only stipulated that the MO should provide clinical and preventive medical care, and visit and survey the outlying areas of his district. Doctors in the field were therefore largely left to their own devices to identify, adapt and coordinate their responsibilities as best they could. There were relatively few restrictions and very little official monitoring, an experience that was universal throughout the Colonial Medical Service regardless of where doctors were posted. As one MO stated '[o]ne is very much on one's own and has to learn to be self-reliant and practical'.[7] Often early on in their careers, officers' only tangible links to central government were the answering of intermittent circular despatches and the supply of the required monthly, quarterly and annual medical reports for submission to the central bureaucracy. There were occasional inspection visits by senior staff, but even during the later period, when senior staff numbers were higher, these were described as unusual and infrequent.[8]

George Maclean reminisced that in the early days of rule in Tanzania an MO 'might find …[themselves] responsible for the public health of a quarter of a million people, or even (although rarely) half a million people'.[9] Raymond Barrett recalled how he was allocated a posting in Uganda in the late 1920s that was 'the size of Yorkshire,'[10] and James Hunter similarly described his first district (West Mengo, Uganda) as having been 'about the size of Wales.'[11] The experience was not an exclusively rural one. A single MO could find himself responsible for a variety of urban institutions — significantly more than a single doctor would ever be expected to supervise at home. In the late 1920s, for example, the MO in charge of the Native Hospital in Nairobi was also in charge of the mental hospital (Mathari) and the large down-town dispensary, not only supervising the patients, but also managing the accounts, supplies and personnel of these facilities.[12] Arthur Cole concisely summed up what must have been the feeling of many young colonial recruits — despite the great amount of administration to be done in outlying stations, the autonomy conferred upon young doctors also brought with it large advantages, not least the 'satisfaction in deciding one's needs for staff, equipment, drugs and even buildings.'[13]

Generalism and Versatility

Closely associated with increased independence was the wider professional remit Colonial doctors were likely to experience. This was an extremely common theme of accounts by officers reflecting on their careers, and was also promoted by the Colonial Office as one of the most attractive job features. Given the meagre distribution of MOs compared to population needs, even during periods of recruitment boom, it is not surprising that the model MO was presented within the recruitment literature as generalist who could carry out a variety of medical procedures.[14] The successful MO needed to have the professional confidence and initiative to perform 'every aspect of medicine in its widest sense',[15] and to possess leadership abilities, so as to manage staff within a large region and promote medical advantages to locals through methods of 'persuasion and influence'.[16]

Accounts by MOs support this official image. Arthur Boase reminisced how the job demanded that he be 'as versatile as a Royal Marine Commando'. He described how his first Ugandan appointment in 1920 caused him daily to face a wide variety of medical problems from bubonic plague to strangulated hernia. In the colonies, '[t]he conjoint title of physician and surgeon was truly earned.'[17] Robert Hennessey likewise recalled his large early responsibilities. After only four months in service he was moved to a station in the Eastern Province of Uganda where staff shortages meant that he was immediately to take on the responsibilities of acting SMO.

> So at the age of 24 I found myself responsible for the local anti-plague measures...detection and control of endemic disease outbreaks, maintenance of public health measures, general care of hospital patients (assisted by an Indian Sub-Assistant Surgeon), emergency surgery, supervision of district dispensaries and various odd jobs (such as attending an execution and certifying that life was extinct).[18]

As the MO was frequently the only point of contact for western medical care in the region, the type of diseases and conditions officers were likely to deal with were by no means restricted to classic tropical diseases.[19] Furthermore, not only did the duties suppose wide clinical and surgical skills, but also the possession of basic laboratory abilities, so that Officers could perform simple analyses and microscopy to diagnose disease. Laboratory facilities were extremely scarce and problems of communication meant samples could not be easily processed remotely.[20]

Diversity and adaptability was not only required in purely medical matters. One of the consistent elements of the career was the way it demanded skills far beyond the scope of those provided by even the broadest medical training — perhaps precisely why so much emphasis was put on character rather than qualifications during the recruitment process. At the beginning of British colonial rule in East Africa the MO needed to be a 'Jack-of-all-trades' with 'soldiering, administration, building and gardening' abilities.[21] But even by the end of the period, versatility was still advertised as one of the pre-requisites of the job. The successful MO was someone who displayed 'adaptability and breadth of outlook, political "flair" and what may be comprehensively described as the art of public relations, as well as pure professional competence.'[22]

These broader spheres of activity were partly created by staff shortages. To support the basic infrastructure, MOs needed to be able to turn their hands to anything and be able to take on the wider duties that have been described as the broader 'social mandate' of Officers' responsibilities.[23] As a symbol of the colonial order, the MO was intrinsically involved with social, economic and political structures of the regime. This fits with a large body of evidence in which MOs described their involvement with local affairs, including the construction of new buildings, the presentation of detailed reports and the resolution of local disputes. This extension of the job was experienced at the more senior levels of the service too, with SMOs and their seniors often actively participating in some of the territorial government bodies.

> ...a senior officer of the Colonial Service is more than just a civil servant...He must have a seat in 'Leg. Co.'[Legislative Council], and even in 'Ex. Co.' [Executive Council] and he must therefore be something of a politician. He will have to take part in debate, explain and defend in the public the work for which he is responsible....He needs to have at his command all the art of

diplomacy as well as ability in administration or skill in his own professional technique.[24]

Naturally, just as the actual breadth of the job depended upon an officer's rank in the service, the character of individual experiences was coloured by the location of a posting. As one commentator of the Colonial Service pointed out, '[s]ome men seem fitted by nature and interests for the bureaucratic life of secretariats; others chafe at urban living and thrive in the bush.'[25] The sort of duties an MO was likely to be involved with therefore were very place specific. An officer posted to the Northern Frontier district of Kenya (the isolated semi-arid region bordering with Ethiopia) needed to be prepared to defend his districts against border raids, so it was stipulated that service in this region approximated 'active service' and required good soldiering ability.[26] In contrast, an officer posted to Mulago, Uganda, after the mid 1920s would invariably become involved with the medical school there and would find clinical and surgical duties supplemented by additional teaching commitments.[27]

This necessity for generalism was regarded as a positive and rewarding aspect of the career.[28] Farnworth Anderson felt grateful that the experience had deterred him from any notions of specialisation he may otherwise have been persuaded to undertake.[29] The variety and emphasis upon every MO's own 'initiative and judgement', was precisely one of the features that made the career so interesting. [30] Within the Colonial Service doctors were told they could expect a 'wider scope for the exercise of their gifts than would be likely to come their way, unless they were exceptionally lucky, in the more settled conditions of home.'[31]

The Pace of Professional Life

If the different accounts of officers are to be believed, having a wide and varied job did not necessarily translate into having an unreasonably overburdened professional life. While some officers described situations where they were overworked and exhausted, others described a comparatively leisurely pace of life, occasionally even expressing frustration that they did not have enough work to fill their hours. The pace of life depended not only upon local conditions of each posting, but also on the personal initiative of individuals.

Whether MOs felt personally challenged for time or not, it was the perception of the medical departments that certainly MOs *ought* to feel busy. One of the constant complaints emanating from the East African dependencies during the pre and the post-World War One periods centred on the lack of personnel and the consequent pressure upon those who were in post. Subsequent historical analysis too has related the slowness of development of interrelated fields, especially research, to the fact that doctors were excessively 'overburdened' with practical duties to the sacrifice of longer-term medical projects.[32] In the early years the lack of resources, coupled with the relatively poor appeal of the East African Colonial Service, created considerable personnel pressures. The effects of the war only made things worse, with fewer people applying for Colonial Medical Service jobs than ever before. Most PMOs despaired at the strains their respective medical departments had to bear. The amount of work a MO was expected to undertake in a district posting was, Gilks (PMO Kenya 1921–33) declared, 'ridiculous': 'no man could possibly undertake the variety of duties and responsibilities which were expected of Medical Officers'.[33] It was on the basis of these and like·complaints, that the subsequent proposed personnel expansion of the medical services in East Africa of the mid 1920s was based.[34] Similarly, one of the reasons given to employ low-grade European Sanitary Officers in Uganda and Tanzania in 1925 was that it was thought increasingly 'impracticable', for MOs to deal with all their local curative and administrative duties as well as attending to preventive measures.[35]

Personal evidence throughout the period supports this picture. A frequent cause of complaint centred on the regular medical safaris to oversee the running of rural dispensaries and provide help for patients needing specialist treatment. These trips were commonly described as being long and demanding, especially because many areas could be accessed only on foot; officers and their entourage were regularly underway for several days, occasionally even weeks, at a time.[36] This strenuous aspect of the job was realised by the Colonial Office who warned potential officers of these hardships in some of their later recruitment literature.[37] Despite the warnings complaints over 'ceaseless travelling' defined much reflection on medical safaris.[38] The pressures on time also meant that doctors regularly grumbled that they had little or no occasion for keeping up to date with new medical developments or expanding any areas of specialist interest they wanted to nurture.[39]

Some MOs saw restrictions in more pecuniary terms as curtailing the amount of private practice they could potentially undertake. If official duties were too heavy the privilege of supplementing wages through attending to private patients became worthless. The right of MOs to undertake private practice was recognised throughout the period in East Africa, although the issue had always been thought to be rather a 'vexed question'.[40] The amount of private practice government officers had depended mostly upon their location. In Kenya with its large settler community opportunities were quite numerous, especially in urban areas. In Tanzania the comparatively small British presence, combined with the numerous Indian Sub-Assistant surgeons competing on the private practice market, meant that opportunities were more limited.[41] A survey taken in Kenya in 1915, asking officers to supply information on the amount of private practice they undertook in their districts, revealed large differences between individual stations in a single country. While some officers replied that their official duties or isolated location precluded them from earning extra income, most reported some supplementary income derived in this way.[42] MOs with ostensibly large private practices often found that bills were frequently·unpaid, undoubtedly because of the expectation that government doctors were meant to provide free health care.[43] Accounts vary, but clearly sufficient officers had enough private practice to be vocally indignant when murmurings were made that the privilege might be taken away. Even if private practice meant that MOs' time became even more pressured, most doctors were unwilling to let the opportunity of extra fees slip.

Another familiar cause of complaint was that staff shortages made it perpetually difficult to arrange leave. Many MOs grumbled about the long tours of service they were required to undertake.[44] MOs were expected to travel to cover for colleagues who had resigned or been invalided. Officers frequently complained that they were not given any advance notice of transfers. As one PMO, Arthur Milne, of Kenya, explained, this was because of the constantly changing requirements of Colonial planning:

> [T]he conditions alter from six months to six months requiring a constant readjustment of the point of view; that the plan formulated say — in November is not the best arrangement to carry out when the officer returns [from leave] sometime in August of the next year. The experience of epidemics alone proves this.[45]

Many memoirs reveal the frequency in which officers were expected to change their posting.[46] 'The posting of MOs from district to district at unpredictable intervals was a disruptive feature of Colonial Service'.[47] This was because home leave, when granted was for several months, too long to leave an area unmanned. MOs had to be moved around 'like pawns'. A process, critics maintained, that did not make for 'efficiency or job satisfaction — or domestic contentment'.[48]

By the time of Service unification in 1934 official policy recognised the advantages of maintaining a sense of continuity in the local setting, though paradoxically the reforms were intended to facilitate inter-territorial movements of staff. New MOs were reminded that they should acquaint themselves with their predecessor's policies and not institute changes that could entail losing the confidence of the local community. Indeed, these considerations were so high on the agenda that in Uganda in 1934 it was made official that any MO wishing to start any new policy in his district would have to obtain specific sanction from head office to do so.[49]

Not everyone had a hard life. Several MOs described how much free time they had and how their clinics were often empty rather than full. Most of the evidence for this relates to the period after the First World War, but if the early diary entries for Clement Baker and Aubrey Hodges are anything to go by, there was plenty of time to go on shooting expeditions, even mid-week. [50] Clare Wiggins similarly recalled how his MO duties at Kisumu in Kenya during the pre war era were 'not heavy'; when he was not on medical safari, most of his duties were completed by 10am each day.[51] The Great War, when many officers were commissioned into the East African forces, seemed especially to entail long periods of inaction, especially as officers were taken away from their regular duties and ordered to wait for casualties to arrive at the special military hospital camps. During this period in East Africa, Carpenter recalled how his peripatetic life as a Captain in the Uganda Medical Service was characterised more by boredom than by anything else.[52]

Evidence of the rather slow pace to professional life can be found throughout the period. Barrett described how during his 1935 posting he was 'far from stretched in routine duties...there was no lack of time and opportunity for exploring this superb district in sightseeing and searching for big game.'[53] As would be expected, however, the location of a posting largely determined how busy it was. Hugh Trowell seemed to have experienced both extremes: while in Kenya, working at Machakos District Hospital in 1929, he was at first daunted by the task he was given as a new recruit responsible for all surgery in the hospital. His fears soon subsided: 'I need not have worried, during my six months the ward had usually only three or four patients and not a single operation was called for.'[54] His next posting to Uganda, in contrast, appears to have been much busier — his description of the working day there offers a dramatic contrast to the experiences at Machakos.[55]

Whether life was busy or not sometimes reflected local native perceptions of the medical services. Government medical care paid very little attention, if any, to local herbal remedies, variolation, magical or voodoo customs, even though it was frequently acknowledged that this medicine would be most easily understood by the largest number of people.[56] The strength of indigenous medicine no doubt helps to explain the distinct lack of enthusiasm some doctors reported in response to their medical efforts for native populations. As late as the 1930s, doctors found antipathy, and sometimes even outright hostility, to treatment.[57] The lack of native interest in colonial medicine can also be better understood when the coercive nature of some of the medical interventions are recognised.[58] Arthur Procter, for example, although proud of the success of his anti-smallpox vaccination campaign at Fort Hall, Kenya in 1925, acknowledged that the vaccinations were carried out 'often unwillingly and by force'.[59] Local resistance was usually displayed through non-attendance at clinics rather than through more aggressive action, although in one reported instance, a sanitary superintendent actually lost his left hand and part of his forearm in a native protest against enforced plague quarantine in the Luwere region of Uganda.[60] In general, opposition had diminished by the end of the period, with favourable reports of the reception of western medicine by African people outstripping unfavourable ones. [61] By 1937 the Kenya Annual Medical Report announced that European medicine was 'thoroughly established throughout the colony'.[62]

Difficulties and Risks

Life, especially in the bush, was sometimes isolated, usually difficult and often risky.[63] Hugh Calwell remembered that mail arrived only once a week to his station, brought by a runner who had to travel for seventy-two hours. This made contact with the outside world very limited and letters from home very welcome.[64] In these terms the differences between rural and urban postings were most pronounced as communications were better in the larger cities.[65] In town there was also a broader and more organised European community; the opportunity for professional debate and the chance to share official duties if the need arose. Clearly, some MOs found district life difficult to grow accustomed to. Indeed this was common enough for the Colonial Office to adopt a policy by the 1930s of grouping colonial officials together in enclaves with other European officers nearby. [66]

It is a common feature of personal reminiscences to mention the basic and primitive facilities that faced officers on their arrival to their post. Not only did the officer usually find that their own standard of living was considerably lower than he would expect at home, but also, that the medical facilities were sparse and rudimentary. The facilities that greeted many MOs on arrival to their stations often took even the most adventurous MOs aback. Farnworth Anderson was dismayed that his house in Teita District, Kenya (in the late 1920s) had a pit latrine, very little furniture and no bath, despite a stunning view.[67] Wiggins similarly described his first impression upon arrival at Kisumu as being unimpressive: with only a 'few grass thatched mud and wattle huts' constituting the Government's headquarters.[68]

Perhaps most difficult were the poor medical facilities in both urban and rural postings. Robert Small on arrival to Jubaland, Kenya, in the first years of the century was dismayed to find the European hospital practically 'useless for its purpose'.[69] By the 1920s descriptions of the operating theatre in the same hospital reveal that, although conditions had improved, by modern European standards conditions were still very poor.

> The operating theatre was just an ordinary room with barely sufficient space to hold the operating table and two or three persons; there was no water laid on and everything ran on paraffin…there were only three of us who dealt with surgery, and when one was operating, another assisted and the third gave the anaesthetic. How terrified I was when I was the anaesthetist![70]

Standards in native hospitals almost always lagged behind the European ones, so it is unsurprising that Trowell also was exasperated by the poor facilities at Nairobi Native Hospital when he was transferred there in 1930.[71] One has to feel some sympathy at William Connell's reaction upon reaching his posting in Songea, Tanzania in 1924: he recorded that he felt 'like crying over the condition of my hospital, which is a dingy hole with 40 horrible native beds.'[72] The dispensaries regularly had very few medicines and medical supplies and even if an MO could get to patients, the use of intermittent or one-off treatments was regarded by many MOs as of little sustained effect.[73] 'Distances were considerable', the earth roads were 'dubious' and the first dispensaries themselves were often only mud huts.[74] By the end of the period the situation had not improved as much as might be expected. Although there was much more of a physical infrastructure in place, MOs still bemoaned the 'the lack of resources both human and material to provide more than an elementary "medical" and "health promoting" service.'[75] Even when initiatives were proposed they often had to be curtailed owing to lack of staff.[76] The scarce resources and comparative isolation meant that in practice officers had to call upon their own resourcefulness to adapt and experiment with what was (and was not) viable medical practice.

The very nature of work in the colonies meant that doctors were exposed, willingly or unwillingly, to dangerous tropical diseases, although after 1900 these decreased. The chances of pursuing a long and healthy career to retirement age, if an officer so desired, were not as remote as they were before 1900. A few doctors in the service of the greater good used themselves as guinea pigs to further their research. James Corson twice infected himself with *Trypanosoma rhodesiense* during his research into sleeping sickness.[77] Many officers caught tropical diseases less willingly and as a result had to be, temporarily or permanently, invalided out of the Service.[78] Illness was a persistent feature of colonial life. Aubrey Hodges, one of the first MOs in East Africa, recorded his numerous sicknesses and was one of the first of a long line of intermittently ailing Colonial MOs.[79] Two of the most common problems appear to have been malaria and tick-borne fever, diseases that attacked all strata of society. Even if officers managed to escape serious illness, their wives often became afflicted. [80]

Many MOs got so sick in the course of their duties that they were forced to retire: for example, Cyril Burges, Arthur Clanchy, Robert Hamilton, Alfred Mackie, Neil McLean, Joseph Ridgway, John Ross, Philip Ross, Douglas Scott, Kenneth Wallington and Charles Wilcocks.[81] A significant number even died while in Service, often, but not always, from tropical diseases.[82] A few passed away in more dramatic circumstances: Ralph Stoney died from an elephant attack in 1905; a buffalo killed Walter Densham in 1907.[83]

The strains put on bodily health by the tropical environment were not the only things that made doctoring in East Africa difficult. The psychological pressures of colonial life were also significant. The tropical climate had long been accepted as being more emotionally challenging than the temperate home environment.[84] A survey in the *BMJ* that looked at the chief causes of invaliding for both members of the military and missionary professions found that nervous disorders, characterised at the time by the fashionable term, neurasthenia, surpassed systemic diseases as a cause of permanent invaliding.[85] Officers who left the Colonial Medical Service because of mental breakdown (perhaps caused as much by the stresses of the job as those of the climate) included Peter Milne and Robert Small.[86] The position of PMO in Tanzania appeared to be particularly ill-fated. The first choice, Hugh Stannus was forced to step down soon after appointment for reasons of ill health. His successor, Arthur Horn, also had to leave before Tanzania officially came under British control in 1919, suffering from a mental breakdown.[87] Even those who were not diagnosed as mentally sick sometimes complained about the routine stresses of their duties, which caused them to lose weight or suffer from persistently interrupted sleep.[88] Attempts to find solace in narcotics were not looked on favourably by the establishment: Harvey Welch was sent home for becoming a drug addict; Ernest Adams also appears to have been involved in an addiction scandal and was invalided out of the service.[89]

Common Complaints

Two common sources of discontent among MOs were low pay, with comparatively remote prospects for promotion, and excessive amount of paperwork associated with the job. Throughout the period contemporary comments were almost uniform in their bitter criticism of colonial medical salaries. An anonymous 'observer' of the East African Medical Service described how 'the pay of the Senior Medical Officers is quite inadequate and the prospects are nil'.[90] Furse admitted that although a single man could live sufficiently well on a Colonial Medical Service salary in East Africa, a man wanting to bring his wife or family with him would 'have to go very carefully indeed unless he has private means'.[91] Combined with this, promotion opportunities were notoriously scarce.[92] This led to the perception, by some at least (despite consistent Colonial Office claims to the contrary), that promotion within the Service was as much to do with the length of service as to the quality of individuals.[93] It was not uncommon for officers to have served for over ten years before being promoted to the rank of SMO, and some officers served fifteen or even twenty years without promotion.[94] When Davey was offered the PMO job in Tanzania, he came out of sick leave to take it up; before this he had not been promoted for seventeen years. Unsurprisingly, he felt he 'could not afford to let this chance go'.[95] Complaints about salary and prospects were so pronounced that the BMA conducted a campaign for improvement on the Colonial Medical Service's behalf (see below). Similarly, attempts were made to reform the amount of administration Colonial MOs were expected to undertake quite early on. [96] As early as 1903 a report was circulated to all colonial governors relating recommendations made by Manson (originally prepared in 1900) over the improvement of medical reports, especially through standardising their presentation and content.[97] MOs still routinely claimed, however, that administration took up inordinate amounts of time. They often found themselves simultaneously having to work on the annual report and the monthly report, as well as compiling local statistics of patient numbers, length of stay and medical profiles, for the blue book returns.[98] Gradual improvements were made towards standardising and reducing medical reporting, but complaints continued throughout the 1930s.[99] The load was considered so oppressive that it was claimed that it interfered with clinical duties and wives were occasionally drawn in informally to assist with the administrative burden.

The role of the British Medical Association

From the 1890s onwards the structure and organization of the Colonial Medical Service was often challenged by external commentators as well as its employees. As the career path solidified, this *ad hoc* questioning of its fundamental purpose was replaced by more specific cavils (emanating almost exclusively from within the Service) over the terms and conditions of employment. Dissatisfaction became much more organised during the twenties and thirties. During this later period East African branches of the BMA vigorously lobbied the Colonial Office for improvement and reform of the East African Medical Service.[100] As the primary channel through which medical professionals in the colonies could appeal directly to the BMA in London, these regional divisions were important in uniting widely dispersed groups of medical practitioners under a single umbrella organisation. Prominent senior East African MOs actively collaborated via their local BMA divisions with the BMA in London to improve their terms of service.[101] The BMA campaigned for improvements in the terms and conditions of employment, most importantly through publishing demands for reform in the influential *BMJ*. Three periods of concerted campaigning for change were conducted by members of the metropolitan BMA: 1) 1919–21 when the BMA petitioned the Colonial Medical Services Committee of the Colonial Office on behalf of its East African members; 2) 1925–26 when it made specific remonstrations over the terms of the new East African Medical Service regulations (*African (East) No.1103*, published March 1925); 3) a wider protest around 1936 that called for improved terms for the Colonial Medical Service in general.[102]

Dissatisfaction was sometimes expressed through the official reports that MOs and their seniors submitted to the central medical departments, but these complaints did not have the political leverage and bargaining power of the more centralised protests organised by the BMA. On several occasions the BMA used the threat of withholding advertisements for the Colonial Medical Service or warnings that it would publish negative reports on the career, as bargaining points for improvement.[103] In 1926, when the right of MOs to private practice was under threat, an explicit warning against the Colonial Medical Service as a career for young graduate doctors was published in the *BMJ*.[104] Central government was quite aware of the significance of the BMA in influencing medical opinion and Furse noted the 'considerable importance' of keeping the Association onside as an aid to recruitment.[105] In a series of editorials and letters in the *BMJ*, the BMA asserted that the poor conditions of service actually discouraged the best doctors from taking up the career. Although this raised the profile and urgency of perceived problems within the Service, it was very much a double-edged sword. The criticisms risked reinforcing an impression that Colonial Service doctors were less competent than their contemporaries back home, or at least were part of an ill-fated organisation. It is ironic that, while the BMA's campaign lessened the appeal of the career to top medical graduates, the Colonial Office was more concerned with recruiting good character types than top–notch candidates.

In describing sources of complaint and dissatisfaction is not intended to suggest that MOs were perpetually unhappy; on the contrary, most memoirs are coloured by genuine fondness and emotional attachment to African life. Even if some of the terms and conditions of employment were problematic, it was acknowledged that many aspects of the lifestyle were highly enjoyable and that the extraordinary experiences conferred rare and valuable opportunities upon colonial doctors. Even when discontentment with the service peaked in the 1920s, evidence suggests that, on the whole, MOs were not seriously unhappy.[106] Recruitment, although never totally adequate indicates that discontent was not a serious disincentive to new candidates. The exotic and adventurous images surrounding colonial life were pervasive enough to guarantee a certain amount of tolerance. It was expected that life would be testing; in fact it was a desire to escape the predictable ordinariness of the home medical profession that enticed many young candidates overseas.

Colonial Medical Service Women

An analysis of colonial medical experiences would be incomplete without specific reference to women officers. Though they were subject to the same pressures and concerns as their male colleagues, their minority experience was necessarily different in some respects. Women were not officially excluded from employment within the Colonial Service (except some branches, such as the Administrative Service), but the traditional, masculine ethos of this government career made it a less appealing option for many female candidates. Not only would women have had to convince an all-male interview panel of their suitability, they had to contend with pervasive beliefs which strongly argued for the long term unsuitability of women for tropical residence.[107] Furthermore, the African Medical

Service, like the Administrative Service, was considered to require characteristics of leadership, resourcefulness, mental stability, and stamina that were mostly identified as masculine traits. Consequently, the few openings available to women within the Colonial Service by the 1920s were principally situated within the nursing or educational services. When medical jobs for women did come up, they were almost exclusively associated with education or maternity and child welfare work, a gendering of duties that was quite typical for women doctors at that time in Britain. [108]

In this context the experiences of the few women MOs during this period are even more remarkable. In Kenya, Uganda and Tanzania between 1893 and 1939 only twelve women (less than three per cent) worked for the Colonial Medical Service. Eleven of these were recruited in the 1920s and 1930s, representing roughly 15 per cent of the total number of female MOs recruited to the Colonial Service during that time. When this is compared to the 2,189 women recruited in the same period for the Empire nursing services it can be seen how comparatively restricted female doctoring opportunities were. Although some places such as the Federated Malay Straits, seemed to be more open to recruiting female MOs than others, women made up only a very small percentage of the colonial medical cohort. Significantly no women held any medical department headships or deputy headships within the period in East Africa and no women obtained the rank of SMO. When women did do exceptionally well it was usually as researchers. This is not a criticism of the part women played, but an acknowledgement that opportunities were few and when they did present themselves, severely curtailed. Although the Assistant Medical Adviser to the Colonial Office, Archibald Smart stated in 1939 that he felt that there was 'increasing scope' for women, even as late as 1949 another official commentator described the prospects for women in the Colonial Services as still being dominated by nursing, clerical and educational vacancies.[109]

The low representation of women within the Colonial Medical Service directly reflected the small chances for women to enter medical school in the early part of the twentieth century. Although medical opportunities had grown since women first began to participate in university medical education in the 1860s and 1870s, it took the shortages of male doctors precipitated by the First World War to sustain women's entry into medicine with any force.[110] Such positions as existed were available at home rather than in the far reaches of the Empire, and there was never an active recruitment drive to attract female medical graduates to the Service. When women doctors did choose colonial careers, they usually worked as missionaries, sometimes accompanying their missionary husbands.[111]

Although women were poorly represented, Uganda appeared to be the most open of the three territories to the recruitment of women. It was there that the first woman MO, Muriel Robertson, was appointed in 1911. It was an auspicious start, as Robertson became widely acknowledged as one of the most important protozoologists of her generation. Significantly, Robertson did not enter the Colonial Medical Service through the usual Colonial Office interview route, but joined after having been as part of the Royal Society's Sleeping Sickness Commission in Uganda. Her period in the Colonial Service lasted only three years, during which time she 'contributed enormously' to the subsequent understanding and elucidation of sleeping sickness.[112] Robertson returned to the United Kingdom after the outbreak of the First World War but continued her research on parasitic protozoa, eventually becoming head of the Department of Protozoology at the Lister Institute (1944), and being elected FRS in 1947.[113]

At least two other women were thought worthy of obituaries: Mary Michael-Shaw, who was a specialist in venereal diseases in women and children, and Mary Turton who had a long and successful career in bacteriology in Uganda before returning to England just before the Second World War.[114] Turton achieved the rank of Senior Pathologist (previously titled Senior Bacteriologist), the highest rank a woman reached in the pre-World War Two East Africa Medical Service. Notably, it was also a woman, Margaret Holliday, who held the first specialist surgical posting made to Mulago Hospital, Uganda in 1926.[115] Predictably, Holliday was appointed expressly to deal with female and infant surgery, in keeping with the conventional remit of women doctors.

Little other evidence of the other women MOs survives. An examination of job titles and other chance mentions within the sources, confirms that most had obstetrical, gynaecological and paediatric duties. By the 1930s exclusion from other medical areas was the cause of some frustration among the female profession and some complaints explicitly addressed this gender-orientated categorisation of duties.[116] Women were occasionally active protestors. An early medical history of Uganda by Albert Cook, recalled how an unnamed woman MO brought a 'bitter indictment' against Mulago medical school for their policy of compulsorily examining women suspected of having venereal disease.[117] Although Cook does not name the MO involved, it was probably Margaret Lamont, who was an employee of the Uganda service in Mulago at that time. As was typical of those who voiced their complaints too vehemently, Lamont left the Service after her protests — those who did not fit to the prevailing ethos were not easily assimilated.

Despite these anomalous examples the Colonial Office itself had remarkable little to say on the woman question. There was very little coordinated action during this period, either from within or without the Service, to improve opportunities for women within the medical corps. When issues did arise they were usually dealt with on a case-by-case basis: such as the protest made by Cecily Twining that she had to resign her position of MO upon marriage.[118] By the 1930s queries was also made (by the National Council of Women of Great Britain) as to why there were no women representatives on the Colonial Appointments Board.[119]

Colonial wives, a number of whom were medically qualified themselves, played a large role in colonial communities. The number of MOs stationed in East Africa who were married to doctors is difficult to quantify, as colonial records do not record the qualifications of spouses. Some medical wives, perhaps finding it difficult to get work with the Colonial Medical Service, registered independently as private practitioners. The Kenya and Tanzania *Government Gazettes* of the period are an informative guide as they regularly published the names of all licensed practitioners resident within their respective countries, with the type of medical practice in which each individual was engaged (private, missionary, government etc.). Many private practitioners listed were women, who shared the surname (and often the same medical school) of men in government service at the time. Examples include, Shona Aitken (wife of William Aitken, Tanzania); Violet Clarke (wife of James Clarke, Kenya); Gwendolen Chataway (wife of James Chataway, Kenya); Maud McNaughton (wife of James McNaughton, Tanzania); Jane Vint (wife of Francis Vint, Kenya); Frances Wilcocks (wife of Charles Wilcocks, Tanzania).

Some of these medically-qualified women became informally involved in local healthcare schemes. Charles Wilcock's wife, Frances, for example, seemed to have been regularly occupied with her husband's district based work, and Peg Wilson had worked informally or on short-term contracts for the Colonial Service since her arrival to join her Colonial Medical Service employed husband Bagster Wilson.[120] Within months of her arrival in 1930, Peg Wilson, who had worked as a doctor in Nepal, was examining blood specimens in the makeshift laboratory in Tabora and in the following years routinely accompanied her husband on medical safaris, conducting inoculations and health examinations. She was so helpful that her husband claimed that when she was ill, his laboratory work doubled. During periods when the annual report was being prepared Wilson described her life as 'entirely coloured' by it and she certainly played an active role in its production. By 1933 Wilson was working formally as a part-time entomologist, and in 1939 she took up a position as a Health Officer, finally being appointed a full MO in 1948. She became an accomplished parasitologist and entomologist, and remained working in Uganda until 1965, when she moved to the Medical Research Council's unit in the Gambia. She stayed there until 1973 and eventually retired at seventy-six years of age.[121]

Not all careers were as dynamic as Peg Wilson's. Some colonial wives found colonial life tiresome and insalubrious, others played a very active part in the districts. Hugh Trowell recalled how his wife, Peggy, accompanied him on some of his medical safaris, and although she did not feel comfortable with medical matters, helped by illustrating some of the public health information booklets issued in Kenya for distribution to African families.[122] Farnworth Anderson, too, remembered how his wife was a regular companion on the medical safari trail.[123] Robert Moffat's wife, Hilda, was 'dragged in' to assist him with his duties, because he found himself too busy to undertake all the paperwork on his own. He was happy to report that she 'really makes a very good amanuensis'.[124] Robert Procter's wife was also active in district medical care and was, along with the Assistant District Commissioner wife, 'recruited to vaccinate' the native inhabitants of Fort Hall, Kenya against smallpox in the early 1920s.[125]

The role of Colonial wives, although not entirely unappreciated, largely remains unexplored within Colonial Service history.[126] Just as men needed to be the right sort, the wives that accompanied them needed to be of the right stamp if they were to endure, and even thrive, among the stresses integral to colonial life. One official wrote how fortuitous it was that the selection procedure, with its reliance on character and interview, was also a means whereby the right sort of wives were also indirectly chosen: '[p]rovidence no doubt arranges that the sort of chap who is the sort of chap they want in the Colonial Service chooses (or is chosen by) the sort of wife he ought to have.'[127] The best sort of woman was described as 'one of the modern out-of-door practical girls that are fortunately becoming so common'.[128]

Life for wives was not easy, with their husbands having more social stimulation and the benefit of professional interaction. Connell commented that, while he was very busy with his duties, he could appreciate that '[i]t is pretty deadly for a woman'.[129] Nevertheless, most wives seem to have had an important part to play in colonial life; even those women who had no interest in pursuing matters medical, often created niches for themselves in society by getting involved with local community projects or educational initiatives.[130]

Women were not readily recruited into the Colonial Medical Service before 1945, but the prospects for women gradually began to improve from the 1930s.[131] Those women who did actually choose the career combated two formidable hurdles: overcoming widespread restrictions over women's entry into medical education; and overriding assumptions that women had no serious contribution to make within the government services other than in the nursing, clerical or education services. As will be discussed in the next chapter, women also had an important social part to play in colonial life. Their presence helped to normalise the otherwise exotic or exceptional experiences of colonial life, contributing to the creation of communities that made life feel, in some important ways like a home-from-home.

*   *   *

As all officers were part of shared administrative structures and communal policies, it is not surprising that MOs perceived and experienced colonial life in a broadly similar way. While individual opinions and perceptions varied, and clear regional differences existed, an ethos emerged that eclipsed the idiosyncratic differences. All MOs were part of the same Service; their professional training, place and employer unified them. All had to work daily within the same hierarchy, they had to follow the same briefs, obey the same regulations and adapt to their departmental decisions over the focus of medicine. This fostered a sense of solidarity, which was enhanced (further than other shared professional identities back home) through the colonial context. Here MOs were not only united through their profession and shared experiences, but also unified by their skin colour and their status as part of the ruling elite. This forged bonds, which went over and above any rivalries that developed. It created and perpetuated a specifically colonial medical identity.

Chapter 8: Medical Recruitment and the Ideals of Empire

[An] "ordinary" personality became magnified and…emotions heightened by the very un-suburban way of life. [1]

A substantial body of historical work has examined from different angles the creation of imperial ruling class and imperial subjects.[2] The question of a specifically colonial medical identity, however, has only recently become the subject of historical scrutiny in its own right.[3] There has been relatively little concentration on the actual *constitution* of colonial group identities, or what they could mean for, or add to, broader medical historical accounts.[4] This is despite the fact that medical historians have regularly, usually implicitly, assumed the importance of common group markers as a means of moulding and perpetuating collective experiences and expectations. This chapter and the next offers an expansive, culturally embedded, description of colonial communities within medical history, based on empirical evidence. The aim is to draw upon and augment the historiographical debates over colonial identity mentioned in the first chapter and to explore the way that certain common themes were manifest in the attitudes and behaviours of colonial doctors. The stereotype of the colonial medical servant is explored and compared to a detailed analysis of 'real' colonial medical profiles.

The Colonial Service Stereotype

Strong correlations exist between Colonial Service stereotypes and the actual make-up of the medical cohort, but the composition of the Medical Service diverged in several important ways from the conventional image of colonial officers during this period. Three important aspects stand out as being fundamental to generalised public perceptions of Colonial Service identity: first, the image that the Service was principally made up of upper-class, or at least upper-middle class, entrants who had attended either Oxford or Cambridge Universities.[5] Second, the idea that the group advocated predominately traditional values based on public school notions of sportsmanship, fair-play, and conservatism — with an over-riding respect for time-honoured practices and a general resistance to innovation or change. Third that Colonial Officers were somehow intrinsically a more adventurous, heroic type, guided in their career choice through an innate spirit of adventure, which differentiated them from their contemporaries at home.

These images partly derived from the character of British officialdom in India, which had a more established tradition of overseas public service than the African Colonial Service. The renowned severity of the entrance examination to the Indian Civil Service meant that recruits were generally drawn from a privileged social group with access to a classical education.[6] Indian Civil Service entrants had typically attended public school and then Oxford University, which remained, above Cambridge, the most popular university for fledgling Indian Civil Service officials until 1939.[7] This image of privilege surrounded high profile ex-colonial officers such as Leonard Woolf and George Orwell. These links fuelled accepted assumptions that Colonial Officers tended to comprise a prosperous, public (i.e. private) school educated social elite.[8]

This dominant impression of entrants is sustained by studies that have profiled members of the various Empire political services. Important works undertaken by Henrika Kuklick about members of the Gold Coast Administrative Service, or Alex McKay with regard to the political cadre stationed in Tibet (who were drawn from the colonial government of India) have confirmed that the colonial type was, by and large, taken from a public school, Oxbridge-educated pool. These individuals were frequently the sons of landed or professional parents and, naturally enough, sported many of their ideological trappings.[9] Data collected by Bruce Berman on the Kenyan Colonial Service between 1919 and 1939 similarly shows that 90 per cent of those officials for whom he could find information were British public school graduates, three quarters of whom had attended Oxford or Cambridge Universities.[10] Works by Kirk-Greene and Crawford also support these specific studies through their broad historical analyses of different spheres of colonial recruitment.[11]

The profile of colonial recruits naturally reflected the policies pursued by Ralph Furse at the Colonial Office, and others in equivalent positions in the Foreign Office or India Office. Furse quite consciously favoured a certain type of recruit (see Chapter 3) and the subjective ideas about character that came into play during the recruitment process, as well as the continuation of many of the tenets of patronage, influenced the class group that was actively recruited. Not only were those who came from good colonial families deemed particularly suitable types, but since full university scholarships were rare before the Second World War, the reliance on Oxbridge as the main recruitment base ensured that candidates were of relatively uniform class origins. Despite these official preoccupations with class and gentility, however, a noteworthy proportion of Colonial MOs came from a broader social and educational background.

The face of the Colonial Service was unfailingly traditional and conservative in outlook. Even if the class origins of the individual members did not always fit with the ideal — as increasingly occurred from the 1930s and 1940s — the traditional ruling class ethos that typified the Colonial Service offered tangible opportunities for the socially ambitious to improve their status.[12] As Kirk-Greene argued in his study of Colonial Service novels, even if the protagonists were from unexceptional middle class backgrounds the career gave them opportunity to elevate themselves in terms of status.[13] The Colonial Service, in reality and fiction, took individuals to places that represented excitement and difference, and increased their professional prestige.[14] Membership of this group also automatically and implicitly enrolled individuals as supporters of its core values, which stemmed from the key public school tradition of *noblesse oblige*. This assumed the right to rule through such traits as heroism, discipline, leadership, self-control, courage, sport, fair-play and a respect for tradition. It was world-view that was politically conservative, any more radical elements within it being silenced for the sake of preserving the status quo.[15] These traditional values were, moreover, associated with certain physical attributes. The successful officer would be a sporting, outdoor type physically able to endure (even relish) the climate and the strenuous life that the colonies presented.[16]

While the image of the physically strong and morally upstanding hero had much of its basis in the public school tradition, many of these class associations in the colonial context were reinforced by ideas of heroism and exoticism found in popular stories of exploration.[17] British popular culture was packed with images directly linking colonialism with adventure and some of these, naturally enough, affected perceptions of Colonial Service officers. Following the big-selling nineteenth-century biographical accounts of Victorian explorers such as Stanley, Livingstone, and Kingsley, a new trend in fictional writing about similar topics took off from the second half of the nineteenth century. Writers such as George Alfred Henty (1832–1902), Rider Haggard (1856–1925), and Edgar Wallace (1875–1932) achieved great popular appeal, as did the influential stories that featured in popular comics of the day, such as *Boy's Own Paper* (launched 1879), or in the Edwardian period *The Magnet* and *The Gem*.[18] Additional to this was the influence of film. By the 1930s, Empire films began to be produced in Britain and America with telling regularity. Pictures such as *Sanders of the River* (1935); *Rhodes of Africa* (1936); *King Solomon's Mines* (1937); *Four Feathers* (1939); *Stanley and Livingstone* (1939) provided forums for escapism (especially from the Depression) and helped to further entrench stereotypical ideas about colonials.[19] Of course more than one colonial type was caricatured in film and popular literature: for every upper-class dynamic hero there was a bumbling buffoon to counterbalance him, and for every ambitious young careerist a dreary misanthropic counterpart immersed in the intricacies of bureaucracy. However, the image of the colonial officer, explorer and missionary as a privileged, healthy and adventurous chap was omnipresent.[20] The stereotype was, moreover, usually derived from collective ideas surrounding the Colonial Administrative Service, which as the biggest branch of the Colonial Service dominated all other impressions of colonial types.[21]

With regard to British East Africa, it is important to acknowledge that many of the archetypical images derive specifically from Kenya. The colony contributed disproportionately to perceptions of colonial life owing to its prominent public profile, directly derived from the large and vocal British settler population. Many quixotic ideas became specifically associated with Kenya owing to its healthy climate, dramatic rolling hills, opportunities for big game hunting and relatively close historical connection with the lives of African explorers such as Livingstone, Stanley and Kirk. These romantic links were important because of the public (and often salacious) rumours surrounding the 'happy valley' that dominated much of the gossip emanating from the country between the 1920s and 1940s. Although these reports were principally about the settler, rather than the official, community, they nevertheless fired popular perceptions of East African life in much more general terms. Images of Kenya during this period frequently depicted colonials *en masse* as part of a gay, decadent community, preoccupied with dinner parties, hunting safaris, champagne breakfasts and sexual excesses. Most importantly, this colonial set were all thought to be having a thoroughly good time, markedly different from their contemporaries in industrial, Depression-ridden, Britain.

This image, which Evelyn Waugh famously described as the colonial life of the 'English Squirearchy', contained some truth. Kenya was, after all, home to many members of the British ruling classes, such as Lord Delamere, Lord Cranworth and Lord Erroll, and no doubt this society did shape the behaviour and expectations of other British groups resident in Kenya. Other colonies had a different social structure and distinctive preoccupations arising from their particular circumstances, but the associations that surrounded Kenya were especially powerful in moulding ideas about colonial East African life. [22]

The stereotype of the Colonial Officer was an amalgamation of numerous ideals of Britishness but, crucially, it was also, differentiated from home society through its celebration of specifically local African influences. Colonial MOs both conformed to, and diverged from, the images of Colonial Service types. In some ways they drew upon and perpetuated popular images, but in other important ways they distanced themselves from them — not least because of their professional associations, which demarcated them as doctors whose immediate aims were humanitarian, rather than politicals who ruled. Even if their collective behaviour upheld many distinctive colonial attitudes, this group, nevertheless, had a subtly distinct identity of their own.

The Constitution of the Colonial Medical Service

In total 424 MOs served in the Colonial Medical Service of British-ruled Kenya, Uganda and Tanzania before World War Two. In some cases the information obtained for this group has been consistently available, in others it has disappeared. It is particularly regrettable that the original Colonial Office P1 (Med.) application forms — except for a handful which have turned up in archives where they officially should not have been — were all destroyed after a fixed period of time through a centralised policy of the Colonial Office.[23] Nevertheless, by cross-referencing *Medical Directory* entries, *Colonial Office Lists* and personal accounts and obituaries, a profile of the staff of the Colonial Medical Service during this period has emerged.

Class profile

Doctors were drawn from a more diverse social group than colonial administrators and they did not necessarily comply with the dominant stereotype of the financially privileged Colonial Service official. A number of MOs mentioned in their memoirs that they came from less well-off family backgrounds; indeed, it seems that the promise of a regular salary and additional allowances actually stimulated some doctors' to choose a colonial career. Occasionally the socially privileged joined the Colonial Medical Service (for example, Drs Fairfax Bell, Arthur Bagshawe and Clinton Manson-Bahr), but their presence did not dominate the East African cadre.[24]

The mixed class background of the Medical Service compared to the Administrative Services is echoed in the work of Mark Harrison who has shown that, between 1859 and 1914, Indian Medical Service recruits were drawn from a broader social grouping than their equivalents in the Indian Civil Service. Interestingly, Harrison also found that the Indian Medical Service doctors came from a less socially elevated background than their medical contemporaries practising in the UK.[25] This accords with the idea that entrance to the Indian and African Medical Services was seen as a means of enhancing social position.[26]

Unsurprisingly, these broad-based class affiliations affected doctors' common perspectives and group identity. Doctors' positions in colonial society were determined not so much by class, as by collective membership of a special status group. Although MOs were an integral part of the colonial ruling classes, they regarded themselves — and their contemporaries in other branches of the Service — as an essentially different group. Very definite divisions formed within colonial society. Officials grouped together with like-minded colleagues, usually in the same branches of the Service as themselves.[27] Doctors were particularly defined through the occupation of medicine, which intimately associated them with a scholarly and scientific profession, rather than a political position with its associated ruling class pageantry and regalia.[28] In some cases these differences were so pronounced as to present an 'ostensive class barrier between the different types of colonial officer', one that was said to have 'fostered mutual hostility' between different Colonial Service groups.[29]

Nationality

Without birth certificates (which were destroyed with the application forms) nationality is difficult to establish. *Medical Directory* and *Colonial Office List* entries list, nearly always state the place from where individuals gained their medical education, but this cannot be used as definitive indicator of nationality, especially as it was fairly common for people to travel to prestigious medical schools. The Colonial Office regulations required all entrants to the Medical Service to be naturalised British citizens, although not necessarily born in Britain; after 1925, it was stipulated that both parents must be European.[30] Confirmation of national origins remains elusive and for some is available only from autobiographical writings or obituaries.

Scotland and Ireland were particularly well represented among the colonial medical profession.[31] As many of the MOs formally identified as Scottish went to Scottish universities, and Irish to Irish ones, it seems likely that educational background gives an indication of nationality. Although the lack of data precludes a formal count of national origins, it is estimated that around a third of all Colonial MOs were Scots and a sixth were Irish (Figure 8.1).

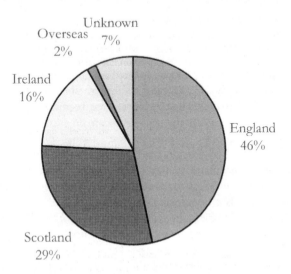

Figure 8.1: National Distribution of MOs' Qualifications

The large proportion of particularly Scots in the Medical Service can be related to their lack of access to the pre-requisite capital, or opportunity, to establish themselves as private practitioners in their home country from the 1880s onwards.[32] Furthermore, the prominent colonial presence of Scots was based on a long established tradition of Scots overseas since the seventeenth century.[33] The large Scottish component of Empire meant that Scots would have been more exposed to the career through the accounts of colonial friends or relatives. Other assessments have been based on more subjective ideas of Scottishness: Derek Dow has suggested that career choices favouring Africa were made by Scots as a means of satisfying a national desire to take on new challenging environments.[34] This idea is given added weight by the popular links between Scots and colonial adventure, as personified by David Livingstone and John Kirk.

Andrew Balfour called upon the combined factors of tough competition at home and an inherent tradition towards adventure in his 1924 colonial recruitment address to Glasgow medical students. Balfour repeated a gloomy forecast made by Sir Humphry Rolleston (1862–1944) that the Scottish medical profession would soon possess a glut of one doctor to every thousand inhabitants. With those sort of prospects at home, Balfour emotively challenged those imbued with the 'blood of the Celt' to take up a Colonial Medical Service career. By following a Scottish tradition of *wanderlust* they were not only being true to their historic pedigree, but were responding with characteristic resourcefulness to the lack of job opportunities at home.[35]

Although British extraction united Colonial Officers, it should be remembered that, within the overall articulation of British identity, there were definite sub-groups, which strongly identified with their Irish or Scottish ancestry (e.g. the Highland dancing societies in East Africa).[36] As Julian Huxley remarked on his tour of British African colonies in 1929: 'the Scots section of every colony is always large and always vocal.'[37]

Education and Qualifications

In total, qualification information has been ascertained for 414 of the 424 MOs who make up this study (98 per cent). Although some MOs attended Oxford or Cambridge, the idea that this was the preferred recruitment base for all Colonial Officers is not applicable to the East African medical cohort. Although Furse strongly favoured Oxbridge recruits for the Colonial Administrative Service, the growth of the medical profession with the London and Scottish medical schools as their seedbeds, meant that the narrow educational preferences that were operable for the political service were untenable for the adequate staffing of the medical one. While both Oxford and Cambridge had offered medical degrees since the thirteenth century, the growth of the Scottish medical schools in the eighteenth century and the London medical schools in the nineteenth century, meant that Oxbridge's importance as a key provider of medical graduates had begun to recede. This was particularly the case of Oxford where the medical school did not achieve prominence until after the Second World War. Cambridge, in comparison, already had, by 1900 a large and successful medical school that offered medical degrees with clinical training in London.[38] Medical education principally developed around London, Cambridge, Edinburgh and Glasgow. As a pragmatic and long overdue acknowledgment that medical students were drawn from this broader base, the Warren Fisher Committee decided in 1930 that the official medical recruitment policy would correspondingly concentrate its attentions accordingly.[39]

Given this trend in medical education, it is unsurprising that only 57 (13 per cent of those for whom qualifications could be ascertained) MOs went to Oxford or Cambridge Universities as undergraduates; only 10 of these officers had been at Oxford. This reflects the lesser emphasis on medical education at Oxford, but it was also partly due to the greater interest in tropical medical education at Cambridge. From 1904 to 1933 Cambridge University held a diploma course in Tropical Medicine and had teaching staff with tropical medical interests.[40] Although most MOs made their career decisions early on, 34 of them had obtained a BA before embarking upon their medical education.

Table 8.1 profiles the spread of highest medical qualifications for the cohort. Significantly, most colonial doctors (45 per cent) had achieved the joint medical bachelors degree (MB, ChB; MB, BS etc.). This indicates that the standard of recruit was generally reasonably high, as the medical and surgical bachelors were commonly regarded as the more difficult and, therefore, prestigious of the medical examinations to take: especially when compared to the qualifications awarded by the medical corporations (i.e. MRCS, LRCP). In part these results only reflect the relative contemporary popularity of the bachelors' degrees; they tally with a sample survey done by Dupree and Crowther of the Scottish medical profession in 1911 that concluded that by far the most popular combination of qualifications for Scottish medical graduates was MB with ChB or CM (86 per cent of their sample).[41]

Highest Medical Qualification	Officer Nos.
Licentiate of the Royal Society of Apothecaries	5
The Conjoint	128
Joint bachelor degree	192
Higher postgraduate degree	84
Other specialist qualification	5
No medical qualification[42]	1
Medical qualification unknown	9
Total of MOs:	424

Table 8.1: MOs Highest Medical Qualifications

Yet, even if medical and surgical bachelors were universally the most popular route into medicine, the result is interesting with regard to the Colonial Service. In a Colonial Office survey of medical qualifications obtained between 1927–29, the Chief Medical Adviser to the Colonial Office, Thomas Stanton, concluded that of the 297 candidates surveyed, 266 held on appointment 'professional qualifications higher than those required to satisfy the standard for admission to medical practice.'[43] This indicates that the medical cadre were more highly qualified than was deemed necessary (or even desirable) for the ideal colonial civil servant.[44] Medical Service recruiters were not looking for top-class candidates, but solid, resourceful and resilient medical men who could be relied upon to represent the Empire in its dispersed locations. As well as being of a higher calibre than is commonly believed, about a fifth of MOs possessed, or went on to acquire, higher postgraduate medical qualifications. Many of these qualifications were obtained during a period of home leave, often based upon observations collected while in East Africa. Plainly, a significant proportion of MOs were keen to extend themselves and to transform their specialist experiences into further medical qualifications.[45]

It is difficult to make any claims about medical school distribution as the information is available for only 152 officers (36 per cent). Of these, the bulk attended London medical schools with the majority coming from St Bartholomew's (28); St Thomas' (24); Guy's and the London Hospital (18 each).

The data fit with those of a (pre-Warren Fisher) Colonial Office investigation, that concluded that Bart's (the largest London Medical School with a reputation as the 'Mother hospital of Empire'.) was the main London supplier of Colonial MOs.[46] With regard to official perceptions of the Colonial Service in general, the predominance of London is interesting. When the Secretary of the London University Appointments Board assessed the reasons why more Oxbridge men than London graduates took up the Colonial Service career he surmised that it was something to do with Londoners' 'naturally unadventurous' characters.[47] Clearly, with regard to medical recruits, this assessment was far off the mark. The dominance of London in the Colonial Medical Service was to be expected however as most medical schools were in London, and these attracted students from all over the country.

A sense of the national distribution of medical training can be gleaned from data pertaining to highest medical qualifications (Table 8.2).

Place of origin of highest qualification	Officer Nos.
London	134
Edinburgh	70
Ireland	67
Cambridge	33
Other Scottish university	29
Glasgow	25
Other provincial English university	21
Oxford	9
Overseas	7
Place of qualification unknown	29
Total of MOs:	424

Table 8.2: Place of Origin of Highest Medical Qualification

Dupree and Crowther have concluded that the most popular Scottish university for medical degrees was Glasgow; followed by Edinburgh and then Aberdeen.[48] This is slightly different to the results found in this analysis of Scottish educated Colonial MOs, who mostly came from Edinburgh. This may reflect tropical medical interests in this university medical school — Edinburgh, was the only Scottish institution to offer the Diploma in Tropical Medicine and Hygiene during this period and from 1901 had a lecturer in Tropical Diseases,

Andrew Davidson.[49] Although London and Edinburgh dominated, provincial university medical schools, such as those at Birmingham, Liverpool and Bristol also figured highly on recruitment profiles, particularly after the 1920s.[50]

The number of MOs with specialist qualifications in Tropical Medicine and Hygiene is surprising: although all Colonial MOs were required to undergo a course in tropical medicine and hygiene before taking up their position, only 230 (54 per cent) of them were listed as possessing the relevant Certificate or Diploma.[51] Although salary incentives were offered to officers who possessed the Diploma in Public Health (when they became MOHs), only 84 officers (20 per cent) seem to have been attracted by this option. This reflects difficulties that were expressed by central government in 1930 over securing candidates with a Diploma in Public Health. Those who had the qualification appeared to view it primarily as a means of entrance to a public health career in the UK, rather than in the colonial context.[52]

Age at Entry & Prior Experience

The mean age of entry to the East African Colonial Medical Service was 30.[53] Since this average is skewed by entrants well over the prescribed age, it is more useful to group recruitment ages into bands.

Age Band	Officers
Band 1: (23–29 years of age)	165
Band 2: (30–39 years of age)	87
Band 3: (40–49 years of age)	18
Band 4: (49+ years of age)	1
Age unknown:	153
Total of MOs:	424

Table 8.3: Age of Entry to East African Medical Service

The commonest age bracket for entry for the Colonial Medical Service was between 23 and 29 years (Table 8.3; 27 was the most common entrance age among that group). This was in line with official age requirements which, although fluctuating, generally required medical candidates to be between 23 and 35.[54] Official policy stated a preference for MOs who had obtained a couple of years' hospital experience before applying for a Medical Service position.[55] Nevertheless, this was not always the case — some MOs joined at 23 on graduation, and sometimes, especially when specialists were needed, much older candidates were appointed. Henry Gordon joined the Colonial Medical Service as a consultant psychiatrist at the ripe age of 65.[56] Particularly before 1930, older experienced candidates were sometimes employed on a temporary basis to fill staff shortfalls.[57] These older recruits were often seconded from other organisations, such as the RAMC or the Royal Society Sleeping Sickness Commission. During the early years of colonial establishment in East Africa older officers who had formerly worked for the Imperial British East Africa Company to the Colonial Service were also employed.[58]

In all, 301 officers (71 per cent) had some documented professional experience before taking up their colonial medical position — although, the figure may be an underestimate, since prior experience is not always mentioned.[59] This high figure does however seem to indicate Colonial Office preference for more professionally mature doctors. Of the 301 known to have previous professional experience, 153 (51 per cent) listed a hospital residency of some sort before they applied to the Colonial Medical Service, and 185 (61 per cent) had military medical experience, usually in the First World War.[60] Many Colonial MOs had formerly worked in Africa or India, or belonged to a colonial family. 120 officers (40 per cent) claimed some such colonial experience, whether in a professional capacity or via the circumstances of their upbringing, supporting the contention that the colonial type was one imbued with a belief in the tradition of Empire.

Most recruits 323 (76 per cent) came to East Africa as their first government appointment — only 70 (16.5 per cent) had been in another branch of the Colonial Medical Service, or in the Indian Medical Service, before appointment in East Africa (54 of this 70 had been previously employed specifically by the Colonial Service). For 47 officers it is not known whether East Africa was their first posting or not.

Length of Service

Start date information has been found for 421 (99 per cent) of MOs and in 347 (83 per cent) cases retirement dates were also found.[61] Once in the medical service, the average length of service was eleven years; close to the minimum length of time an officer had to serve before qualifying for a gratuity. Since the average is skewed by very long and very short periods of service, it is again useful to look at the data in different bands (Table 8.4).

A large proportion of entrants saw the Colonial Medical Service, as the recruiters would have wished, as a long-term career.[62] The spread of figures between long and short service is remarkably even: 181 Officers stayed under ten years, while 167 stayed for ten years or more. It appears that the Colonial Medical Service selection methods were remarkably accurate in terms of suitability: over a 46-year period only 19 officers left the service after a year or less. The longest serving officer was Cliff Braimbridge who was in East Africa for 36 years. The figures should be used with some caution as they do not differentiate between officers who left the Colonial Medical Service was and those who transferred to a colony outside Kenya, Uganda and Tanzania. Many senior officers transferred to other colonial dependencies later in their careers. Officers such as John Buchanan and William Lamborn had extremely lengthy Colonial Service careers, although they spent large proportions of them in other territories.

Length of Service Band	Officer Nos.
Band 1: (0–2 years service)	74
Band 2: (3–9 years service)	107
Band 3: (10–19 years service)	85
Band 4: (20–29 years service)	74
Band 5: (30+ years service)	8
Length of service unknown:	76
Total	424

Table 8.4: Length of Service in East Africa

Honours and Fellowships

Brief mention should be made on the subject of awards and fellowships. In 1938 Charles Jeffries was able to encourage prospective recruits that 'every New Year and Birthday Honours List contains the names of numerous members of the Service'.[63] This claim is certainly borne out by the evidence, as 86 (20 per cent) of MOs received a formal decoration or honour from the British Government for their services to Empire. The most common decoration was the CMG (Companionship of the Order of St. Michael and St. George), followed by the Companionship of the Imperial Service Order; some officers were also knighted or received an OBE (Order of the British Empire) for their services. Notably, no KCMG (Knight Commander) or GCMG (Knight's Grand Cross) were awarded to any of the officers profiled in this study. This is not entirely surprising, as these decorations, were usually conferred only upon Governors or very senior officials. Service in World War One also meant that a significant number of officers (72) received military titles, clasps or honours: usually orders of chivalry such as those of St. Michael or St. George. These were typically gained either in the Boer War or the African campaigns of World War One.

Another important marker of professional recognition was the award of a Fellowship of prestigious bodies such as Royal Colleges of Physicians or Surgeons in England, Ireland and Scotland. 41 (ten per cent) MOs achieved Fellowships of Royal Colleges.[64] A couple of important medical researchers, namely Percy Garnham and Muriel Robertson, were awarded the prestigious FRS.

Titles and honours conferred by the State were tangible symbols of inclusion into the imperial system. The awards bestowed a uniquely British tribute and were a visible encouragement to conform to the conservative, class ideals of imperial governance. The fifth of MOs who were awarded such accolades were physical reminders to their colleagues of the whole group's ultimate allegiance to the British monarch, and helped to promote a sense of common belonging and collective participation for colonials in the far-flung corners of Empire. David

Cannadine has made a similar point: the British honours system in the colonial context, he argued, 'created and projected an ordered, unified, hierarchical picture of Empire'.[65] Fellowships were a conferral of professional honour, normally based upon scientific knowledge. They were an important way of accrediting work done in the colonial locations by tying MOs into the prestigious accolades system of the home country.

*   *   *

The collective identity of Colonial MOs built on their shared profiles. Although individual experiences were necessarily distinct, rationales varied, and circumstances changed, the medical cohort embodied similarities that bound them together above their differences. Most entered the career under 30 years of age, and it was usually their first Colonial Service posting. This was, by and large, a young, impressionable group whose subsequent careers became inextricably bound to their shared early initiation to Africa. Most officers were from mixed class backgrounds and they had all completed a broadly similar medical training. The bulk had professional medical experience in other spheres; several came from colonial backgrounds; they were also, it should not be forgotten, mostly men. Within this group there were, of course, many sub-groups. People formed local communities united by their common nationalities, age bands, *alma mater*, as well as regional posting and personal interests. Yet, over and beyond the bonds created through backgrounds and origins, came broader, further reaching, ideological similarities that were articulated after MOs were established *in situ* as government officials. These ideologies were drawn from their shared conceptions and experiences of government service, their membership of the (tropical) medical profession, their implicit ideas of racial superiority, and, most importantly, their distinctive expressions of ultra-British, and yet specifically British East African, behaviour.

Chapter 9: Colonial Medical Communities

In lonely stations, far from the restraints of European public opinion and supported by no lavish remuneration, the officer must remain dignified and incorruptible. Moreover, with whatever margin of individual qualities, the members of this increasing corps must share the same standard of conduct and manners sufficiently to allow them to understand one another. They must act, when dispersed over wide and tested regions, upon similar principles and in pursuit of the same almost unspoken purposes.[1]

A tacit sense of kinship between Colonial MOs was informed by a desire to present a united front. This desire fostered and encouraged group loyalty, stifled dissenting voices and created in the colonial setting an environment that was based on traditional notions of Britishness but was also adapted to be uniquely British-East African. Furthermore, the distinctiveness of this cadre was particularly intense, as it was drawn from several sources each with strong and established identities. Members of the Colonial Medical Service were not only members of the white ruling class minority, they were British citizens, and mostly male. Moreover, their identity was overlaid by employment by a single agency (the Colonial Medical Service) and membership of a distinct profession (medicine), with closely converging tropical medical interests. The colonial medical identity, it is argued, transcended the individuality of those who made up the group.

A colonial medical identity developed partly because of the distance from centralised control that most Colonial Officers experienced. This, coupled with a cumbersome Civil Service bureaucracy, meant that dialogue between the ruling centre and the colonial periphery was notoriously slow.[2] A notable gap existed between central government and field officers, which created powerful circumstances, as Philip Curtin has argued, for those 'on the spot' to develop perspectives different from their contemporaries back home.[3]

Even if MOs could expect to enjoy a considerable amount of professional independence in the field with relatively little accountability — this did not preclude (indeed it strengthened the need for) the existence of further-reaching, shared ideologies. Living in widely dispersed communities, as a racial minority in an alien place, MOs quite naturally identified with others in similar situations to themselves

Service Loyalty

Most obviously, MOs were united by their membership of the Colonial Service. Employment by this single agency enrolled employees as part of the new governing classes in Africa while including them in a long established British tradition. This differentiated Officers from other sectors of colonial society, such as the religious missions, or those that owned large farms. MOs' 'right' to be in Africa was validated through their government employment. They were part of a sturdy administrative tradition connected by implication, if not directly, to a continuous line of British service overseas originating in India in the sixteenth century. Regardless of the extent to which individuals connected spiritually or professionally with their place of posting, their ultimate rationale for being there, and therefore, their critical allegiance (if they wanted to keep their jobs), had to be with the British Government they served.[4]

The Colonial Office quite self-consciously used the rhetoric of collective belonging as a means of encouraging uniform behaviour in its employees. Official circulars issued by the Colonial Office to Colonial Service officers often used rigorous, emotive language to emphasise the importance of maintaining standards of conduct in the field for the sake of the collective propriety of the Service as well as of individual integrity. [5] Civil service tradition provided the rationale for officers to set a good example to their colleagues: both in loyalty to those that had served before them and as a precedent to those that would serve after them.

Absorption into the Colonial Service tradition can be identified from the very earliest stages of recruitment. The selection system was centrally devised to facilitate continuity of attitude among officers. Furse was quite explicit that he was looking to recruit types that would uphold prestige and cultivate collective pride in the institution, which he felt had hitherto not had the public recognition it deserved.[6] A sense of common culture and privileged belonging was encouraged by channelling all applications through the same uniform paths and aiming to select types in accordance with conservative ideals and selection via interview. Generally most officers actively wanted to be in the Service and felt honoured to have been chosen. No officers (who left memoirs) gave any indication that they had been forced to join the Service against their will or that it was in any way a career of which to be ashamed.

Collective rituals were undergone before embarkation. The most emblematic rite of passage to the exotic life was the obligatory trip to the tropical outfitters. Many MOs recalled the money they spent on tropical paraphernalia before they went away and numerous advice books listed the lengthy (so-called!) minimum kit necessary for those venturing abroad.[7] Philip Mitchell, former Tanzanian District Officer (later governor of Uganda), provided one of the best examples of this pre-departure experience that typified most colonial departures:

> We bought...vast pith helmets, spine pads, cholera belts and the Lord alone knows how much other junk....You could buy anything a man really needed,

at half the prices paid in London, in the general stores of any African colony — but again, nobody told us that, in London; and if we had been told we would not have believed it. For the truth is, we all felt like a lot of young Stanleys and Spekes and the more exotic and peculiar the things we bought, the more we felt like intrepid explorers bound on some romantic 'Mission to the Interior'.[8]

Once on the ship to East Africa officers would have felt part of a shared adventure. The sea voyage provided an extended opportunity to meet fellow doctors about to start colonial service (or rejoin after leave). The voyage also afforded an opportunity to meet officers in other branches of the Colonial Service. Arthur Williams remembered that on his outward trip '[n]early all passengers were in some East African Service or other'.[9] It was undoubtedly a socially very useful trip and many of these early acquaintances endured throughout subsequent careers.[10]

Early shared experiences helped to nurture a sense of pride and belonging. The Colonial Office itself was well aware that '[t]he most important training was thought to take place during the early years of Colonial Service' and saw the benefits of recruiting officers while relatively young when they were unlikely to have well developed separate (or even contrary) ideological commitments.[11] If Service ideas were imbibed while young, they were more likely to engage people with the whole ethos of the Colonial Service.

As soon as the new appointees arrived in East Africa they were made to feel part of an organised establishment — although it was impressed upon the new arrivals that they were unmistakably juniors within that group. The idea that officers had to look to their seniors for examples of social and professional conduct was tacitly accepted, and mentoring (usually at one of the main hospitals in the nearest urban centre) was the most popular way of showing young officers the ropes.[12] Early conventions of arrival would involve meeting with a senior official, and then discussing over a sundowner, fundamental bureaucratic requirements as well as 'the peculiarities of the organisation'.[13] In Kenya, new MOs were given typed-up notes telling them how to prepare food, appoint suitable servants and take precautions against the disease and the sun.[14] In some ways, these were unremarkable, routine, welcoming procedures, except that they were crucially connected to the somewhat rigid expectations of Service conduct and requirements. Young officers were effectively introduced to accepted norms of behaviour and attitude — a period of orientation that one MO wryly recalled as having been one of both 'acclimatisation and indoctrination'.[15]

Colonial Service Officers were all subject to the same rules and regulations and all had their colonial careers assessed via a regular system of confidential reports.[16] Officers shared an institutional experience and one that was quite conscious of its prominent role in the shaping of official British (and African) history. The Colonial Service provided new recruits with a formidable ideological framework; one that they would not have benefited from had they gone to Africa to seek their fortunes independently. Many features of daily life were seen to and regulated by this protective body. Employees' housing was provided and furnished by the Public Works Department, officers were recommended to join the nearest European club (even if they then moved into the outlying districts) and everyone was issued with regulations establishing codes of behaviour.[17] If the Colonial Officer was allotted a district posting, the community in which he lived was called the *boma* (Swahili for stockade or enclosure). Many officers identified this as the most important social unit of the district-based Colonial Service, with officials from various branches of the Service forming a European enclave physically distinct from the African communities around them.[18] It was around the *boma* that mutually identifying communities developed, not only forging friendships and lifelong loyalties; it was also the site of acrimonious internal feuds and rivalries.[19]

Despite personal and professional disputes, accord and unity were the Colonial Service's over-riding strength. Senior officials actively pursued a policy that suppressed certain types of treachery and discord and purged undesirables. An unspoken distinction operated between *acceptable* and *unacceptable* complaints. Acceptable complaints were pursued through customary pathways, which for MOs was their local branch of the BMA. It was tolerable for officers to agitate for improved terms and conditions of service; seeking these ends was perceived as being for the collective good. This was quite different from individual insubordination or misconduct that, in contrast, was dealt with summarily and, often, heavy-handedly. The examples are numerous: when Hugh Trowell complained about the effectiveness of medical safaris he was threatened with a posting to the remote desert region of Kenya, the Northern Frontier District; when Margaret Lamont complained about the policy of enforced venereal disease examinations of African women, she was dismissed; Harvey Welch and Ernest Adams were 'got rid of' because their alcohol and drug addictions.[20] Above all else, the Colonial Service worked towards presenting a united and decorous front.

Other historians have commented upon the tendency for self-regulation within colonial societies.[21] The East African Medical Service was really no special case in this regard and the evident culture of self-censorship was linked to the intrinsic conservatism of the Colonial Service as a whole. As one commentator noted: 'the *esprit de corps* of the Colonial Service, or red tape, as it is sometimes termed, is so rigid and dangerous to the prospects of those who transgress its canons that seldom indeed is there friction.'[22] This is not to say that everyone accepted blindly the rule and attitudes of the Colonial Office. People *did* complain, and were further united in their shared frustration. But ultimately most felt aggrieved by such a formidable institution such as the Colonial Service. Percy Garnham (one of the most famous malariologists to come out of the East African Medical Service) summed up what must have been the feelings of many. He (privately) bemoaned:

> [The] tone of the Service, which necessitates (for advancement within it), a blind devotion to doctrines and theories to which one personally is completely averse. (in [*sic*] order to be looked upon with favour, one must subscribe blindly to the prevailing doctrine, just as a Nazi must in Germany or a fascist in Italy).[23]

Employees' identification with the Colonial Service usually stayed with them long after they had retired. In the United Kingdom, the Corona Club, an official Colonial Service and Colonial Office club was established in 1900 to provide a setting in which current and retired officers could share their colonial experiences. The Corona Club had a membership that grew from over a thousand in 1905, to over four thousand by 1958 and, although it was not characterised by plentiful meetings, it provided an important focal point for individuals who had been (or were) part of the ruling classes of Empire.[24] Between 1948 and 1962 the club published a journal, *Corona*, the delivery of which was looked forward to by officers in outstations and provided further tangible evidence of their collective membership of a group.

Other forms of media served consciously to tie Colonial Service employees together. In 1932 the BBC began broadcasting to Africa and other parts of Empire via the Empire Service, the forerunner of the BBC World Service. These programmes connected officers in the localities with others in similar situations to themselves; they also actively promoted the Colonial Service by broadcasting the speeches of the annual Colonial Service dinner of the Corona Club.[25] Other schemes looked after colonial officers in their retirement. The Osborne Convalescent Home on the Isle of Wight provided facilities for ex-colonial officers and in 1967 the Overseas Pensioners Association was established.[26]

The Colonial Service, in short, deliberately nurtured a group culture. Recalcitrant individuals were mostly silenced by dismissal or by allocation to a less desirable posting. This discouraged individual freedom of expression, but it brought with it large social and experiential rewards — not least, membership of a prestigious ruling class, support from British government and, at the height of Empire, the implicit support of the British people. Before World War Two, officers felt little need to doubt that they were undertaking good and worthy government duties. Doctors were clearly influenced by their strong Colonial Service identity, but their membership of the medical fraternity provided them with another important mutual reference point.

Professional Unification

Colonial Officers associated at a general level with all their Colonial Service colleagues, but naturally migrated towards the same vocational corps as themselves. Even in areas where Europeans were widely dispersed, the Colonial Officer identified with his or her counterparts in other regions; if this was not always practicable (as it often was not) the option remained for the isolated individual to identify himself or herself with the profession that they officially represented. Just as the District Officer (DO) became the symbol of regional authority, embodied in a single individual, so the doctor became the symbol, for many Europeans and Africans, of health and (western) medical adeptness.[27] In colonial society, officers frequently found themselves in situations where they were the only administrator, doctor or veterinarian for miles around — although these single representatives of the various Service branches, may all have lived together in the same *boma*. Personal identity became profoundly, and often interchangeably, linked to their professional standing; creating a situation that made it 'difficult for an officer to get away from an atmosphere of "shop"', unable to 'leave his work behind him when he quits his office in the evening.'[28]

Arguably, this professional identification was particularly strong in the case of medicine. Doctors were reminded through the Hippocratic Oath that they were part of a sacred fraternity, bound together under the same codes of conduct and terms of reference. Medicine, like the church, was seen to be a vocational calling and however far apart different doctors might find themselves, they were ultimately all seen as individual representatives of the ancient Aesculapian tradition. They were also, significantly, tied together ideologically through their participation in formative training in tropical medicine and hygiene.

The course in tropical medicine and hygiene that MOs were required to undertake, regardless of posting, prepared colonial doctors for a generic tropical medical world.[29] By formally training doctors in the new and developing specialism, the British colonial government was effectively producing the first official messengers of metropolitan-taught tropical medicine, a subject that was ignored in most medical school and university courses.[30] The official sponsorship of tropical medical training marked the point where government began to exert influence over the type of knowledge that official doctors would be using. The establishment of special institutions to train officers was, in the wider perspective, an initiative to unite all MOs in a common purpose. This additionally aligned the Colonial Medical Service with a certain amount of medico-scientific modernity, and nurtured group allegiances based upon shared participation in a new and developing field. This project, above all, allowed government to oversee the training of MOs who were to be dispersed throughout Empire. It gave them some sort of theoretical control over the way Britain would be medically represented abroad and ensured that all doctors were trained to believe in collective and common goals within the broad framework of British colonial policy.[31] Uniformity was an important stabilising element in a geographically and culturally diverse Empire. In the medical sphere at least, this homogeneity of approach was chiefly achieved by channelling all appointees through specialist training at a specialist training facility.

The curriculum of the London School in the early days centred more upon clinical training than laboratory work.[32] The core textbook was Manson's *Tropical Diseases: A Manual of the Diseases of Warm Climates* (1898). Protozoology and helminthology were initially seen as more essential than bacteriology, which was not added to the syllabus until 1913.[33] It was only after 1919 that the curriculum began to include detailed instruction on tropical hygiene. Even after improvements to the curriculum, many officers found the tropical medical instruction poor and of only limited relevance, but relevant or not, collective participation on the course had vital symbolic power.[34]

The establishment of the London school was a politically centralising move, but it also offered a reasonably cost-effective solution to a problem that had been expressed within the medical press for some time. With an estimated one in five British medical graduates heading for a career in the tropics, there had been calls for a special training to unite Colonial MOs since the end of the nineteenth century.[35] This shared inter-territorial involvement in a growing area of expertise was actively promoted by the Colonial Office and its supporters as making the

Colonial Service career an attractive one for ambitious young doctors and furthermore resulted, by the 1920s, in the emergence of colonial scientific communities beginning to develop autonomously from Britain.[36]

The BMA actively promoted its branches as a means of locally nurturing a sense of common cause.[37] It explicitly hoped, through branch meetings and widespread distribution of the *BMJ*, to include the colonies in a feeling of common 'kinship' with the home countries. Doctors were to gain strength from being part of a wider professional group that went over and above the 'distance which divides one part of the Empire from another'.[38] Furthermore, not only did BMA branch meetings foster a sense of inclusion with the British medical profession at large, they also created a forum in which local identity, 'unity and vitality' could be celebrated.[39] Although membership of the local branches of the BMA was open to all members of the medical profession, whether private practitioners, commercial doctors or missionaries, government doctors were particularly prominent with many Colonial MOs serving as BMA branch presidents.[40] The local branch was usually the first point of referral for Colonial Service complaints and it frequently acted as an arbitrator between the profession and the government.

One of the most important stages of the development of a scientific community in East Africa was the establishment in 1923 of the *Kenya Medical Journal (KMJ)*.[41] This periodical had originally been intended solely for Colonial Medical Service staff in Kenya: to give them a forum in which to share their professional ideas, but also to act as a unifying force to doctors posted far and wide within the region. The *KMJ* reported meetings of the local branches of the BMA, made announcements of particular interest to Medical Service staff and detailed officers' movements to, from, and within the colony. In fact, the journal quickly became more generalist in its remit and expanded beyond the borders of Kenya to represent the broader European medical community throughout East Africa, including private and missionary doctors.[42] The MO responsible for setting up and editing the journal was Christopher Wilson, a man of outspoken and candid opinions, who went on, in his retirement in Kenya, to write two political works on the country. With the benefit of hindsight, it was entirely characteristic for him to have started a publication that gave voice to local opinions.[43] Over time the newsy format subsided and became replaced with the more serious professional tone, with an emphasis on publishing local research findings that still survives today.[44] Significantly, in the period covered by this study, Colonial Medical Staff featured prominently amongst its editors, even after it had broadened its sphere to become a mouthpiece for the East African medical profession at large.[45] Officers also used this journal to report local findings or the results of trials.

The *EAMJ* was not the only medical journal available to East African medical profession. Colonial medical departments gradually developed small libraries stocking relevant books and journals that allowed doctors to keep abreast of major international medical developments.[46] Journals were sometimes distributed through the central secretariat to MOs in outstations and, so far as geographical restrictions allowed, an informal culture of book and periodical swapping existed between doctors.[47] Indeed, intellectual isolation sometimes made colonial doctors all the more conscious of the need for access to contemporary medical literature.[48] About half of the monthly circulation of the *Sleeping Sickness Bulletin* went to doctors in Africa,[49] and many MOs used their periods of home leave as important opportunities to refresh their professional knowledge and gain supplementary qualifications.[50]

In so far as homogeneity of medical beliefs can be determined as a unifying force, the evidence suggests that pre-World War Two MOs found themselves in an unusual situation. On one hand, they identified strongly with the contemporary medical profession of which they were a part; while on the other, they were significantly distanced from it, both physically and mentally. The establishment of the *KMJ* and of local branches of the BMA show that successful attempts were made to nurture feelings of colonial medical belonging, but doctors nevertheless found themselves both socially and professionally in a much freer space than they were likely to have experienced back home. As Driver has argued in the case of field experiences of early geographers, doctors found themselves — in terms of their daily work and intellectual development — in a position that was characterised by very little outside interference.[51] This meant that MOs often embodied more diffuse ideas than may have been acceptable back home. A curious situation developed with doctors simultaneously aligning themselves with the modernity of modern tropical medicine, while frequently perpetuating old-fashioned medical ideas, particularly about disease causation.

Operating at the very heart of the field, Colonial Service doctors were among the few interpreters of the state of African health and medicine to the outside world; they were often the first to see unusual cases and the first to judge the efficacy of medical procedures. They also had access to the biggest trial group — the diseased African population — and so were able to compare and contrast treatments and theories of infection. It is clear from the high proportion of MOs who published scientific papers, that many identified themselves as tropical medical experts despite the generalist nature of their official duties.[52] MOs commonly mentioned their 'almost limitless' access to topics for further research or investigation that were caused by the circumstances of their everyday duties.[53] When writing their own histories, some MOs identified themselves as part of a long line of (field-based) tropical medical pioneers.[54]

As most MOs were employed as clinical generalists, any specific research interests arose out of the circumstances of their job; for example, involvement in a particular disease survey, participation in the work of a local laboratory, or simply a brief from senior officers to work in a particular area of tropical medicine.[55] This research was sometimes recognised internationally: a number of MOs in Kenya, Tanzania and Uganda were awarded the prestigious North Persian Forces Memorial Medal. This award was given for the best piece of original work in tropical medicine for the year and holders included many officers employed in the East African Medical Service: William Hood Dye (1924 and 1927); Farnworth Anderson (1930); Neil McLean (1931); Henry Burke-Gaffney (1932) and Arthur Forbes Brown (1935).[56] Clearly, despite a scarcity of research facilities and a lack of access to metropolitan knowledge, many MOs had worthwhile professional information to impart. This is also indicated by the large number who continued their tropical medical interests in subsequent careers, after retirement from the Colonial Service.[57]

Intriguingly, despite these prevalent associations with modernity, colonial medical beliefs often also incorporated a decidedly more old fashioned approach to tropical health. Particularly tenacious was the belief that there was something inherent in the tropical climate and lifestyle that could exert a pernicious long-term effect on Europeans. These views were becoming increasingly untenable in the UK, but right until the late 1930s, medical debate about health in Africa regularly assumed (and actively engaged with) ideas about health and its relationship to climate.[58] There seemed to be no internal contradiction in most people's minds between these two ways of thinking about the world: indeed, some biomedical explanations seemed to fit quite naturally with earlier models. Many objective scientific theories implicitly still relied upon a generalised idea of Africa and its peoples as being inherently pathological. The nature of these associations changed as the period progressed. By the 1920s and 1930s, colonial attitudes had begun to re-orientate towards public health education, and ideas of civic responsibility, rather than continuing notions of Africa being inherently disease-provoking. It was felt that, with better education and training, Africans could learn to help themselves towards better health. Importantly, however, this idea was still based on colonialist assumptions that felt no especial need to take seriously traditional African medical practices, and did very little to research into medical techniques that might be more culturally applicable to the African tradition. It was naturally assumed that the western medical approach was the best and most universally desirable medical tradition.[59]

The colonies provided an important, yet isolated space for doctors to work. The limited facilities and distance from central control, allowed medicine to develop along independent lines and put Colonial MOs in an intermediary world between tradition and modernity. Yet, whatever the ambiguities expressed in the colonial situation, it is clear that the official line promulgated by colonial governing bodies, was to associate the career with active participation in tropical medical research. Although before the 1930s systematic investment in locally based research was negligible, it is clear that the intention to involve MOs had been there since the very beginning of the period. As early as 1897 one of the first recommendations made between Manson and Chamberlain was that MOs were to be encouraged to write special papers on tropical diseases that they had encountered, which were to be appended to the annual medical reports of each colony.[60] In 1912 the standing orders of the Uganda Medical Department made this hope explicit. The written regulations expressed the formal expectation that all MOs would take 'a specially active interest in the investigation, treatment and prevention of such diseases as are endemic, epidemic or unduly prevalent in the Uganda Protectorate'. It went on to stress the importance of individuals making collections and bionomic studies of insects that were possibly implicated in the transmission of disease to man.[61] As the Colonial Medical Service grew (along with tropical medicine), the emphasis put upon developing specialist interests among its employees also expanded. By the 1920s the Colonial Office was pushing a recruitment line that a Service career might make a tangible difference to doctors' research ambitions.[62] It was emphasised that individuals would have more opportunities to undertake pioneering research, with more professional independence than was normally available in the home environment.[63]

One additional point indicates an important element of the specifically medical aspects of this group's identity: the way MOs differentiated themselves from other groups of Colonial Service workers. Despite the emphasis on working together 'with as little friction as possible' with officials in other departments, MOs clearly did distinguish themselves from other Colonial Service members and owing to the nature of their duties, MOs held a certain amount of power in some spheres of Colonial Service activity. [64] They represented the principal guardians of all government employees' health, and as part of their official role found themselves drafted in as experts when the central colonial government had to make certain personnel decisions. MOs issued health certificates that were often the sole basis for the decision whether officers were invalided out of the Colonial Service. Doctors also had an important say in which officials were most physiologically or psychologically ready for leave. This power within the community, meant that 'the lordly DC could not always ride roughshod over the humble MO'; indeed members of the other Colonial Services needed to keep MOs onside in the eventuality that they needed a medical certificate for themselves or their families. As John Carman tellingly remembered, the doctor could 'usually find a good excuse' for withholding a medical certificate if he so wanted.[65]

The ways in which Colonial MOs identified with their membership of the medical profession did not necessarily override their identification with other aspects of their collective group culture, but rather it was a vital component of their complex group identity. Community spirit between colonials was also fostered through their collective attitudes and behaviour; these sometimes went beyond affiliations determined by their profession or their shared involvement in governmental service. Some of the attitudes that MOs espoused were expressions of a group culture of whiteness, one that bound people together through shared allegiance to certain aspects of British culture.

Attitudes and Conduct

Colonial behaviour conformed to certain conventions. These were expressed in the way officers related to the people they ruled, the accepted modes of conduct that were required between fellow European colonials, their recreational interests, their conceptions of family life and their ideas about their new tropical home. Although individuals necessarily held different opinions, the evidence nevertheless presents a striking uniformity of attitude.

All colonials, whether settlers, missionaries or government officials, were ultimately bound together by their skin colour. This firmly identified them as members of the ruling class with a dominant socio-political role as officials, overseers or converters. Mutual racial identification, however, had particularly strong connotations within the medical sphere since it was often through the language of medicine that racial segregation was justified and African people were described in (inferior) contrast to their 'civilised' rulers.

Unlike the Indian Civil and Medical Services, all Colonial Officers had to be British either by birth or naturalisation. Justification for the debarment of indigenous people was often articulated in rather general terms: they did not have the 'character' for effective public service. Africans had no written culture, and their society was arranged in a sufficiently dissimilar way to European society for British rulers to assume a lack of fit between the two systems. It was felt that, until a point where Africans were trained in western models of governance and social policy, they were unable effectively to participate in the government process — except at a very low level.

The racial policy of the Colonial Office was so strong during this period that even those with medical qualifications registrable in the UK were sidelined to subordinate posts within the Medical Department if they were not of Caucasian extraction. An Indian doctor, Sakharam Bhagwat, was listed in the *Medical Directory* as working as an Assistant Surgeon in the Uganda Medical Department between 1913–20. Yet he possessed medical qualifications equivalent to his higher-ranking white contemporaries; he received his BSc at Bombay (1902), LRCP, LRCS (Edinburgh, 1908) and LRFPS (Glasgow, 1908) and had written scientific articles including one published in the *BMJ*.[66] Although he was a registered licensed private practitioner in Uganda, presumably working for the local Asian population, he was only given a subordinate position in the Colonial Medical Service.[67] In contrast, a white doctor, Alexander Lester, who had received his medical qualifications (MB, BS) in Bombay, had a long career as a member of the Colonial Medical Service in Tanzania and Uganda from 1924 onwards despite having no British qualifications.

Doctors naturally subscribed to certain ubiquitous ideas about race that characterised white attitudes in general, although the odd exception can be found.[68] Typically, '[t]here was little or no social intermingling between the different races' in the period before the Second World War.[69] In contrast to West Africa, which developed a less rigid demarcation between Africans and Europeans, because of the emerging British-educated African elite, East African society was resolutely segregationist in its approach to social, political and economic affairs. Africans were rarely entertained in European homes, and if friendships developed between the races it was invariably within the confines of a master-servant relationship.[70] Colonial Officers in particular, with their role intimately connected to governance, had little scope, compared, for example, to missionaries, to transgress the unspoken social boundaries.[71]

One of the things that physically delineated Europeans from their African counterparts was the inequity of facilities established by the colonial governments for different racial groups. While hospitals built for Africans were in a poor state, the European hospitals received higher subsidies and greater attention was paid to their facilities. Town planning schemes also prioritised European enclaves rather than native quarters; as Julian Huxley remarked on his trip to Kenya in 1929 '[t]he Europeans have as much air, view and space as they need; but behind this attractive façade is a slum.'[72] The specifically medical demarcation of the racial 'other' has been the subject of much medical historical study.[73] Popular associations came to surround the indigenous populations, identifying them with the principal sites of disease and characterising them as the location of unwholesome behaviour. The African people came to represent the inverse of the values and behaviour that the white community supposedly represented. To the modern eye, these categorisations embody crude and unfair generalisations. At the time they acted as a critical opposite against which the white community could define itself. When social anxieties developed in Kenya over black men raping or molesting white women (the 'black peril'), active debate and coverage of racial issues united the white community through their shared perception of the risks to which the African population exposed them.[74] It was an entirely logical reaction, perhaps, to categorise what was culturally, scientifically and epistemologically confusing as the inverse of what the colonisers saw themselves to represent.[75] Beliefs were often so embedded that their supporters did not make a conscious decision to subscribe to them. Colonial society in this pre-1939 period had many rigid ideas about 'proper' collective behaviour and it was unquestioningly assumed that the colonisers and the colonised would not mingle.

Aside from differences of skin colour, there were differences in social status that affected the way colonials behaved and informed their collective attitudes. As Terence Ranger has pointed out, even white agriculturists in Africa saw themselves more as upper-class settler farmers than peasants.[76] Perhaps precisely because equivalent class ideals were becoming increasingly out-moded in Britain, they were increasingly celebrated and magnified in the colonial setting.[77] In 1939, Charles Jeffries could still describe the career as 'a Service in which you are treated as a gentleman by gentlemen'.[78] In general these idealised values referred back to a rural aristocratic model rather than to any more modern conceptions of the urban entrepreneurial spirit and, even if anachronistic, they were thought to be attractive features of colonial society. The colonies symbolised the last bastion of an old British social system. This image certainly influenced attitudes towards Colonial Service recruitment positively, but it also informed opinion of those resident within the colonies — as one old Kenyan colonial told another '[w]hy should I retire to England? In this country I am somebody; in England I would only be a number on a door.'[79]

This is not to say that there were no criticisms of this image. Opinions were voiced that Empire was too intrinsically conservative and resistant to change or self-reflection. All government employees had to slot ideologically into an established system, with a primary objective to master 'their section of the machine', a notion that, while it offered some autonomy of action, also left very little room for innovation or flair.[80] Other critics felt that the overwhelming public school ethos contributed to the development of inward looking colonial type 'which is innocently, but none the less insolently, Narcissistic — it takes itself for pattern and cannot trouble to see that any other types could be really admirable.'[81] These proved to be resilient themes in later criticisms of the Colonial Service; even when describing administrative officers in the 1960s, Colonial Service commentator Robert Heussler lamented that 'today's administrators…perfect and transfer more than they design and build'.[82]

Despite these, and other, criticisms the conservative ethos of the socially privileged predominated. Everything that was possible was done to make the colonial setting a place that physically, socially and culturally conjured up home. Even in the smallest stations, British traditions were upheld. The monarch's birthday was celebrated, British public holidays were adhered to and ceremonies were put on to welcome governors and visiting dignitaries. Caledonian and St. George's dinners were regularly held from the turn of the century, as well as the Old Etonian dinner held on 4 June each year at the Norfolk Hotel, opened in 1904 and alleged to be the 'Claridge's of Nairobi'.[83] The pages of the contemporary Government Gazettes of each respective territory reveal the type of occasions organised by these 'micro' British communities. [84] Announcements of sporting events, dinner dances, race-meetings, agricultural and horticultural shows all point towards the reproduction of middle and upper-middle class Britain.

Naturally enough, the main social centres were the large towns. European Clubs were established in Nairobi, Entebbe and Dar Es Salaam, and became important sites of social mingling. As prominent members of the European community, MOs commonly met there and used them for social gatherings. Other groups also developed around churches, the YMCA, the Rotary club and voluntary organisations.[85] Even those colonials posted to more isolated stations were encouraged to build a home from home; advice existed on how to keep an English country garden, and the small communities that formed around *bomas* held their own local events and dinner parties.[86] One of the primary undertakings of the British administration was to 'institute the comforts of home, to establish a visual and social environment which resembled England as much as possible in order to provide a sense of security and demonstration of English "civilization"'.[87] What the location lacked in art galleries and theatre, it made up for in abundance of sporting events, social opportunities and wildlife.[88] In 1911 Nairobi was said to be a town that was 'one of the best equipped with pastimes in the world', with opportunities for dances, films, sports and clubs.[89] Dar Es Salaam was described as cheap to live in while possessing a cinema and two European clubs; Tabora (Tanzania) was said to have a good lending library, a decent club, and held popular film events once a fortnight.[90] One of the most evocative images of relaxed civility, however, has to be that given by Frederick Treves, describing his trip to Uganda around 1910:

> Entebbe is the administrative capital of Uganda. It is as unlike a capital as any place can well be, while as for administration it must be that kind which is associated with a deckchair, a shady verandah, the chink of ice in a glass, and the curling smoke of a cigar. Entebbe, as being the prettiest and most charming town on the lake, would seem to be concerned more with her appearances than with the cares of state....Entebbe, indeed, gives the impression of being a place of leisure, a summer lake resort where no more business is undertaken than is absolutely necessary.[91]

Although facilities clearly got better once an administrative infrastructure was established in the second half of the period, from the earliest colonial times attempts were made by resident Europeans to bring to tropical Africa the better features of home. Sport was one of the most important aspects of British life to be transported to the colonies.[92] Indeed, this became a notably important part of the colonial identity and many MOs were praised for their outstanding sporting abilities.[93] Descriptions of colonial life invariably invoked sporting opportunities as one of the most dynamic features of colonial life.[94]

Another way that Britishness was expressed was through the strict codes of social behaviour that developed in the colonial locations. These naturally enough mirrored conventions back home, but the stress put upon formality in the bush was remarkably persistent, despite its obvious inappropriateness in a tropical climate with dispersed European society. Dressing for dinner, for example, was a standard ritual 'in the most isolated outposts as well as its social centers[sic.], for parties or when dining alone', and would have also acted as a visual marker of distinctions of race, gender and social rank.[95] A colonial medical wife described the three stages that comprised the local social etiquette for greeting new *boma* arrivals: firstly 'calling' (usually just leaving a calling card), then the sundowner (an evening drink) and lastly, the dinner invitation. The dinner would be a formal occasion with evening dress, seating plans organised by rank, and the best silver, glass and china the hostess could muster.[96] It was generally accepted that new colonial arrivals, including MOs, would call upon their seniors very soon after their arrival in a colony.[97]

To some MOs this emphasis upon protocol seemed decidedly old-fashioned. Hunter and his wife, who arrived in Uganda during the late 1930s, found themselves immersed in a world of social etiquette to which they had not been used at home: '[w]e were not used to the full ritual of calling cards, visitors-books with P.P.e. entries etc. and dressing for dinner so regularly; sitting by strict order of precedence at dinner parties.'[98] Margaret Wilson, characterful wife of MO Bagster Wilson, and doctor in her own right, described in her Tanzanian diary their social calendar in June 1933. It provides an impressive example of a colonial schedule:

> Last Friday we were hard at it in the Lab. till 8pm…Sat. am the same. Then D[onald Bagster] and I went for a Swim. Returned and Nicholls from Amani came to have a drink. Rushed into evening clothes. People arrived for dinner, grapefruit, kidney soup, fillet of beef, golden cream, cheese fondue. Then off to dance at the Club and stayed until 2.30am when my feet refused to function anymore, ending up with a wild Polka with D. Went to Gombero in the Afternoon. Walked for 3 hours before breakfast and saw three buffalo, wart hog, water buck, duiker and steenbok. We are going again next week with our rifles.[99]

Clothing was an obvious way in which social principles were visually upheld. Women were particularly advised to dress appropriately. One piece of sartorial advice recommended that women pack for their trip at least 'two or three evening dresses of crêpe de chine, satin and velvet'.[100] The MO wife, Mrs Bödeker, 'one of those women who kept up standards despite everything', allegedly bought with her to Kenya a 'large variety of hats…trimmed with osprey and veiling to match a selection of gowns in the high fashion of the day.'[101] This was quite in keeping with expectations, even if the exigencies imposed by local circumstances meant that decorous and formal behaviour had to occasionally be put to one side, for example while on a medical safari, or trekking through the bush. Dressing for dinner meant that people were always coming back to their civilised roots by the evening. Keeping up standards was, however, not just about distancing European communities from the behaviour of the natives, it was also thought to be good for morale. Women, by keeping themselves decent, were doing important work for both themselves and their husbands in terms of keeping up standards:

> As for finery it is as important for your morale as for your husband's. It is all too easy, in hot countries, to become used to faded cottons, dim linens of indeterminate colour and pattern and crumpled voiles. First thing you know, you are wearing them once too often, and that is the beginning of the Sad Story of the Slut. If there is any doubt, there is no doubt. Into the basket![102]

It was imperative for officers' careers that they subscribed to these and other common ideas of propriety. Social gatherings were an important chance to network and much of the valuable experience officers gained was 'socially effected, at dinner tables or at clubs'.[103] The sundowner particularly was seen as a chance for younger officers to be introduced to the codes of conduct within colonial life.[104] Clearly some MOs found these social requirements rather trying — Farnworth Anderson complained of the many unspoken directives such as 'regulation dress' and 'regulation refreshment' (whisky) at sundowner time — but in general officers acknowledged the advantages of conformity more than they resisted it, and even came to enjoy the social aspects of their work.[105]

After 1919, when European women (usually in their capacity as wives) increasingly became a feature of colonial life, one of the ways that colonials made their new environment more like home was through instituting 'normal' rituals of British family life. The replication of middle-England was so successful, that Julian Huxley evocatively described Kenya in 1929 as 'suburbia unrestrained'.[106] The first European marriage in Nairobi is said to have been that of an MO, Clare Wiggins, in 1904.[107] Gradually thereafter it became more common for officers to marry in Africa. Many Colonial Officers' wives had children in the colonies, and many children were schooled there, usually in Kenya, which had the best schooling facilities in East Africa.

One widely perceived corollary of the increased presence of women in the colonial location was an erosion of relations between Europeans and Africans. Before the arrival of European women, concubinage was recognised (if unmentioned) as one of the perks of the job. Indeed it was so overt that the government felt impelled to issue a circular directive in 1909 reminding officers of the inappropriateness of this behaviour.[108] The arrival of European women has been regarded by many historians as marking a period of increased tensions between white and black communities with the significant hardening of racial boundaries.[109] These women brought with them new moral codes and an emphasis on etiquette and decorum; they instituted home-grown standards and upheld the moral tone.

Yet vitally, among all this ritual and archetypical British behaviour, lay continually reiterated expressions of difference. Difference was what ultimately made the colonial experience exciting and helped make up for perceived deficiencies in terms of employment or pay. It aligned officers with an evocative history of travel and exploration and made them living examples of an imperial genre of adventure within popular literature and (in the later period) film. New recruits arrived 'bursting with zeal to start this Sanders of the River business' and the archetype continued to inform the way the group's identity was expressed.[110] There was no necessary internal contradiction in this double embracing of both similarity and difference. On one hand, colonial officials expressed their identity through reference to their shared roots, while on the other, they stood together because of their shared place-specific experiences. Colonial African identity embraced both historic ideas of adventure and embedded ideas of British conduct and decorum; as one contemporary commentator put it, it combined expressions of 'individual spirit and enterprise' with a 'desire to establish British culture and civilisation'.[111] Even exaggerated Britishness made Africa a different enclave.[112]

One of the most obvious things that made colonial life distinctive was the climate. This necessitated the adoption of various health regimens to ensure salubrity. These routines were endorsed by the medical profession and were seen as essential to a successful colonial life. Much health advice centred on the ill-effects of the sun. Wearing spine-pads, cholera belts or topees (sun helmets) was recommended. Regimens involved drinking alcohol only after sun down, bathing at certain times of the day and avoiding certain foods. As Lord Cranworth advised those contemplating a life in Kenya: 'although a hairy chest peeping through an unbuttoned shirt is picturesque and gives the air of a pioneer, in reality the less surface exposed to the sun the better.' Above all Europeans in the East African tropical world were advised to adhere to the maxim 'keep the spirits up, the bowels open, and wear flannel next to the skin.'[113]

Many contemporary descriptions expressed this combination of the strangely familiar, yet ultimately unique, nature of the colonial experience. Calwell remembered how the house he had in Ushirombo, Tanzania, although infested with white ants, with only petrol boxes for bookcases, a grass roof and a pit latrine, nevertheless had beautiful rose bushes planted around the verandah.[114] This in many ways was the key of colonial life; it could replicate a nostalgic vision of aristocratic land owning classes back home, while also being crucially and exotically different. The memories of Rex Surridge, who started in 1923 in the Tanzanian Colonial Administrative Service, illustrate the contrast aptly; on walking through his *boma* for the first time he found:

> ...carnations, roses and violets in bloom, a lovely running stream and a glorious climate. So good, indeed, that many Europeans and Asians had settled in the area; there was a country club with golf course and tennis courts, and even a few horses—plus the odd lion.[115]

Big game hunting particularly seemed to sum up this difference — while conforming to a public school sporting ethos, it also was an undeniably unusual pastime for most British. It neatly encapsulated the romantic associations of African adventure and its essential difference within easily understandable terms of reference. Within East Africa, particularly, hunting was a fundamental part of the colonial identity and the majority of officers regularly participated in the sport.[116]

Finally, language reflected and reinforced behaviour. It was common for Colonial Officers to learn Kiswahili, but the specific manner in which they did went far beyond the mere pragmatics of facilitating communication with the communities they ruled. Some officers learnt local African dialects, but attention throughout East Africa was focused upon learning Kiswahili — not least because Colonial Office terms of employment included a salary incentive (the language allowance) to those who had passed appropriate examinations.[117] This led to a situation whereby some officers took standard language examinations even though they were posted to districts were Kiswahili was not widely spoken; a smattering of Kiswahili became a marker of European colonial identity irrespective of its actual applicability.[118] If Bernard Cohn's argument for the European interest in learning Indian languages (during the consolidation of power of the British East India Company) is followed, then this drive to take on language could be seen as a further attempt to appropriate culture in such a way as to confirm European superiority.[119]

In the East Africa context colonials used African language to define not only themselves, but also their relationships with indigenous people. One contemporary account described the variant used by Europeans as 'kitchen Swahili'. This guide advised prospective students to descend from the 'mountain heights of linguistic precision' — the best way for them to converse with the *wa-shenzi* (backward peoples)' was to use an imprecise hybrid of language.[120] Kitchen Swahili was a crude pidgin, made by stringing together various essential Swahili nouns and verbs, interspersed with English.[121] It was used not only to communicate with Africans, but also to bind together European communities in a mutual code. When colonials spoke to each other they typically littered their regular speech with Kiswahili words that implied shared understanding and mutual recognition and rudimentary African language ability became an important part of a shared colonial expression. John Carmen affectionately remembered the motto he constructed with his colonial medical workmate, Cliff Braimbridge: 'Hakuna Pesa Nyingi, Lakini Tunaona sana La Vie' ('we haven't got much money, but we do see life').[122] The very way this phrase was conceptualised, using a hybrid of Kiswahili and French, celebrated shared educational roots (i.e. it assumed a knowledge of French) while referring also to their acquaintance with a new language derived specifically from the colonial location.

Colonials adopted certain emblematic behaviours that bound them together as a group. As well as physically converging, as often as they could, at clubs, dinner parties and sporting events, they were also bound, despite geographical distances, by uniformity of approach and attitude. There was a remarkable convergence of ideas; ones that harked back to a bygone British age while celebrating the new challenges thrown up by the colonial situation. Many of these factors were not unique to the colonial medical experience, but they did inform the identity of the group. Combined with other group loyalties, a very distinctive group identity emerged among East African colonial doctors.

*   *   *

Officers had to adhere to uniform conditions of Service, and they were constrained in many of their actions by the power of the Colonial Office. They were also united with other members of the medical community through their shared training and professional perspective and, riding above all these vocational affiliations, they were closely tied to the white colonial community in general. At the heart of these converging group commitments lay a tacit acceptance of the priority that had to be afforded to the local, East African, experiences.[123]

All these different factors demanded allegiance. If at one level colonials stood shoulder-to-shoulder in support of the imperial mission, or in support of keeping out undesirables from their community (there were protests in East Africa against Jewish immigrants, Austro-German refugees and poor whites[124]), at another level society was split into numerous localised allegiances, stemming from the affiliations that developed around the *boma*, the district, or through professional ties.[125] Local loyalties were expressed in numerous ways: MOs, for example, were reprimanded for associating too closely with members of other colonial groups, even missionaries.[126] Settlers and Government officials were said to fall into two distinct camps, invariably in direct opposition to each other.[127] Often these rivalries were played out on sports fields through the Settler versus Official cricket, football and rugby matches that became a regular feature of colonial life. Each colonial group had its own subtle version of identity. Whether settlers, missionaries or conscript doctors, they drew upon common experiences and made distinctions between themselves and other groups.[128] The fact that each European group, including MOs, can be reduced to common denominators of local allegiance still acknowledges the need to work within an overarching colonial identity.

MOs were a distinct sub-group working within the broader definitional frameworks of government service culture, medicine and colonialism. Of course there was no absolute homogeneity, people did speak their minds and individuals did go against convention. But, crucially, the factors of their employment and situation tended to militate against change and favoured preserving the status quo. This resulted in a preoccupation with maintaining cultural norms and the presentation of a united front, even if the group as a whole did not actually constitute one.

Chapter 10: Conclusion

Everyone must strike a balance for himself. He must weigh up, perhaps, the satisfaction of pioneering against the deprivation of "cultural amenities"; the pleasures of warmth and sunshine against the trials of mosquitoes and sweat; the relief from queues and washing-up against the interruption of family life and the bogy of "two establishments"; the stimulation of seeing new countries and meeting with unfamiliar people against the parochialism of small-station "shop". It has been said, with as much truth (or half truth) as is to be found in most epigrams, that the Colonial Service is the only profession in which one can live the life of a country gentleman on the salary of a civil servant. The fact is if you like the sort of life the Colonial Service has to offer you will like the Colonial Service.[1]

This work draws together common strands within East African colonial medical careers before World War Two. It considers Colonial Office selection criteria; the motives for doctors to apply for governmental careers; the organisation of the Medical Service within three British territories (and the impact of this organisation upon typical 'in-field' experiences); and finally, how common points of reference, based upon shared professional as well as social and cultural affiliations, helped to create a colonial medical identity.

This is only one part of the multi-faceted history of the Colonial Medical Service. The perspective focuses upon personal experiences and perceptions rather than examining the development of medical policies or tracing the course of tropical medical advancements.[2] It has necessarily prioritised the cultural and social aspects of the Colonial Medical Service encounter over political, scientific and economic ones. This book has made no claim to offer a complete picture of colonial medical practice; it scrutinises things from the European perspective and concentrates upon no more than the most persistent, official and popular, ideas that impacted upon colonial medical lives.

This approach highlights the general over the particular. Although Africanists have been eager (and correctly so) to celebrate the long-overlooked histories of individual African countries, their worthy projects should not be confused with the aims of this one. One of the most striking aspects of this period was the way that sub-Saharan Africa was lumped together in both the official and popular imagination as a single entity, and was dealt with in conspicuously uniform terms by one governing body, the Colonial Office. This in turn affected the behaviour and attitudes of British personnel stationed there and, for better or worse, these government participants acted out their role essentially as cultural attachés of colonialism. Colonial Office policies recurrently emphasised generalisations over the African continent more than the specificities of each region. This tendency towards over-simplification was borne of a long tradition that enjoyed rhetorically evocative descriptions of Empire that usually paid little heed to intra-continental differences.[3] It assumed the intrinsic 'rightness' of the established precedents that guided Colonial Service priorities. The Service was seen as a single career rather than numerous diverse local careers. Officers could not apply to work in a particular country within the Colonial Service (although they could express a preference), so that in applying for a Medical Service job, a desire to participate in colonial life was expected to take precedence over any attraction to a particular country. Tellingly, most official policy directives were issued under blanket headings such as 'Africa East' or 'Africa West' and serve as further evidence that, in the official mindset at least, African colonial dependencies were often grouped together *en masse*. Needless to say, to the career was more important than its location. As both the unification of the East African Medical Service in 1921 and the Colonial Medical Service in 1934 show, there was an ongoing desire to standardise personnel management as far as possible and encourage transfers between the colonies. From the time when MOs applied for their jobs until their careers ended, the official policies directed them towards improving the workability of the bureaucracy; the objective was to strive towards uniformity and similarity before individuality and distinctiveness could be considered.

Officers were selected based upon certain ideas of good colonial types; they were attracted to colonial life because of certain commonly perceived advantages and stereotypes. Once selected and in position, officers found that they worked within the official limitations of one powerful parent institution as well as within the tacit cultural boundaries of a highly conservative Empire. An exploration of these broad frameworks does not challenge the individual characters of the countries or the particularities of individual colonial experiences. Indeed, once in the location, people often emphasised and celebrated their place-specific experiences, alongside expressions of their Britishness (Chapter 9). What is interesting is that ideas of supposed Britishness were as generalised and selectively used as were widespread ideas of the African continent. Colonials frequently defined their identity through associations that embraced concepts of home as much as a recognition of African-situated difference. The colonial experience was, it has been argued, a hybrid of these two ideologies.

There are ways, of course, that this study could have been broadened; chapters could, for example, have looked more precisely at the scientific identity of the medical cohort. How did the content of the tropical diploma courses offered in London, Liverpool, Cambridge and Edinburgh impact upon policies and practices transported to the tropical world?[4] More, too, could be said on the issue of how scientific research fitted into the way officers saw themselves. The growth of scientific identity, although touched upon in Chapter 9, could also have been traced in relation to the development of laboratory medicine in Kenya, Uganda and Tanzania.[5] It would have been interesting to chart the development of research interests in fields such as malariology or parasitology, and to analyse how these interests influenced the development of colonial medical practice and the scientific self-image of the colonial medical community. Certainly, individual research contributions from the East African field contributed substantially to advances within tropical medical science during the colonial period.[6] In the analysis presented here individual contributions have been surrendered in favour of looking at the universal features of the job.[7]

The period covered by this study was one in which medicine in the colonies changed considerably. Important country-specific developments include the development of medical education for Africans in Uganda, the growth of interest in public health, and the history of campaigns against prevalent tropical diseases such as sleeping sickness or malaria.[8] This work does not closely examine the reception of medical initiatives by the African communities, although there is evidence to suggest that they were not always gratefully or passively received. No doubt, if some of the theories were applied to the arguments presented here, it would also be found that African resistance and negotiation was a factor in influencing the way that MOs behaved and the types of practices that they embodied.[9] These approaches, however, have not been the main focus of this work. An exploration of the colonial medical identity provides a lens through which to view the assumptions, expectations and, sometimes, contradictions that informed the experiences of government medical staff during this period. However uneasily an exploration of exclusively European relationships with the colonies may sit within our post-colonial consciences, it can still be acknowledged as part of the colonial story.

The Post-War Period

To complete the picture, brief mention needs to be made of the developments that occurred in the Colonial Medical Service after World War Two. Ann Beck described the situation that the East African Medical Service found itself in by 1939 as 'vulnerable' and under massive financial stress. She describes how the Service gradually shifted towards a more modern approach, with more official focus placed upon public health programmes and the sponsorship of field-based scientific research.[10] Central office in London faced many problems: most importantly the manpower pressures and financial stresses created by World War Two. In an active attempt to avoid repeating the severe recruitment problems that the Service experienced during World War One, the Colonial Office made every effort in its publicity to emphasise that officers could serve their country through membership of the Colonial Service as well as joining the fighting ranks.[11] Despite these efforts there was still a considerable reduction in medical recruitment during the war years and in 1942 it came almost to a standstill. To make up this deficit, MOs in Africa were not allowed to leave their posts or were transferred to active war service. Many who were due for retirement were retained in service.[12] After the war the urgent need for new recruits quickly meant that the entry requirement of the Diploma of Tropical Medicine and Hygiene was waived for new MOs. It became normal instead for MOs to take the course when on leave, usually after their first tour of duty.[13] Although there was a brief resurgence in the popularity of the career after the second war, competition from other careers also became more pronounced in this period and there were worries that the Colonial Service would be under-staffed.[14] Crisis point did not arrive, however, and by 1946 the Colonial Service had grown considerably, with just under three thousand appointments across the board.[15] Yet, the career was still, despite Furse's best efforts, regarded as having a relatively low profile (largely caused by the uncompetitive terms offered) when compared to other public services.[16] With increasing moves towards independence in the colonies, the British Colonial Service was reorganised in 1954 under the title of Her Majesties Overseas Civil Service (HMOCS). In 1966 the Colonial Office was merged with Commonwealth Relations Office, which in turn became part of the Foreign Office. This effectively signalled the end of the Colonial Service, although some of its aims and functions lived on in a reduced HMOCS right up until the handing over of Hong Kong to China in 1997.[17]

By the 1940s the Colonial Service was quite different to the organisation it had been at the turn of the century. Colonial policy in general was beginning to move away from notions of native-administration and indirect rule, and looked instead towards setting up systems of local government. Working within this changed emphasis, plans were centrally developed between 1943 and 1954 for the expansion and progressive development of the Colonial Service. In 1943 Furse presented a new post-war plan for the training and preparation of candidates. Additionally, the Colonial Development and Welfare Acts of 1940 and 1945 abolished the principle that the colonies should be financially self-supporting. Instead these acts decreed that a proportion of crown monies should be expressly laid aside for the development of colonial societies in general and for the training of new officers in particular. In the second act of 1945 a grant of £1.5 million was earmarked for a ten-year training programme.[18] The 1946 government White Paper entitled the *Organization of the Colonial Service*, gives a feel for the new priorities: key points included financing the training of experts to work in the colonies and 'co-ordinating the distribution of staff so that the available resources are disposed to the best advantages of the colonies as a whole.'[19] It warned that in the colonies 'the younger generation will expect a place in Native Administrations, with a freer hand in their control.' The government spoke of 'the fundamental change to be expected'; not only did Britain have to acknowledge the need to allow native peoples to actively participate in their own governance, but they saw that they could no longer pursue policies and actions solely 'according to what seems best to us'.[20] Partnership rather than trusteeship was the order of the day; development was pursued, but for the first time with an insight into probable independence.[21]

From the 1930s onwards pictures of economic productivity, with bright cocoa groves, banana plantations and rubber forests, gradually replaced the images of Empire conjured up by the title of Stanley's *In Darkest Africa* as important visual representations of the continent.[22] The idea of development became more pronounced (albeit voiced in terms of *mutual* benefit). The notion of nonreciprocated aid was raised for the first time. Widespread educational initiatives were introduced. The new emphasis also affected the way native populations perceived their colonial rulers. Local populations began participating actively, with more power than ever previously, in the course of their own country's medical development.

Clearly, this new language of colonialism would have affected officers' behaviour and their collective perceptions of their role. These changes also fundamentally altered the ethos of the Colonial Service, but in other ways, the Service continued to be predicated upon essentially conservative establishment ideals — especially in the way it was organised. Furse remained in charge of recruitment until 1948 and his succession by his brother-in-law, Francis Newbolt — who held the position as Director of Recruitment until 1954 — did very little to radically alter prevailing attitudes and expectations. In fact, the increased regularisation and bureaucratisation of the Colonial Service that characterised the post-World War Two period in general could be seen to have actually reinforced ideas of conformity above any broadening of attitudes to embrace examples of entrepreneurial sprit. A 1951 description of the duties of a District MO stipulated as 'essential' that he should 'regard himself as one of a group of workers who are all directing their energies towards the same end.'[23] In the days when the fate of Empire seemed much less sure, it was more vital than ever that officers should group together and present a united front. Old values were in retreat and officers whose careers spanned the pre and post World War Two periods complained about their demise. As one administrative officer reminisced on return to his old posting in Anglo-Egyptian Sudan, 'nothing is now taken for granted. Prestige has gone, it has to be earned anew.'[24]

Yet, despite these feelings of change and mounting insecurity, which the Medical Service experienced with as much force as any of the other branches of the Colonial Service, a new confidence came to characterise the colonial medical endeavour. Medicine came to be increasingly seen as the one defensible, even humanitarian, aspect of colonialism.[25] This period saw a revolution in the control of infectious disease with major repercussions for the tropical world: the development of DDT and other insecticides; the introduction of synthetic anti-malarials; improved treatment of sleeping sickness; effective drugs for the therapy of schistosomiasis and other helminthic diseases; the use of sulphones for leprosy, potent antituberculosis compounds and antibiotics for many other common bacterial diseases; and the development for the first time of an effective yellow fever vaccine. A new self-assurance profoundly affected the way the post-war generation of MOs perceived themselves; not least as these medical developments provided officers with a new powerful armoury with which to enact their role.

Many of the MOs that have informed this work's findings served in the East African forces during the Second World War and then continued their colonial careers right through until independence.[26] Some went on to prominent positions in other colonial dependencies,[27] while others went back to their home countries and used their specialised tropical knowledge there either in a consultancy or teaching capacity.[28] A couple of East African MOs even went into prominent governmental positions in London, using their on-the-ground experiences to inform the direction of future colonial medical policies.[29] Interestingly, several

MOs found themselves unable to adjust to urban life in Britain and returned to East Africa for their retirement, either temporarily or permanently.[30]

The colonial career put doctors, administrators, lawyers and policemen in a location that heavily influenced their perception of the world. It was an experience that informed their subsequent careers, and associated them with an important historical period, one that many officers considered to signal the last real phase of British power and greatness. Even those colonial servants that did not return to their place of posting for any length of time usually saw their career experiences as in some way self-defining.[31] Officers (and not only medical ones) felt their colonial careers provided experiences that were worth preserving for posterity, as witnessed by the ample contributions to the archives that exist at Rhodes House and (during the later period) at the Bristol Empire and Commonwealth Museum. Colonial experiences were also kept alive at Corona club events, and through the Overseas Pensioners Association. Membership of the Colonial Service symbolised something more than just a run-of-the-mill job — it involved its members in a personal as well as professional journey, it elevated their status and made them integral participants in governance. It united career and place in an identity that was immensely evocative and enduring.

Career, Place and Identity

This examination of the colonial medical identity hopes to have placed an important aspect of British culture within a broader historical context. Colonial Medical Service recruitment policies have been laid out, and the conditions and criteria that officially governed the careers of doctors in the East African Service have been analysed. Through outlining the official and non-official selection criteria, the reasons why doctors might have applied for the job, and typical in-field career experiences some important cultural assumptions have been uncovered — especially how closely ideas of government service were related to broader conceptions of Africa as well as ideas of Britishness.

The profile that has been presented reveals a subtly distinctive sub-set of the colonial identity. Membership of the medical fraternity delicately influenced the terms of reference for the Medical Service cohort and made them distinct from their other Service colleagues. It drew doctors together in professional bonds and codes of conduct that were separate from their Service obligations, and gave them respected professional forums in which to express themselves, independent of their rank within the Service. It also gave them access to another system of professional recognition: one in which they could elevate their status by gaining extra medical qualifications, specialist publications or honorary Fellowships. Most importantly, being part of the colonial medical endeavour meant that MOs were involved, almost by default, in the new medico-scientific field of tropical medicine — a new specialism that at that time prioritised in-field experiences and observations over metropolitan-based research. It seems fitting that the remit of this study spans the period of the East African colonial medical career from its roots within early medical exploration (Robert Moffat, the first Ugandan PMO, was Livingstone's wife's nephew[32]) to the scientific modernity encapsulated by the grandson of the father of tropical medicine (Manson-Bahr who joined the Service in 1939 was the grandson of Patrick Manson).[33] Although during this period East Africa was never a major colonial medical research centre in its own right, the fact that the story can be traced from Livingstone to Manson-Bahr, says something about the symbolic associations of the place, linking the traditions of medicine and adventure in the pre-World War One period with medical and scientific modernity of World War Two.

The medical careers of 424 colonial doctors have been investigated for this book to ascertain their education, backgrounds and motivation. These findings were analysed in the context of colonial identity, to gauge the conformity of MOs to prevalent ideas, and to elucidate how they used specifically medical aspects of the identity to define themselves further. Above all, although it had expressions unique to its own group, the medical identity ultimately relied upon the symbolic capital that Empire gave all members of the colonising classes. The identity was intimately related to place and celebrated the distinctiveness of colonial life over and above other unifying features. The colonial place, in this case, Eastern Africa, offered the means to enact a certain way of life.

The Colonial Service was an occupation that embodied certain class standards and to successfully enjoy the career staff had largely to conform to these views. Perhaps more than many other medical careers offered at the time, it encapsulated a desire to leave Britain and do something different, something that carried evocative associations and offered a chance, often for people of modest class backgrounds, to participate in an exciting and worthwhile venture.

Before the outbreak of the Second World War, the African experience was still loaded with popular allure, professional challenge, personal development and escape from the ills of modern life. Career and place became intimately connected precisely because of the different experiences it gave them. As Margaret Trowell, wife of Hugh Trowell, reminisced, even though MOs and their families often felt homesick during their first tour of duty, after returning home to England they were just as often shocked to find that they had less in common with their former friends than they had presumed. They found, just as many others had done, that they had become Africa's 'willing prisoners' and even though they recognised that some aspects of the colonial life were undoubtedly hard, they soon longed 'to be again with people who share the same joke or even the same grumbles' and to be part of their like-minded communities.[34] The whole experience became deeply embedded in people's memories. It represented a period when people felt sure of their imperial role, and believed in their mission, albeit in an Empire that progressively became obsolete. It allowed, moreover, an escape from British life, during a time when professional options to live abroad were relatively scarce.

As this book has concentrated on personal medical experiences, it seems fitting to give some of the final words to a MO Robert Hennessey, whose career in Uganda spanned 26 years, in many ways epitomised the most successful of colonial medical servants. After finishing his career at the Director of the Service in Uganda, he joined the Wellcome Laboratories of Tropical Medicine in London, becoming Head of Research in 1958 and Assistant Research Director from 1967–70.[35] His memoirs are a rich source; they provide his reasons for joining the Service, the premium put upon locally-gained experiences, the articulation of the differences of African life, and the genuine attachment that he formed with both

East Africa as a place and the tropical medical interests that presented themselves. In short, he embodied many aspects of the colonial personality for which this study has argued. His words speak for himself, but also could speak for many others, for they encapsulate, as does his career, some aspects of the very essence of *being* a Colonial MO.

> About ten weeks later [after appointment] I landed at Mombasa and underwent a kind of enchantment. I suppose my early addiction to the works of Ballantyne, Henty, Marryat and the like was a predisposing factor. My imagination had taken me to places like those I was now seeing, and I was ready to be captivated by reality. Landscape, vegetation, people, animals, light, sound, smells—all the ingredients of the scene combined to produce a powerful impact and what turned out to be a lasting attachment.[36]

Even though, physically, groups of officers were often posted far apart from each other '[p]aradoxically the bush which separated them was the very thing that held them together'.[37] More than the employment opportunities, the scientific advantages, or the promise of a sundowner on the verandah after a day on medical safari, the Colonial Medical Service provided scope for doing medicine in the service of Empire.

Appendix 1

Heads of the Medical Departments

NB: Between 1903–08 the medical departments of Kenya and Uganda were run together under the directorship of one Principal Medical Officer: first, Robert Moffat, who had previously been in charge of Uganda Medical Department, and second, James Will who for a short period at the end of his joint directorship led the Kenya Medical Department.

Kenya:

July 1895–1903	Walter Halliburton Macdonald [IBEAC since 1892] (*b*.1859–*d*.1916)
April 1903–04	Robert Unwin Moffat [IBEAC since 1891] (*b*.1866–*d*.1947)
February 1904–09	James Will (*b*.18?–*d*.19?)
February 1909–21	Arthur Dawson Milne (*b*.1867–*d*.1932)
February 1921–33	John Langton Gilks (*b*.1880–*d*.1971)
November 1933–41	Albert Rutherford Paterson (*b*.1885–*d*.1959)

Uganda:

January 1898–1904	Robert Unwin Moffat (*b*.1866–*d*.1947)
February 1904–08	James Will (*b*.18?–*d*.19?)
September 1908–19	Aubrey Dallas Percival Hodges (*b*.1861–*d*.1946)
February 1919–22	Clare Aveling Wiggins (*b*.1876–*d*.1965)
August 1922–23	John Hope Reford *Acting* PMO
July 1923–28	John Hope Reford (*b*.1873–*d*.1957)
January 1928–33	Gerald Joseph Keane (*b*.1880–*d*.1943)
March 1933–41	William Henry Kauntze (*b*.1887–*d*.1947)

Tanzania:

1917–19	Arthur Horn (*b*.1871–*d*.1943)
October 1919–24	John Bernard Davey (*b*.1875–*d*.1967)
December 1924–32	John Owen Shircore (*b*.1882–*d*.1953)
January 1932–35	Albert Harold Owen (*b*.1880–*d*.1936)
March 1935–45	Ralph Roylance Scott (*b*.1893–*d*.1978)

Appendix 2

Service Dates of MOs Kenya, Uganda & Tanzania: 1893–1939

[NB: service dates spent in other colonial territories are not listed.]

Adams jnr., Frederick Vasey: Tanzania (1928–36)
Adams, Ernest Beadon: Kenya (1903–06)
Aitken, William John: Tanzania (1926–?)
Allen, George Vance: Kenya (1921–27)
Anderson, Theodore Farnworth: Kenya (1928–45; 1949–57)
Ansorge, William John: Uganda (1895–98)
Archibald, Robert George: Uganda (1906–08)
Armstrong, James Septimus: Tanzania (1925–36)
Auden, Francis Thomas: Kenya (1919–22)
Austin, Thomas Aitken: Tanzania (1939–43)
Bagshawe, Arthur William Garrard: Uganda (1900–08)
Baker, Clement John: Uganda (1903–22)
Baker, Henry Hugh: Kenya (1908–09)
Balfe, Basil George Hamilton: Tanzania (1939–?)
Barnetson, William: Uganda (1936–62)
Barrett, Raymond Edward: Uganda (1928–55)
Bartlett, James Henry: Kenya (1937–53)
Bateman, George Stanley: Uganda (1913–37)
Bateman, George William Barthrop: Uganda (1937–50)
Bateman, Herbert Raymond: Uganda (1908–10)
Battson, Alfred Ansell: Kenya (1926–1929); Uganda (1929–?)
Bayon, Enrico Pietro Giorgio: Uganda (1907–10)
Bell, David: Kenya (1926–49)
Bell, Fairfax: Tanzania (1935–60)
Bell, Philip Shaw: Tanzania (1926–38)
Beven, John Osmonde: Kenya (1921–27)
Black, John Jamieson: Uganda (1930–?)
Blackwood, Archibald McAllister: Tanzania (1919–39)
Blomfield, Douglas Miles: Kenya (1936–?)
Boase, Arthur Joseph: Uganda (1924–58)
Bödeker, Henry Albert: Uganda (1899–02); Kenya (1902–13, 1914–18 & 1920)
Boon, Alfred Henry: Kenya (1919–20)
Bowden, James William: Kenya (1929–31)
Bowles, Roger Vincent: Uganda (1928–33)
Braimbridge, Clifford Viney: Kenya (1920–56)
Branch, Stanley: Uganda (1900–03)
Breeks, Charles Wilkinson: Tanzania (1921–22)
Brennan, Charles Henry : Kenya (1921–36)
Briscoe, Ralph Cay: Kenya (1920–36)
Broadbent, Marcus Stanley Reuss: Kenya (1929–32)

Brooks, John Edward: Uganda (1921–24)
Brown, Arthur Forbes: Uganda (1928–50)
Brown, John Scott: Uganda (1929–?)
Buchanan, John Cecil Rankin: Tanzania (1925–28, 1931–36); Uganda (1943–45)
Bullen, Walter Alexander: Kenya (1926–?)
Burfield, George Alfred: Tanzania (1939–?)
Burges, Cyril Philips: Uganda (1924–25)
Burke-Gaffney, Henry Joseph O'Donnell: Tanzania (1925–46)
Burton, Edward: Uganda (1930–?)
Bury, Raymond: Tanzania (1930–33)
Butler, George Guy: Tanzania (1920–25)
Caddick, Charles John: Kenya (1922–31)
Caldwell, John Colin: Uganda (1921–31)
Caldwell, John McCormick: Uganda (1939–55)
Callanan, John Charles Joseph: Kenya (1921–46)
Calwell, Hugh Gault: Tanzania (1930–48)
Campbell, John McPhail: Kenya (1923–30); Tanzania (1930–38)
Carman, John Ambrose: Kenya (1926–51)
Carothers, John Colin Dixon: Kenya (1929–50)
Carpenter, Geoffrey Douglas Hale: Uganda (1910–30)
Chapman, Wallace Milne: Kenya (1937–39)
Chataway, James Harold Herbert: Kenya (1926–?)
Chell, George Russell Haines: Kenya (1908–23); Uganda (1923–33)
Cherrett, Bertham Walter: Kenya (1910–18)
Chevallier, Claude Lionel: Kenya (1901–23)
Chilton, Noel: Tanzania (1929–?)
Cimino, Hugo Gerard: Uganda (1921–23)
Clanchy, Arthur Daniel: Uganda (1913 only)
Clark, Ernest Malcolm: Kenya (1937–61)
Clark, James McKillican: Kenya (1916–18); Tanzania (1918–27)
Clarke, Madeleine Harvey: Tanzania (1927–32)
Clearkin, Peter Alphonus: Kenya (1916–25); Tanzania (1925–32)
Clemmey, Albert Victor: Tanzania (1928–?)
Cobb, Geoffrey Francis: Kenya (1938 only)
Cobbe, Thomas Jacob: Uganda (1910–12)
Cochrane, Thomas Saville: Kenya (1926–27)
Coghlan, Bernard Augustine: Tanzania (1926–?)
Cole, Arthur Claud Ely: Tanzania (1938–60)
Cole, Harry Arnold: Kenya (1926–30)
Collar, Frank: Kenya (1913–15)
Collyns, John Moore: Uganda (1906–27)
Connell, William Kerr: Tanzania (1924–46)
Connolly, Patrick Paul Daly: Kenya (1926–46)
Cook, Ernest Neville: Uganda (1926–36)
Cooke, Eric Robert Nathaniel: Kenya (1939–51)
Cormack, Robert Pairman: Uganda (1926–28); Kenya (1928–45)
Corson, James Frederick: Tanzania (1925–39)

Cowen, Charles Edmund: Kenya (1930–36)

Cowin, Philip John: Uganda (1930–?)

Crawford, Robert Phillips: Tanzania (1919–20)

Crichton, Arthur John Moncrieffe: Tanzania (1920–22)

Cronyn, Hugh Desmond: Kenya (1931 only)

Cumming, Patrick Grant: Kenya (1926 only)

Dakers, Bernard William: Kenya (1920–25)

Davey, John Bernard: Tanzania (1919–24, 1941–43)

Davies, Cyril Sims: Kenya (1929–32)

Davies, Henry Norman: Tanzania (1926–58)

Davies, John Rodyn: Kenya (1925–38)

Davison, Eric Alan: Kenya (1921–24)

De Boer, Henry Speldewinde: Kenya (1920–31); Uganda (1933–38, 1942–47)

De Smidt, Frank Philip Gilbert: Kenya (1926–36)

Dennard, Leslie David: Uganda (1924–37)

Densham, Walter Arnold: Uganda (1905–07)

Dickson, Robert Francis Goldrick: Kenya (1928–33)

Doble, Francis Carminow: Uganda (1913–17)

Dodds, Horatius Bonar: Kenya (1903–05)

Donald, David: Kenya (1899–00)

Donnison, Cyril Percy: Kenya (1925–28)

Dowdeswell, Roland Melville: Kenya (1930–50)

Drake-Brockman, Ralph Evelyn: Uganda (1900–02); Kenya (1902–04)

Drury, Graham Dru: Kenya (1929–46)

Duke, Herbert Lyndhurst: Uganda (1910–36)

Dunderdale, Geoffrey: Kenya (1913–16)

Dunlop, Ronald Yorston: Uganda (1935–46)

Dye, William Hood: Tanzania (1925–34); Uganda (1934–?)

Earl, John Cecil St George: Uganda (1923–43)

Eccles Davies, Sidney Richard: Uganda (1920–23)

Edmond, John James Balmanno: Tanzania (1922–33)

Edmundson, Kenneth: Tanzania (1928–53)

Edwards, Charles Stanstay: Kenya (1911 only)

Enzer, John: Kenya (1925–?)

Esler, Alexander Rentoul: Kenya (1924–38)

Fairbairn, Harold: Tanzania (1925–51)

Fisher, Harold Mayston: Tanzania (1919–46)

Fisher, Richard William Middleton: Kenya (1906–07)

Fisher, Vicars Maddison: Kenya (1919–33)

Fitzpatrick, Owen: Tanzania (1923–26)

Fleming, Alan McKinstry: Uganda (1929–33)

Floyd, Henry Gilbert: Uganda (1931–?)

Foley, Edwin John: Tanzania (1937–?)

Follitt, Harold Harold Baily: Tanzania (1928–31)

Forbes, John: Kenya (1921–37)

Forrest, Stanley: Uganda (1925–39); Tanzania (1939–?)

Forster, Arthur Frost: Kenya (1907–10)

Fraser, Alexander Donald: Uganda (1908–11)
Freeman, Frank Percy: Uganda (1924–30)
Freeth, Arthur Causton: Uganda (1924–30)
Gallagher, Gerald Hugh: Tanzania (1920–21)
Garde, Alfred Jervoise: Uganda (1931–35)
Garnett, Donald Goddard: Uganda (1924–27)
Garnham, Percy Cyril Claude: Kenya (1925–47)
Gibbon, Geoffrey McKay: Uganda (1938–?)
Gilkes, Humphrey Arthur: Uganda (1939–?)
Gilks, John Langton: Kenya (1909–33)
Goldie, Walter Leigh Mackinnon: Kenya (1905–08)
Goodliffe, John Henry: Uganda (1905–21)
Gordon, Henry Laing: Kenya (1931–37)
Graham, John Wallace: Tanzania (1925–35)
Gray, Arthur Claypon Horner: Uganda (1904–09)
Gray, John Macfarlane: Uganda (1925–33)
Grieve, Ian Martin Donaldson: Kenya (1929–31)
Griffin, Robert George: Uganda (1921–30)
Guinness, Ernest Whitmore Newton: Kenya (1920–22)
Hailstone, John Edward: Uganda (1909–29)
Hale, George Samuel: Kenya (1926–51)
Hamilton, Henry Fleming: Kenya (1918–19)
Hamilton, Robert: Kenya (1911–14)
Haran, James Augustine: Kenya (1898–20)
Hargreaves, George McNeill: Kenya (1928–34)
Harkness, John: Tanzania (1927–?)
Harley-Mason, Robert John: Kenya (1921–48)
Harris, Brian Poulett: Kenya (1936–?)
Hartley, Evelyn Francis: Kenya (1938–?)
Haworth, Wallace Ellwood: Tanzania (1920–24)
Haynes, William Secretan: Kenya (1937–?)
Heard, William Haughton: Kenya (1912–18)
Heisch, Ronald Brodie: Kenya (1939–64)
Helme, Arthur Crofts de Beetham: Tanzania (1935–38)
Henderson, Frederick Louis: Kenya (1904–37)
Hennessey, Robert Samuel Fleming: Uganda (1929–44, 1949–55)
Herridge, Margaret Alex Lindsay: Kenya (1930–37)
Hinde, Sidney Langford: Kenya (1895–15)
Hodges, Aubrey Dallas Percival: Uganda (1898–19)
Holliday, Margaret: Uganda (1926–33)
Holmes, Gerald: Uganda (1930–?)
Horn, Arthur: Tanzania (1917–19)
Horowitz, Eric Mark: Kenya (1935–38)
Howat, Clarence Hugh: Tanzania (1931 only)
Howell, Alan Taylor: Kenya (1926–47)
Hunter, James Kellock: Uganda (1938–58)
Hunter, Ronald Nelson: Kenya (1921–34)

Hutchinson, William John: Kenya (1926–29)
Hutton, Philip William: Uganda (1937–61)
Hyder, Ronald Ingham: Uganda (1930 only)
Ievers, Charles Langley: Tanzania (1918–32)
Irwin, Henry Francis George: Kenya (1935–38)
James, William Robert Wallace: Kenya (1906–07); Uganda (1908–10)
Jarvis, John Fulford: Tanzania (1936–?)
Jewell, Norman Parsons: Kenya (1914–32)
Jobson, Eric William Charles: Kenya (1924–39); Tanzania (1939–?)
Johnson, John Taylor Connell: Kenya (1898–1912)
Johnstone, Frederick John Carlyle: Kenya (1921–44)
Kanulse, WH: Kenya (1920 only)
Kauntze, William Henry: Kenya (1916–33); Uganda (1933–41)
Keane, Gerald Joseph: Uganda (1908–32)
Keigwin, George John Williams: Tanzania (1917–18)
Kelly, William Patrick: Uganda (1921–24)
Kerr, Walter Gifford: Kenya (1938–?)
Kingdon, Alfred Thomas Lock: Uganda (1923–26)
Laird, William John: Kenya (1928–29)
Lamborn, William Alfred Stedwell: Tanzania (1917–18)
Lamont, Margaret Marion Traill: Uganda (1922–23)
Lanceley, James Leslie: Uganda (1938–61)
Lane, George: Uganda (1904–21)
Langan, Thomas: Tanzania (1925–31)
Langton, Edward Athol Clarence: Tanzania (1919–21); Uganda (1921–37)
Latham, Donald Victor: Tanzania (1925–46)
Lawlor, Mary Kathleen: Uganda (1926–29)
Lawson, Thomas Labatt: Uganda (1939 only)
Lee, Sydney William Timpson: Uganda (1922–34)
Lester, Alexander Reginald: Tanzania (1924–34); Uganda (1934–?)
Leys, Norman Maclean: Kenya (1904–13)
Lindsey, Eric Craigie: Kenya (1906–09)
Liston, James Malcolm: Kenya (1935–47)
Lockhart, Frederick Ramsdale: Tanzania (1924–39); Kenya (1939–?)
Loewenthal, Leonard Joseph Alphonse: Uganda (1931–?)
Louw, Graham: Uganda (1925–?)
Lowsley, Lionel Dewe: Uganda (1902–12); Kenya (1912–16)
Lumb, Thomas Fletcher: Kenya (1909–23)
Lumsden, Kenneth: Uganda (1925–28)
Lutze-Wallace, Cyril Randolph: Tanzania (1918–26); Uganda (1926–38)
Macdonald, James Stirling: Tanzania (1921–23)
Macdonald, Walter Halli Burton: Kenya (1895–1908)
Macgregor, George Alistair: Tanzania (1938–52)
Mackay, Arthur George: Uganda (1930–39); Tanzania (1939–?)
Mackay, Roderick: Tanzania (1925–44)
Mackie, Alfred Scott: Kenya (1919–29); Tanzania (1929–33)
Mackinnon, Archibald Donald: Uganda (1894–97)

Mackinnon, John McPhail: Kenya (1913–16)

Maclean, Alan Hector: Uganda (1925–?)

Maclean, George: Tanzania (1921–42)

Maclennan, Norman Macpherson: Kenya (1927–30; 1945–?)

Macleod, Nicol Campbell: Uganda (1924–39)

Macmillan, Hector Alasdair: Kenya (1929–32)

Macmillan, Robert James Alan: Uganda (1913–32)

Macpherson, James Simpson: Uganda (1894–02)

Macqueen, Malcolm Donaldson: Uganda (1926–32)

Madge, John Bristo Culley: Tanzania (1928–32)

Mann, Harold Edward: Kenya (1895–1904)

Manson-Bahr, Philip Edmund Clinton: Tanzania (1939–40, 1946–48); Kenya (1953–62)

Marshall, Claude Herbert: Uganda (1908–34)

Martin, Kenneth Allan Thomas: Kenya (1925–49)

Massey, Thomas Hunter: Kenya (1913–34)

Maxwell, Edward Christopher Wood: Kenya (1930–32)

McConnell, Robert Ernest: Uganda (1910–23)

McDaniel, James: Uganda (1929–32)

McDonald, James Hector: Tanzania (1926–?)

McElroy, Robert Samuel: Uganda (1924–38); Tanzania (1938–47); Kenya (1947–?)

McFiggans, Robert: Kenya (1926–53)

McKenzie, Alan: Tanzania (1925–?)

McLean, Neil: Kenya (1926–47)

McNaughton, James Garvie: Tanzania (1920–27)

McQuillan, Cecil James: Tanzania (1927–?)

Meade-King, William Thomas Pearse: Uganda (1913–14)

Meek, Andrew Inglis: Tanzania (1922–38)

Michael-Shaw, Mary: Kenya (1928–34)

Middleton, Ian Cameron: Tanzania (1929–40)

Miller, Frederick Richard Lanfear: Kenya (1924–31)

Milne, Arthur Dawson: Uganda (1898–1903); Kenya (1904–21)

Milne, Hugh Campbell de Burgh: Kenya (1938–?)

Milne, Peter: Kenya (1923–34)

Mitchell, Andrew Henry: Kenya (1922 only)

Mitchell, James John: Uganda (1927–?)

Mitchell, John Phimister: Uganda (1924–45)

Moffat, Robert Unwin: Uganda (1892–1906); Kenya/Uganda (1903–06)

Morley, Arthur Harold: Tanzania (1938–50)

Morrough, Alexander MacCarthy: Uganda (1900–02; 1905–07)

Mostert, Henrik van Reenen: Tanzania (1926–c.29)

Mouat, Alexander: Kenya (1909–15)

Mowat, Allan Henry: Uganda (1931–?)

Murcott, Evangel Howard: Kenya (1939–53)

Murphy, Michael Francis: Kenya (1920 only)

Murray, Douglas: Uganda (1930–39)

Murray, Gerard John: Uganda (1937–39)

Neill, James Hood: Kenya (1919–20); Uganda (1920–28); Kenya (1928–36)

Neilson, Harry Ross: Uganda (1912–34)

Newton, Alexander Stafford: Tanzania (1925–35)

Nixon, Robert: Tanzania (1921–?)

Noble, George Strachan Park: Tanzania (1925–?)

Noble, Herbert Arthur Edward: Uganda (1903–04)

Nolan, Thomas Henry: Uganda (1924–?)

Nunan, Patrick Francis: Kenya (1913–23); Tanzania (1923–25); Kenya (1925–35)

O'Connell, John Mary: Kenya (1918 only)

Owen Pritchard, William: Kenya (1903–20); Tanzania (1920–23)

Owen, Albert Harold: Uganda (1912–22); Tanzania (1922–35)

Owen, Hugh Brindley: Uganda (1908–33)

Paget, Alfred James Merrick: Uganda (1899–1900) Kenya, (1900–04)

Parry, James Hales: Tanzania (1919–39)

Paterson, Albert Rutherford: Kenya (1920–41)

Paterson, William Lyle: Kenya (1928–30)

Peacock, Norman Bligh: Kenya (1920–22); Uganda (1923–32)

Peacock, William Luddington: Uganda (1915–32)

Peake, Howard Livingstone: Kenya (1937–c.39)

Pelly, Huntley Nevins: Uganda (1921–24)

Philip, Charles Robert: Kenya (1925–51, 1952–54)

Philips, Claude Hollingworth: Tanzania (1920–?)

Philp, Horace Robert Andrew: Kenya (1921–22)

Pirie, James Hunter Harvey: Kenya (1913–18)

Plum, Denis: Tanzania (1926–1929); Uganda (1929–33); Kenya (1933–?)

Pooley, George Henry: Uganda (1901–04)

Pope, George William: Kenya (1920–24)

Powell, George Maurice Caleb: Tanzania (1938–?)

Pownall, Graham Steinmetz: Uganda (c.1901–c.03)

Preston, Philip Geoffrey: Kenya (1929–?)

Price, Raymond Herbert: Kenya (1906 only)

Procter, Robert Arthur Welsford: Kenya (1921–39)

Pugh, John: Kenya (1910–1924); Tanzania (1924–30)

Quin, Joseph Archibald: Uganda (1920–21)

Radford, William John: Kenya (1898–20)

Rainsford, Cecil Ross Carthy: Uganda (1930–42)

Rawson, Philip Hugh: Uganda (1921–25)

Reford, John Hope: Uganda (1907–28)

Reid, Charles Barrington Balfour: Tanzania (1919–28); Kenya (1928–38)

Rendle, Anstruther Cardew: Uganda (1906–18); Kenya (1919–21); Uganda (1921–24)

Reynolds, John David: Uganda (1924–47)

Ridgway, Joseph Chamney Atkinson: Uganda (1912–13)

Rigby, Edward Pim: Kenya (1939–62)

Roberts, Clifford Ellis: Uganda (1927–39)

Roberts, Maiben Albert William: Kenya (1929–42)

Robertson, Alexander: Kenya (1907–14)

Robertson, James Dick: Kenya (1930–34)
Robertson, Muriel: Uganda (1911–14)
Ross, Gilbert Matheson: Kenya (1924–26)
Ross, John Alexander: Kenya (1921–28)
Ross, Percival: Kenya (1926–?)
Ross, Philip Hedgeland: Uganda (1903–06); Kenya (1906–20)
Russell, Edmund Neptune: Kenya (1913–15)
Sanderson, Iain: Tanzania (1925–38)
Scott, Douglas Somerville: Tanzania (1918–24); Kenya (1926–31)
Scott, Ralph Roylance: Tanzania (1919–45)
Searle, Charles Frederick: Kenya (1939–?)
Sells, Lionel: Uganda (1907–19)
Semple, John Mervyn: Tanzania (1922–24); Uganda (1934–?)
Sharp, Leonard Ernest Steigenberger: Uganda (1922–24); Uganda (1927–29)
Shelley, Horace Minton: Tanzania (1939–47)
Shelton, Charles Frank: Tanzania (1921–39); Uganda (1939–?)
Shircore, John Owen: Uganda (1908); Kenya (1913–19); Tanzania (1919-32)
Simpson, Francis Odell: Uganda (1919–23)
Skan, Douglas Alkins: Tanzania (1926–39)
Skelton, Dudley Sheridan: Tanzania (1920–22)
Sloan, Gerrard Andrew: Uganda (1925–30)
Sly, Edwin: Uganda (1901–03)
Small, Francis Victor: Uganda (1924–30)
Small, Robert: Kenya (1906–18)
Smith, William Harden: Tanzania (1935–39); Kenya (1939–?)
Snell, Douglas Goddard: Uganda (1936–62)
Spearman, Barugh: Uganda (1912–20)
Speirs, Robert Charles: Tanzania (1925–?)
Spence, Reginald Westmore: Kenya (1913–18)
Spicer, John Robert Colquhoun: Uganda (1930–?)
Steel, Cecil Richard: Tanzania (1925–34)
Stone, Philip Hartley: Kenya (1937–?)
Stones, Robert Yelverton: Tanzania (1921–22)
Stoney, Ralph: Uganda (1899–1905)
Stott, Hugh: Kenya (1939–?)
Strathairn, George Cecil: Uganda (1903–20)
Suffern, Thomas Henry: Tanzania (1917–31)
Swarbreck, Allan Beaumont: Kenya (1929–31)
Talwrn-Jones, Gwilym Ambrose: Uganda (1930–32)
Tatchell, Philip Hemsley: Tanzania (1937–?)
Taylor, John Archibald: Uganda (1908–23)
Taylor, Robert Stanley: Uganda (1914–22)
Theis, Stanley Edward: Tanzania (1927–?)
Thomas, James Douglas Sanby: Kenya (1928–31)
Thomson, Alexander Gray: Kenya (1925–35)
Thomson, James Hutcheon: Kenya (1913–23); Tanzania (1923–28)
Tibbles, Joseph Russell: Kenya (1926–28)

Tichborne, Charles Roger Hobart: Tanzania (1918–28)
Tilling, Harold William: Kenya (c.1931–?)
Timms, Charles Gordon: Uganda (1922 only)
Timms, Geoffrey Lowe: Kenya (1936–60)
Tonking, Harold Denis: Kenya (1927–36)
Tothill, Walter Vincent: Tanzania (1920–22)
Treliving, Joyce Mary: Kenya (1934–35)
Trim, Edwin Alfred: Kenya (1927–59)
Trowell, Hubert Carey: Kenya (1929–35); Uganda (1935–60)
Tudhope, William: Kenya (1913–16)
Tulloch, Forbes Manson Grant: Uganda (1904–06)
Turner, Hugh Nelson: Kenya (1929–?)
Turton, Mary: Uganda (1921–36)
Twining, Cicely Norah: Kenya (1928–31)
Twining, Helen Mary: Uganda (1929–32)
Uffmann, Karl Herman Henry: Kenya (1905–07); Uganda (1907–08)
Van Derwert, James Alexander Henry: Tanzania (1920–23)
Van Someren, Robert Abraham Logan: Uganda (1905–25)
Van Someren, Victor Gurner Logan: Kenya (1912–22)
Vassallo, Salvator Michael: Uganda (1919–25)
Vint, Francis William: Kenya (1927–?)
Walker, Gerald: Kenya (1919–22)
Walker, John Walker: Tanzania (1929–?)
Walker, Sydney Robert: Uganda (1898–04); Kenya (1904–06)
Wallace, James Montague: Uganda (1929–34)
Wallington, Kenneth Tratman King: Kenya (1921–32); Uganda (1932–34)
Waters, Edward John Wynstone: Uganda (1900–02); Kenya (1902–c.07)
Watkins-Pitchford, Henry Otley: Kenya (1935–?)
Webb, William Leslie: Uganda (1913–33)
Welch, Harvey Henry Vincent: Kenya (1913–25)
Welch, Thomas Burges: Kenya (1920 only)
Wetherell, Marmaduke Cordeux: Kenya (1920–21)
White, Walter Croker Poole: Kenya (1906–10)
Wiggins, Clare Aveling: Kenya (1901–09); Uganda (1909–23)
Wilcocks, Charles: Tanzania (1927–37)
Wilkin, Bertram Osbourne: Tanzania (1925–54)
Wilkins, Arthur James Walker: Kenya (1928–31)
Wilkinson, Wallace: Kenya (1925–?)
Will, James: Kenya/Uganda (1904–09)
Willans, Norman Jeune: Uganda (1928–?)
Williams, Arthur Donald John Bedward: Kenya (1912–33)
Williams, Arthur Warriner: Uganda (1931–61)
Williams, Gwilym Ambrose: Tanzania (1921–32)
Williams, Neville Scott: Uganda (1914–26)
Williamson, John: Tanzania (1925–?)
Willmott, Leslie Arthur: Tanzania (1925–33)
Wilson, Christopher James: Kenya (1911–28)

Wilson, Donald Bagster: Tanzania (1929–60)
Wilson, Douglas Edward: Tanzania (1928–42)
Wilson, George Alexander: Tanzania (1933–?)
Wilson, Gerald Richard Courtenay: Tanzania (1919–39)
Wilson, William Arthur: Uganda (1931–?)
Wiltshire, Henry Goodwill: Uganda (1936–?)
Wiseman, Robert Howitt: Kenya (1934–?)
Wright, Frederick James: Kenya (1936–53)
Young, George Campbell: Kenya (1930 only)
Young, William Arthur: Tanzania (1936–?)

NB Moffat and Will were both serving Kenya and Uganda *simultaneously* during their periods as PMO of both medical departments.

Appendix 3

Obituary and Biographical Entry Index

Allen, GV, *BMJ*, iv, 1970, p.183
Allen, GV, *The Times*, 14 July 1970, p.10
Archibald, RG, *BMJ*, i, 1953, pp.1112–3; p.1169; p.1337
Archibald, RG, *The Times*, 5 May 1953, p.8, 7 May p.10 & 12 May p.8
Armstrong, JS, *EAMJ*, 13, 1936–37, pp.58–9
Armstrong, JS, *Tanganyika Territory Government Gazette*, 17 April 1936, p.203
Bagshawe, AWG, *Lancet*, i, 1950, pp.693–4
Baker, CJ, *Lancet*, ii, 1922, p.1251
Baker, CJ, *BMJ*, ii, 1922, p.491
Baker, CJ, *Uganda Protectorate Government Gazette*, 31 August 1922
Bartlett, JH, *EAMJ*, 30, 1953, p.493
Bateman, HR, Robert Drew, *Commissioned Officers in the Medical Services of the British Army: 1660–1960*, London, The Wellcome Historical Medical Library, 1968, p.28
Bateman, HR, *BMJ*, i, 1961, pp.1324–5
Bayon, HPG, *BMJ*, ii, 1952, pp.1260–1
Bell, D, *BMJ*, i, 1967, p.573
Bell, F, *BMJ*, i, 1972, p.450
Bödeker, HA, *EAMJ*, 17, 1940–41, pp.171–2
Braimbridge, CV, *Lancet*, i, 1964, p.279
Braimbridge, CV, *EAMJ*, 41, 1964, p.31
Brooks, JE, Robert Drew, *Commissioned Officers in the Medical Services of the British Army: 1660–1960*, London, The Wellcome Historical Medical Library, 1968, p.148
Buchanan, J, *BMJ*, 2, 1976, p.841
Burke Gaffney, HJ O'D, *BMJ*, i, 1973, p.360
Burke Gaffney, HJ O'D, *Lancet*, i, 1973, p.273
Burke Gaffney, *The Times*, 6 February 1973, p.16
Burkitt, RW, *EAMJ*, 24, 1947, p.105
Bury, R, *Tanganyika Territory Government Gazette*, 6 October 1933, p.605
Caldwell, JM, *BMJ*, 2, 1955, p.1147
Carman, JA, *BMJ*, 308, 1994, p.1234
Carothers, JCD, *BMJ*, 300, 1990, p.1010
Carpenter, GDH, *Lancet*, i, 1953, pp.300–1
Carpenter, GDH, *BMJ*, i, 1953, pp.406–7
Carpenter, GDH, *The Times*, 31 January 1953, p.8
Cherrett, BW, *East Africa Protectorate Official Gazette*, 6 November 1918, p.953
Clarke, JB, *EAMJ*, 31, 1954, p.75
Clearkin, PA, *BMJ*, ii, 1971, p.53
Cole, ACE, *BMJ*, 299, 1989, p.1519
Connell, WK, *BMJ*, ii, 1952, pp.1263–4
Connell, WK, *EAMJ*, 30, 1953, p.44
Cook, AR, *Lancet*, i, 1951, pp.1021–2

Cook, AR, *EAMJ,* 11, 1934–35, p.1

Cook, EN, *BMJ,* ii, 1959, pp.1049–50

Cormack, RP, *EAMJ,* 31, 1954, p.186

Corson, JF, *Lancet,* ii, 1963, p.1073

Corson, JF, *BMJ,* ii, 1963, p.1343

Davey, JB, *BMJ,* iii, 1967, p.743

De Boer, HS, *BMJ,* i, 1957, pp.1533–4

Densham, WA, *East Africa & Uganda Protectorate Government Gazette,* 1 July 1907, p.232

Donnison, CP, *BMJ,* i, 1958, p.463

Dowdeswell, RM, *BMJ,* ii, 1956, p.305

Edmond, JJB, *Tanganyika Territory Government Gazette,* 7 July 1933, p.405

Evans, A.M., *EAMJ,* 14, 1937–38, pp.209–10

Fleming, AM, *EAMJ,* 28, 1951, p.473

Furse, R, *The Times,* 5 October 1973, p.21

Garde, AJ, *Uganda Protectorate Government Gazette,* 31 October 1935, p.386

Garnham, PCC, *Who's Who,* 1994–95, p.548

Gilks, JL, *BMJ,* iii, 1971, p.538

Gilks, JL, *The Times,* 21 August 1971, p.12

Goodliffe, JH, *Uganda Protectorate Government Gazette,* 15 December 1922

Gordon, HL, *EAMJ,* 24, 1947, pp.313–14

Graham, JW, *Tanganyika Territory Government Gazette,* 2 August 1935, p.431

Gray, ACH, Robert Drew, *Commissioned Officers in the Medical Services of the British Army: 1660–1960,* London, The Wellcome Historical Medical Library, 1968, p.44

Gray, ACH, *BMJ,* i, 1963, p.1483

Gray, ACH, *The Times,* 30 April 1963, p.16

Harley-Mason, RJ, *EAMJ,* 54, 1977, p.513

Heard, WH, *East Africa Protectorate Government Gazette,* 27 November 1918, p.1014

Heisch, RB, *BMJ,* iii, 1969, p.722

Hennessey, RSF, *BMJ,* 299, 1989, pp.176–7

Hodges, ADP, *BMJ,* i, 1946, p.933

Hodges, ADP, *EAMJ,* 23, 1946, pp.289–90

Horowitz, EM, *BMJ,* 308, 1994, p.130

Hunter, JK, *BMJ,* 309, 1994, p.870

Ievers, CL, *BMJ,* ii, 1965, pp.948–9

Johnstone, FC, *EAMJ,* 25, 1948, pp.18–19

Kauntze, WH, Richard R. Trail (ed.), *Munk's Roll,* 1968, pp.222–3

Kauntze, WH, *BMJ,* ii, 1947, pp.797–8

Kauntze, WH, *Lancet,* ii, 1947, p.741

Kauntze, WH, *EAMJ,* 24, 1947, p.425

Keane, GJ, Robert Drew, *Commissioned Officers in the Medical Services of the British Army: 1660–1960,* London, The Wellcome Historical Medical Library, 1968, p.85

Lamborn, WAS, *BMJ,* ii, 1959, pp.310–11

Langton, EAC, *EAMJ,* 14, 1937–8, pp.138–9

Langton, EAC, *Uganda Protectorate Government Gazette,* 31 May 1937, p.225

Latham, DV, *EAMJ,* 31, 1954, p.33

Low, GC, *BMJ,* ii, 1952, pp.341–2

MacDonald, WH, *East Africa Protectorate Official Gazette*, 1 March 1916, p.154
MacDonald, WH, *BMJ*, i, 1916, p.222
Mackay, R, *BMJ*, ii, 1966, p.1145
Mackie, AS, *BMJ*, ii, 1959, p.1262
Manson-Bahr, P, *BMJ*, 314, 1997, pp.609–10
Mann, H, *East Africa & Uganda Protectorate Government Gazette*, 1 June 1904, p.189
Marshall, CH, *EAMJ*, 34, 1957, p.280
Massey, TH, *EAMJ*, 11, 1934–35, p.142
McFiggans, R, *EAMJ*, 37, 1960, p.119
McLean, N, *BMJ*, i, 1955, p.917
Michael-Shaw, M, *BMJ*, ii, 1963, p.1343
Milne, AD, *KEAMJ*, 1931–2, pp.359–60
Mitchell, JP, *Lancet*, i, 1962, p.1134
Morley, AH, *BMJ*, 295, 1987, p.220
O'Connell, JM, *East Africa Protectorate Government Gazette*, 23 November 1918, p.974
Owen, AH, *EAMJ*, 11, 1934–35, pp.363–4
Owen, AH, *EAMJ*, 12, 1935–36, p.322
Paterson, AR, *BMJ*, ii, 1959, p.1025; p.1263
Philp, HRA, *BMJ*, i, 1957, p.172
Pugh, J, *BMJ*, i, 1972, p.450
Reford, JH, *The Times*, 15 November 1957, p.13
Reynolds, JD, *EAMJ*, 34, 1957, p.512
Roberts, CE, *BMJ, ii*, 1961, pp.966–7
Robertson, M, *The Times*, 22 June 1973, p.18
Ross, PH, *KEAMJ*, 1929–30, p.149
Shircore, JO, *Lancet*, ii, 1953, p.94
Shircore, JO, *The Times*, 30 June 1953, p.8
Shircore, JO, *EAMJ*, 30, 1953, pp.355–6
Skelton, DS, Robert Drew, *Commissioned Officers in the Medical Services of the British Army: 1660–1960*, London, The Wellcome Historical Medical Library, 1968, pp.38–9
Snell, DG, *BMJ*, 294, 1987, p.1896
Spence, RW, *East Africa Protectorate Government Gazette*, 29 May 1918, p.465
Stones, RY, *BMJ, ii*, 1961, pp.966–7
Stoney, R, *East Africa & Uganda Protectorate Government Gazette*, 15 November 1905, p.373
Tothill, WV, *BMJ*, i, 1958, p.1043
Thomson, JH, *EAMJ*, 5, 1928–29, p.411
Thomson, JH, *Tanganyika Territory Government Gazette*, 30 November 1928, p.738
Trim, EA, *EAMJ*, 46, 1969, p.533
Trowell, HC, *BMJ*, 299, 1989, p.453
Tulloch, FMG, Robert Drew, *Commissioned Officers in the Medical Services of the British Army: 1660–1960*, London, The Wellcome Historical Medical Library, 1968, p.46
Turton, M, *BMJ*, ii, 1958, p.1048
Turton, M, *The Times*, 14 October 1958, p.13
Vassallo, SM, *BMJ*, ii, 1953, p.445

Wiggins, CA, *BMJ*, i, 1966, pp.363–4
Wiggins, CA, *The Times*, 9 July 1965, p.14
Williams, A, *The Times*, September 2005, p.71
Williams, ADJB, *EAMJ*, 15, 1938–39, p.190
Williams, ADJB, *BMJ*, i, 1958, p.1421
Wilcocks, C, *BMJ*, i, 1977, p.847
Wilson, CJ, *BMJ*, i, 1956, p.692
Wilson, CJ, *EAMJ*, 5, 1928–29, p.312 [Presentation dinner speech]
Wilson, CJ, *The Times*, 18 February 1956, p.10
Wilson, DB, *BMJ*, i, 1961, pp.134–5
Wilson, DB, *Lancet*, i, 1961, p.177
Wilson, DB, *EAMJ*, 38, 1961, p.126
Wilson, DE, *EAMJ*, 25, 1948, p.294
Wright, FJ, *BMJ*, 313, 1996, p.556

Notes

Explanatory Notes (pp.xiii-xiv)

[1] A Kirk-Greene, *On Crown Service: A History of HM Colonial and Overseas Civil Services, 1837–1997*, London, 1999, p.38, table 2.8 'Distribution of the Colonial Service in British Tropical Africa, c.1939'

[2] This is the earliest published regional staff list I have found. In the same year, 1914, Somaliland had two and Zanzibar had five Medical Department members. Foreign and Commonwealth Office, *East African Staff List*, London, 1914

[3] C Jeffries, *Partners For Progress: The Men and Women of the Colonial Service*, London, 1949, p.26

[4] That is the only secondary source; there have been several participants' memoirs and histories. A Beck, *A History of the British Medical Administration of East Africa: 1900–1950*, Cambridge, MA, 1999 [1970]

[5] Jeffries, *Partners For Progress*, p.24

Chapter 1: Introduction (pp.1-14)

[1] W Ormsby-Gore, 'Foreword' in C Jeffries, *The Colonial Empire and its Civil Service*, Cambridge, London, 1938, pp.vii–xi, p.x

[2] RHL/MSS.Afr.s.1872/153a AW Williams, 'Detailed Memoranda on Experiences in the Colonial Medical Service in Uganda and Tanganyika, 1931-1949', [n.d. c.1983], p.1

[3] RHL/MSS.Afr.s.1872/9 RE Barrett, 'Memorandum on Experiences in the Colonial Medical Service in East Africa, 1928–55', 1983, p.1

[4] RHL/MSS.Afr.s.1653, TF Anderson, *Reminiscences by T Farnworth Anderson*, Book I, Kenya, 1973, p.14

[5] The medical history of East Africa has been traced elsewhere. See DF Clyde, *History of the Medical Services of Tanganyika*, Dar Es Salaam, 1962; A Beck, *A History of the British Medical Administration of East Africa: 1900–1950*, Cambridge, MA, 1999 [1970]; JA Carman, *A Medical History of the Colony and Protectorate of Kenya: a Personal Memoir*, London, 1976; WD Foster, *The Early History of Scientific Medicine in Uganda*, Nairobi, 1970; O Ransford, *Bid the Sickness Cease: Disease in the History of Black Africa*, London, 1983. There are also numerous detailed studies of specific health initiatives. E.g., J Iliffe, *East African Doctors: a History of the Modern Profession*, Cambridge, 1999; KA Hoppe, *Sleeping Sickness Control in British East Africa, 1900–1960*, Westport, CT, 2003.

[6] Much has been written on the colonial identity, but very little on the specifically medical manifestations. One recent exception is MP Sutphen and B Andrews (eds.), *Medicine and the Colonial Identity*, London, 2003.

[7] The India Office governed British affairs in India (the Indian Civil Service was established in 1858). The Sudanese and Egyptian Services remained governed by the Foreign Office throughout the period (the Sudan Political Service was established in 1899, the Egyptian Civil Service in 1882)

[8] R Hyam, 'The Colonial Office Mind 1900–1914', *Journal of Imperial and Commonwealth History*, 8, 1979, pp.30–55, p.39

[9] T Clark, 'Chalk and Cheese? The Colonial and Diplomatic Services,' in J Smith (ed.), *Administering Empire: The British Colonial Service in Retrospect*, London, 1999, pp.49–59

[10] C Parkinson, *The Colonial Office From Within, 1909–1945*, London, 1947, pp.99–100

[11] C Jeffries, *Partners For Progress: The Men and Women of the Colonial Service*, London, 1949, pp.59–60

[12] For fuller description of colonial government structures see Jeffries, *Colonial Empire*, pp.93–104

[13] Kirk-Greene has identified the first official usage of the label 'Colonial Service' as occurring in 1837. A Kirk-Greene, *On Crown Service: A History of HM Colonial and Overseas Civil Services, 1837–1997*, London, 1999, p.8; Parkinson, *Colonial Office From Within*, p.17

[14] Kirk-Greene, *On Crown Service*, p.11; p.16

[15] HJO'D Burke-Gaffney, 'The History of Medicine in the African Countries', *Medical History*, 12, 1968, pp.31–41, pp.33–4

[16] See H Power, *Tropical Medicine in the Twentieth Century. A History of the Liverpool School of Tropical Medicine*, 1999

[17] 'Instruction in Tropical Diseases,' *BMJ*, i, 1895, p.771

[18] Parkinson, *Colonial Office From Within*, p.25, p.57

[19] Jeffries, *Colonial Empire*, pp.16–17

[20] Cmd.939 *Report of the Departmental Committee Appointed by the Secretary of State for the Colonies to Enquire into the Colonial Medical Services*, London, 1920, p.6

[21] *Ibid.*, pp.3-4

[22] Jeffries, *Colonial Empire*, pp.43–4

[23] Jeffries, *Partners For Progress*, pp.41–58

[24] A Kirk-Greene, *A Biographical Dictionary of the British Colonial Service, 1939–1966*, London, 1991, pp.v–vi

[25] For more on this development of a uniform identity through discipline, see M Foucault, *Discipline and Punish: The Birth of the Prison*, trans. Alan Sheridan. New York, NY, 1977

[26] Arthur Milne named John Smith (arrived 1876 in Mombassa to work in Uganda) as the first British MO in the region. Smith was followed two years later by the (then unqualified— although he later qualified from Edinburgh University), Dr Felkin. AD Milne, 'The Rise of the Colonial Medical Service', *Kenya and East African Medical Journal*, 5, 1928–9, pp.50–8, pp.50–2

[27] Mackinnon was one of the earliest members of the IBEAC (1888–91) but temporarily moved to India, as a civil surgeon (1893–4). He returned to Uganda in 1894 as a MO, once British rule had been formally established there. 'Archibald Mackinnon', *Who Was Who, 1929–1940*, Vol. III, London, 1967 [1941], pp.871–2; Beck, *History of British Medical Administration*, p.8

[28] Ansorge was officially appointed in 1895.

[29] Milne, 'The Rise of the Colonial Medical Service', p.53

[30] JL Gilks, 'The Medical Department and the Health Organization in Kenya, 1909–1933', *East African Medical Journal*, 9, 1932–3, pp.340–54, p.345

[31] KNA/MOH/1/5517 untitled document [History of British Medical Administration in East Africa], [n.d. *c.*.1909]; Milne, 'The Rise of the Colonial Medical Service', p.55; although another source gives this date of amalgamation of railway and government medical services as 1903. KNA/MOH/1/5517 History of British Medical Administration; HA Bödeker, 'Some Sidelights on Early Medical History in East Africa', *East African Medical Journal*, 12, 1935–36, pp.100–7, p.105

[32] A Hicks, 'Forty Years of the British Medical Association (Kenya Branch)', *East African Medical Journal*, 38, 1961, pp.43–53, p.43

[33] Milne, 'The Rise of the Colonial Medical Service', p.56

[34] *Ibid.*, pp.56–7

[35] KNA/MOH/1/5517 History of British Medical Administration

[36] M Worboys, 'Colonial Medicine' in R Cooter and J Pickstone (eds.), *Medicine in the Twentieth Century*, Amsterdam, 2000, pp.67–80, p.70

[37] Beck specifies 1918 as this turning point. Beck, *History of British Medical Administration*, p.200

[38] Worboys, 'Colonial Medicine', p.70

[39] Headrick has argued for the decisive role of technological, industrial and medical innovations in the nineteenth-century European conquest of Africa. DR Headrick, *The Tools of Empire: Technology and European Expansion in the Nineteenth Century*, Oxford, 1981

[40] WD Foster, 'The Mengo Medical School, Uganda' in EE Sabben-Clare, DJ Bradley and K Kirkwood (eds.), *Health in Tropical Africa During the Colonial Period*, Oxford, 1980, pp.172–6, p.172

[41] KNA/MOH/1/5517 History of British Medical Administration

[42] Carman, *Medical History of Kenya*, p.6

[43] For the early development of medical infrastructure in German-ruled Tanganyika see A Beck, 'The Role of Medicine in German East Africa,' *Bulletin for the History of Medicine*, 45, 1971, pp.170–8, p.171; WU Eckart, *Medizin und Kolonialimperialismus, Deutschland, 1884–1945*, München, 1997

[44] Tanganyika Territory, *Annual Medical Report, 1919*, Dar Es Salaam, 1920, p.12 quoted in E Ferguson, *Colonialism, Health and Medicine in Tanganyika, 1885–1961*, Unpublished Research Paper, Dar Es Salaam, 1974, p.21

[45] Clyde, *History of the Medical Services of Tanganyika*, pp.103–4; R Titmuss, B Abel-Smith, G Macdonald, AW Williams, CH Wood, *The Health Services of Tanganyika: A Report to the Government*, London, 1964, p.2

[46] Lord Cranworth, 'The Public School Boy in East Africa', *National Review.*, 336, 1911, pp.992–1000; D Hall, 'Settlers' Problems in Kenya', *Journal of Royal Society of Arts*, 78, 1930, pp.406–23, p.416

[47] Although estimates have varied to as high as 300,000. B Langlands, 'The Sleeping Sickness Epidemic of Uganda, 1900–1920', Paper presented at Makerere University, May 1967 cited in M Lyons, *The Colonial Disease: A Social History of Sleeping Sickness in Northern Zaire, 1900–1940*, Cambridge, 2002 [1992], p.71

[48] Hoppe, *Sleeping Sickness Control in British East Africa*

[49] RHL/MSS.Brit.Emp.r.4, PA Clearkin, *Ramblings and Recollections of a Colonial Doctor 1913–58*, Book II, Durban, 1967, p.165

[50] 'Papers Relating to the Close Union of Kenya, Uganda and the Tanganyika Territory, 1931; Joint Select Committee on Closer Union of East Africa', *Parliamentary Papers*, 7, 1930–1

[51] Jeffries, *Partners For Progress*, p.30

[52] NA/CO/533/662 'East Africa Medical Staff Regulations', 1926-7

[53] KNA/MOH/1/3906 Circular Despatch: 'Administration Decentralisation Scheme', 3 August 1922

[54] KNA/MOH/1/3580 Circular Despatch: to all Heads of Departments, Senior Commissioners and Resident Commissioners, 16 October 1925

[55] NA/CO/737/11 'Memorandum on Native Policy in East Africa', *Special Supplement Tanganyika Territory Government Gazette*, 27 June 1930, pp.1–12 This reiterated the policy declaration originally made by the Duke of Devonshire in a 1923 white paper on East Africa [cmd.1922]

[56] B Berman and J Lonsdale, *Unhappy Valley: Conflict in Kenya and Africa, Book 1: State and Class*, London, 1992, pp.160–1

[57] AA Boahen (ed.), *Africa Under Colonial Domination 1880–1935*, Berkeley, CA, 1990, pp.142–52, p.147

[58] J Iliffe, *A Modern History of Tanganyika*, Cambridge, 1994 [1979], pp.322–5

[59] 'Information as to Colonial Appointments', *Colonial Office List*, London, 1908, pp.443–6, p.443

[60] Lord Passfield, address to the Corona Club, 1930 quoted in Jeffries, *Colonial Empire*, p.68

[61] Exceptional to this is the work of Anthony Kirk-Greene. His works are numerous, but of special significance see: *On Crown Service, Britain's Imperial Administrators, 1858-1966*, London, 2000; *Symbol of Authority*, London, 2005. Before this the only general histories of the Colonial Service were A Bertram, *The Colonial Service*, Cambridge, 1930; Jeffries, *Colonial Empire*. There were a few specific Colonial Service histories including GP West (ed.), *A History of the Overseas Veterinary Services*, London, 1973; DM Anderson and D Killingray (eds.), *Policing the Empire: Government, Authority and Control: 1830-1940*, Manchester, 1991

[62] R Schram, *A History of the Nigerian Health Services*, Ibadan, 1971; C Baker, 'The Government Medical Service in Malawi: an Administrative History, 1891–1974', *Medical History*, 1976, 20,

pp.296–311; A Bayoumi, *The History of the Sudan Health Services*, Nairobi, 1979; H Bell, *Frontiers of Medicine in the Anglo-Egyptian Sudan*, Oxford, 1999

63 DG Crawford, *A History of the Indian Medical Service, 1600-1913*, 1914; DG Crawford, *Roll of the Indian Medical Service, 1615–1930*, London, 1930; M Harrison, *Public Health in British India: Anglo-Indian Preventative Medicine 1859–1914*, Cambridge, 1994; the African medical cohort is briefly mentioned in J Farley, *Bilharzia: A History of Imperial Tropical Medicine*, Cambridge, 2003 [1991], pp.17–29; DM Haynes, *Imperial Medicine: Patrick Manson and the Conquest of Tropical Disease*, Philadelphia, PA, 2001, pp.128–38

64 A Beck, 'Problems of British Medical Administration in East Africa Between 1900–1930,' *Bulletin of the History of Medicine*, 36, 1962, pp.275–83; A Beck, 'Native Medical Services in British East Africa and Native Patterns of Society' in *Verhandlungen des XX Internationalen Kongresses für Geschichte der Medizin*, Hildesheim, 1968, pp.870–5; Beck, *History of British Medical Administration*; Beck, 'The Role of Medicine in German East Africa'; A Beck, 'Medical Administration and Medical Research in Developing Countries: Remarks on their History in Colonial East Africa', *Bulletin of the History of Medicine*, 46, 1972, pp.349–58; A Beck, 'The State and Medical Research. British Government Policy Toward Tropical Medicine in East Africa' in *Proceedings of the XXIII International Congress of the History of Medicine*, Vol. 1, 1974, pp.488–93; A Beck, *Medicine, Tradition and Development in Kenya and Tanzania, 1920–1970*, Waltham, MA, 1981

65 Beck, *History of British Medical Administration*, p.208

66 *Ibid.*, p.206

67 EW Said, *Orientalism: Western Conceptions of the Orient*, Harmondsworth, 1995 [1978]; D Cannadine, *Ornamentalism: How the British Saw Their Empire*, Harmondsworth, 2001. See also EW Said, *Culture and Imperialism*, London, 1993.

68 E Hobsbawn and T Ranger (eds.), *The Invention of Tradition*, Cambridge, 2002 [1983]

69 T Ranger, 'The Invention of Tradition in Colonial Africa' in *Ibid.*, pp.211–62; M Sahlins, 'Goodbye to *Tristes Tropes*: Ethnography in the Context of Modern World History', *The Journal of Modern History*, 65, 1993, pp.1–25

70 See K Tidrick, *Empire and the English Character*, London, 1990; C Hall, *Civilising Subjects: Metropole and Colony in the English Imagination, 1830–1867*, Cambridge, 2002

71 Driver has argued that there still is a romanticised reverence to the 'exotic' and deference to exploration within contemporary culture. F Driver, *Geography Militant: Cultures of Exploration and Empire*, Oxford, 2001, pp.199–219

72 P Brantlinger, 'Victorians and Africans: The Genealogy of the Myth of the Dark Continent', *Critical Inquiry*, 1985, 12, pp.166–203; JM MacKenzie, *Propaganda and Empire: the Manipulation of British Public Opinion, 1880–1960*, Manchester, 1997 [1986]; D Spurr, *The Rhetoric of Empire: Colonial Discourse in Journalism, Travel Writing and Imperial Administration*, Durham, NC, 1993

73 Driver has similarly argued for the status of explorers in the nineteenth century as also being based on a long tradition. Driver, *Geography Militant*, p.9

74 Although, naturally, the growth of field-based expertise, was still reliant upon home institutions for funding, support and validation as well as reliant upon home-based traditions and fashions to extend their popularity.

75 R Hyam, 'The Colonial Office Mind'; R Macleod (ed.), *Government and Expertise: Specialists, Administrators and Professionals 1860–1919*, Cambridge, 1983. To a lesser extent Haynes has done this for imperial medicine. Haynes, *Imperial Medicine*

76 A McKay, *Tibet and the British Raj: The Frontier Cadre, 1904–1947*, Richmond, Surrey, 1997; H Kuklick, *The Imperial Bureaucrat: The Colonial Administrative Service in the Gold Coast, 1920–1939*, Stanford, CA, 1979

77 D Kennedy, *Islands of White: Settler Society and Culture in Kenya and Southern Rhodesia, 1890–1939*, Durham, NC, 1987, p.181; see also his work on the formation of colonial enclaves: D Kennedy, *The Magic Mountains: Hill Stations and the British Raj*, Berkeley, CA, 1996.

[78] Furthermore, Kennedy argues that the success and perpetuation of these ideas partly depended upon the complicity and acceptance of these cultural expressions as either normal or desirable, by both the colonial rulers and the ruled. Kennedy, *Islands of White*, esp. pp.167–92.

[79] *Ibid.*, pp.109–27

[80] *Ibid.*, p.8

[81] Vaughan, *Curing Their Ills*, esp. pp.200–7. Similar issues have also been examined by P Curtin, 'Medical Knowledge and Urban Planning in Tropical Africa' *American Historical Review*, 90, 1985, pp.594-613; W Anderson, 'Immunities of Empire: Race, Disease, and the New Tropical Medicine, 1900-1920' *Bulletin of the History of Medicine*, 70, 1996, pp. 94-118. This idea owes much to M Douglas, *Purity and Danger: an Analysis of Concepts of Pollution*, London, 1966.

[82] Vaughan, *Curing Their Ills*, pp.155–79

[83] W Anderson, *The Cultivation of Whiteness: Science, Health and Racial Destiny in Australia*, New York, NY, 2003

[84] Arnold, *Colonizing the Body*; Bell, *Frontiers of Medicine*; D Gordon, 'A Sword of Empire? Medicine and Colonialism at King William's Town, Xhosaland, 1856–91' in Sutphen and Andrews (eds.), *Medicine and Colonial Identity*, pp.41–60

[85] This idea can be related to ideas expounded by Sahlins over the 'performance' of culture in which we all participate. Sahlins, *Culture in Practice*. Likewise it echoes the disciplined nature of subjects, as expounded by Foucault, *Discipline and Punish*, 1977.

[86] RB Inden, *Imagining India*, London, 2000 [1990]; For filmed images see K Dunn, 'Lights…Camera…Africa: Images of Africa and Africans in Western Popular Films of the 1930s', *African Studies Review*, 39, 1996, pp. 149–75.

[87] For a tremendously important resource see the oral history archive at the British Empire and Commonwealth Museum, Bristol. This is sure-fire testament that ex-colonials relished talking about their lives and evidences the similarities in their experiences. For details of the holdings see, British Empire and Commonwealth Museum, *Voices and Echoes: A Catalogue of Oral History Holdings of the British Empire and Commonwealth Museum*, Bristol, 1999 [1998].

Chapter 2: Recruitment into the Colonial Medical Service (pp.15-31)

[1] RHL/MSS.Brit.Emp.s.415, Furse Papers, Memorandum: Furse to Lord Milner, 18 June 1918

[2] This comment is specifically about the Medical Service, although the structural criticisms could have been applied to any Service branches. S Squire Sprigge, *Medicine and the Public*, London, 1905, p.110

[3] W Ormsby-Gore, 'Foreword' in C Jeffries, *The Colonial Empire and its Civil Service*, Cambridge, 1938, pp.vii–xi, p.vii

[4] R Furse, *Aucuparius: Recollections of a Recruiting Officer*, Oxford, 1962, p.221. He went on to say 'I wanted it [the Colonial Service] to take a place comparable to the Indian Civil Service in the public imagination.' *Ibid.*, p.222

[5] Perhaps this unhappy university result influenced Furse's continued stress on the importance of values imbibed at school. *Ibid.*, pp.9–10.

[6] R Heussler, *Yesterday's Rulers: The Making of the British Colonial Service*, New York, NY, 1963, p.14

[7] 'Ralph Furse', *The Times*, 5th October 1973, p.21; 'Sir Ralph Dolignon Furse' Lord Blake and CS Nicholls (eds.), *Dictionary of National Biography 1971–80*, Oxford, 1986, pp.327–8

[8] Furse, *Aucuparius*, p.240

[9] For a nice description of how the system worked see P Mitchell, 'Forty Years Back' in A Kirk-Greene, *Glimpses of Empire: A Corona Anthology*, London, 2001, pp.278–80, p.278

[10] *Miscellaneous No.99: Colonial Medical Appointments*, London, 1921 [29th Ed.], p.4. NA/CO/612/2 Circular Despatch: 'On the Use of Influence Among Government Officers', *Uganda Protectorate Government Gazette*, 31 July 1911, pp.301–2; NA/CO/542/5 Chamberlain,

published letter: 'The Issue of Colonial Officers' Promotion by Irregular Means', *East Africa Protectorate Government Gazette.*, 15 August 1911, pp.373–4 [a reiteration of an original despatch, 18 December 1897]

[11] Report of the Warren Fisher Committee, 1931 quoted in Furse, *Aucuparius,* p.240

[12] *Ibid.*, p.224. Furthermore, after Furse's retirement, his brother-in-law Francis Newbolt succeeded, continuing his policies until 1954.

[13] 'Anything in the nature of recruiting or 'touting' for men must be avoided…it is an honour to be chosen.' RHL/MSS.Brit.Emp.s.415, Furse Papers, Furse, 'Confidential No.38: Recruitment and Training of Colonial Civil Servants', Colonial Office Conference, 1927, p. 13. '[A]dvertisement in the press, save in the case of an exceptionally attractive or unusual vacancy, should only be used as a last resort. It would normally be guaranteed to attract a mass of rubbish, and so few nuggets as to make sifting the scrap-heap a waste of time.' Furse, *Aucuparius,* p.224

[14] The earliest included *Miscellaneous No.117: Legal Appointments*; *Miscellaneous No.115: Colonial Police Appointments*; *Eastern No.85: Hong Kong, Straits Settlements and the Federated Malay States Police Probationers*; *Miscellaneous No.99*; *African (West) No.678: West African Medical Staff*; *African No.775: Regulations for the Employment of Officers in the East Africa, Uganda and Somaliland Protectorates*; *African No.839: Pensions and Gratuities (East Africa)*; *African (West) No.748 West African Pensions Laws*

[15] The earliest complete example I have found is *Miscellaneous No.99*, 1921. This was the 29th edition, so presuming it was updated yearly, this indicates that these memoranda had been produced since the early 1890s. The *Colonial Office List* of 1899 provides earliest mention of a separate memorandum for medical appointments.

[16] The Eastern cadetships were pre-eminent because they were separately recruited with their own entrance examinations. Mitchell, 'Forty Years Back', p.278

[17] For a (medical) example of the form see NA/CO/822/23/3 Vacancy Form, Tanganyika Territory, 27 August 1930.

[18] These 'Schedules of Offices' were published at the beginning of the 'Green Books', the first of which was to appear for the Colonial Medical Service in 1936. Even though a position may only be listed once, this did not mean that several people could not be appointed to that position. E.g., *Colonial Medical Service List*, London, 1936, pp.2–8; for the policy on using these schedules see NA/CO/850/106/5 Circular Dispatch: W Ormsby-Gore to all Colonies and Protectorates, 5 May 1937

[19] 'Information as to Colonial Appointments', *Colonial Office List*, London, 1899, pp.346–8, p.346

[20] NA/CO/877/3/37175 Circular: 'Recommendation of Local Candidates by East African and Northern Rhodesian Governments', 1 August 1924

[21] E.g., the advice of the Claude Chevallier, acting PMO Kenya, to an interested local European applicant based in East Africa, Dr Wand. KNA/MOH/1/9940 Chevallier to Wand, 27 September 1920

[22] A cadetship was won through a competitive examination, which, until the mid 1920s was the same as that taken by Home and Indian Civil Service candidates. Competitive examinations for the police forces of Ceylon, Malaya and Hong Kong were discarded in 1924 (in favour of a literacy test and then personal selection); in 1927 the customs service of Malaya also joined this group. Furse, *Aucuparius,* p. 147

[23] 'P' for Patronage and then later (conveniently) for Personnel.

[24] This phrase was retained in recruitment literature throughout the period. NA/CO/877/15/17 Colonial Service Application [Form] (P1)[n.d. *c.* 1930]; 'Information as to Colonial Appointments', *Colonial Office List*, 1899, p.348; *Colonial Service Recruitment No.3: Information Regarding the Colonial Medical Service*, London, 1935, p.6

[25] Furse, *Aucuparius,* p.230

[26] *Miscellaneous No.99*, 1921, p.4; *Colonial Service Recruitment No.3*, p.7

[27] 'Information as to Colonial Appointments', *Colonial Office List*, 1899, p.348; This is reiterated, in slightly different words, in the later period: *Colonial Service Recruitment No.3*, p.7

[28] It was an informal policy that the Secretary of State did not always confirm all Colonial Service appointments. In the 1920s Furse described Churchill as having been incredibly hands-off. Once broadly satisfied with Colonial Service recruitment, Churchill declared that submissions no longer needed his confirmatory signature. Furse, while grateful for the confidence put in him, felt that this would have looked unprofessional, and arranged with Private Secretary, Edward Marsh that submissions would continue to be made and come back autographed (even though Marsh was faking Churchill's signature). Furse, *Aucuparius*, p.83

[29] The Appointments Board interviewed all candidates to the Colonial Administrative Service, but 'expert advisors' conducted interviews for the specialist and technical services. NA/CO/877/8/2, 'Colonial Service Appointments Board: Composition, Function and Methods of Procedure', [n.d.*c*.1931]

[30] Furse, *Aucuparius*, p.224; NA/CO/877/4/4 'London University Appointments Board: General Correspondence', 1927–9

[31] NA/CO/877/3/57672 Memorandum: 'Question of Minimum Age Limits for Candidates for Appointment to Tropical Africa', 6 April 1925

[32] *Colonial Service Recruitment No.1: The Colonial Service, General Information Regarding Colonial Appointments*, London, 1936, p.8, pp.12–13

[33] Although in the late 1920s and early 1930s Major Hutchinson went on a tour of certain provincial universities and medical schools to publicise the Colonial Service, these less established universities were never given as much attention as the core three mentioned above. NA/CO/877/7/8 'Visit by Major Hutchinson to Scottish Universities and to Liverpool University to Encourage Recruits', February 1930. NA/CO/877/8/18 Furse, 'Progress Report for the Appointments Department, No.1', 1 July 1931, p.6

[34] *Colonial Service Recruitment No.1*, p.28

[35] NA/CO/877/1/18180 'Openings for University men in the Colonies', 13th April 1921; See also A Kirk-Greene, 'Taking Canada into Partnership in the 'White Man's Burden': The British Colonial Service and the Dominions Selection Scheme of 1923', *Canadian Journal of African Studies*, 15, 1981, pp.33-54.

[36] NA/CO/877/2/38125 'Canadian University Candidates, Central Dominion Selection Committee', August 1922

[37] This was the Tropical African Services Course, held initially at the Imperial Institute, London and, from 1926, at Oxford and Cambridge. Furse, *Aucuparius*, pp.151–2

[38] For example, a Forestry Course (1925), Colonial Agricultural Scholarships (1925) and Veterinary Scholarships (1929); A Kirk-Greene, *On Crown Service: A History of HM Colonial and Overseas Civil Services, 1837–1997*, London, 1999, pp.27–8

[39] Although this was not stipulated in the Colonial Office medical recruitment pamphlets until the 1931 edition, it was mentioned as early 1920 in 'Information as to Colonial Appointments', *Colonial Office List*, London, 1920, pp.552–62, p.560. Practically all 'policy-forming' positions in the British Colonial Service were held by whites, contrasted with the more liberal French and Dutch Colonial Service policies see LA Mills, 'Methods of Appointment and Training in the British and Dutch Colonial Civil Service', *American Political Science Review*, 33, 1939, pp.465–72, p.466

[40] Although some police and customs appointments were open to school-leavers and could be taken as young as 19 and, as previously mentioned, the entrance age to the Colonial Administrative Service was lowered to 21 ½

[41] '[A] University degree is an advantage in nearly all cases, especially if taken with honours, and in many instances…is essential', *Colonial Service Recruitment No.1*, p.11

[42] 'Information as to Colonial Appointments', *Colonial Office List*, 1920, p.552; This remained within the published guidelines until 1931, *Colonial Service Recruitment No.3A: The Colonial Service. Information for the use of Candidates for Appointment to the Colonial Medical Service*, London, 1931, p.7

[43] 'Information as to Colonial Appointments', *Colonial Office List*, 1920, p.560; Also NA/CO/323/999/4 'Marriage Restrictions: Terms of Appointment for Colonial Service', 1928

[44] 'Information as to Colonial Appointments', *Colonial Office List*, 1899, p.347

[45] 'Information as to Colonial Appointments', *Colonial Office List*, 1908, pp.443–6, p.445

[46] Except when new medical departments were established. When Britain was awarded the mandate for Tanzanian rule the senior positions in its medical department were drawn from experienced personnel of other parts of Empire.

[47] NA/CO/850/71/9 'Draft Advertisement: His Majesty's Colonial Medical Service', 11 January 1936

[48] A Balfour, 'Vistas and Visions: Some Aspects of the Colonial Medical Services', *Glasgow Medical Journal*, 6, 1924, pp.353–74; AGH Smart, 'An Impression of Life in the Colonial Medical Service', *St. Thomas' Hospital Gazette*, 37, 1939, pp.123–6

[49] NA/CO/877/7/8 'Visit by Major Hutchinson'; NA/CO/877/8/18 Furse, 'Progress Report for the Appointments Department, No.1', p.6

[50] Although it was agreed that liaison officers in London would be useful for other Service branches. NA/CO/877/8/8 'Scheme for Liaison Between the Colonial Office and the Colleges of London University', 1931

[51] *Miscellaneous No.99: Colonial Medical Appointments*, 1923 [31st Ed.], p.2

[52] Squire Sprigge, *Medicine and the Public*, p.119

[53] Foreign and Commonwealth Office, *East African Staff List*, London, 1914

[54] H Bell, *Frontiers of Medicine in the Anglo-Egyptian Sudan, 1899–1940*, Oxford, 1999, pp.39–40. One 1912 estimate was that the Sudan Medical Service was 'the most highly qualified Service in the world', HC Squires, *The Sudan Medical Service, an Experiment in Social Medicine*, London, 1958, p.14

[55] Harrison has argued for the relative unpopularity of the Indian Medical Service as a medical career choice before 1914, this was certainly true, but it seems to have still been more prestigious than the Colonial Medical Service. M Harrison, *Public Health in British India: Anglo-Indian Preventative Medicine 1859–1914*, Cambridge, 1994, pp.27–35

[56] Unless the candidate was a woman doctor, in which case the best opportunities seemed to be in the Malayan Medical Service.

[57] Furse tabulated the number of appointments which the Appointments Department dealt with between 1919–50, but no expressions of interest are noted however, so although it can be seen how many applicants failed the medical examination or withdrew, summarily rejected applicants are not recorded. Furse, *Aucuparius*, Appendix 1

[58] RHL/MSS.Brit.Emp.s.415, Furse Papers, 'Second Memorandum for the Warren Fisher Committee', January 1929

[59] RHL/MSS.Brit.Emp.s.415, Furse Papers, Memorandum: 'On the Difficulty of Obtaining Candidates for the Colonial Medical Service', March 1931

[60] KNA/MOH/3/246 P Ross, Application (P1 Med.), 1925; KNA/MOH/3/247 N Maclennan, Application (P1 Med.), 1925

[61] 'Medical Appointments in the Colonies', *BMJ*, i, 1891, p.770

[62] *African (East) No.1105: Information for the Use of Candidates to Appointments in the East African Medical Service*, London, 1925, p.8. There had been other earlier medical advisers to the Colonial Office, most famously Manson, but their appointment was not systematic until 1926 and slightly different in remit. Manson, as Consulting Physician for the Colonial Office had to conduct medical examinations of Service candidates as well as advise on policy.

[63] 'Information as to Colonial Appointments', *Colonial Office List*, 1899, p.347

[64] *Miscellaneous No.99*, 1921, p.3

[65] *Colonial Service Recruitment No.3*, p.4

[66] *Miscellaneous No.99*, 1921, p.5

[67] The appointee was not eligible for pension rights, but could claim a gratuity payment of £200 upon satisfactory completion of their engagement. *Ibid.*, p.3

[68] E.g., Ernest Cooke (first employed aged 44); Geoffrey Gibbon (37); Frank de Smidt (37). No mention of this scheme is made in any of the recruitment literature after 1930.

[69] Although MOs did not need to be British born. Unlike the Colonial Administrative Service where, although candidates need not be the children of British subjects (just European) on both sides, they needed to have been born in the UK. NA/CO/877/4/12 'Appointment of Naturalised Colonial Service Subjects to the Colonial Service', 16 August 1927

[70] At least, this is the first reference I have found. The East African, West African and Malayan Medical Services and the Eastern Police Services were the only ones in the Colonial Service to formally declare that racial origins would be a bar from appointment, until it was decided to change the wording in all recruitment memoranda in 1936. NA/CO/877/13/22 'Eligibility of Indians for Colonial Service', 1936; also see NA/CO/537/910, 'Admission of Asiatics to the Medical Service', 1923; for information on the early position of the East African Medical Service see *African (East) No.1105*, p.8

[71] NA/CO/877/1/43122 Minutes: 'Applications by Natives of India for Appointments in the Colonial Service', 5 October 1921. One agenda item was a letter from PL Gupta (MB, ChB, DPH, FRCS) from Gwalior State, India (17 August 1923). Gupta enquired whether there were likely to be any vacancies suitable for him either in the West or East African Medical Services. After discussion of the letter it was decided that 'any such appointment would be undesirable' and, although Gupta should not be explicitly rejected on racial grounds, he was effectively ineligible because of them. It was subsequently confirmed that the Colonial Office policy of refusal, without making any open declarations over racial ineligibility, was the best one to continue pursuing at present.

[72] 'Will you please state of what nationality you believe the applicant and his father respectively to be, and give the grounds on which you base this belief?' NA/CO/877/15/17 Referees' Statement, (P.7), [n.d., c.1937]

[73] 'Information as to Colonial Appointments', *Colonial Office List*, 1899, p.347; [Cmd.939] *Report of the Departmental Committee Appointed by the Secretary of State for the Colonies to Enquire into the Colonial Medical Services*, London, 1920, p.4

[74] Jeffries, *Colonial Empire*, p.150

[75] *Colonial Service Recruitment No.3A*, p.6

[76] Since the 1885 Medical Amendment Act this was the minimum legal medical qualification. 'Information as to Colonial Appointments', *Colonial Office List*, 1899, p.347; *Miscellaneous No.99*, 1923, p.3

[77] Or the equivalent 'triple' from the Scottish Corporations: LRCS (Ed.), LRCP (Ed.) & LRFPS (Glas.).

[78] Jeffries, *Colonial Empire*, pp.76–7; also see NA/CO/850/12/13 'Circular Dispatch to Colonial Governors', November 1932

[79] NA/877/9/2 Memorandum: 'Reciprocity with the British Dominions and with Foreign Countries', October 1930

[80] 'Dr Isabel Hill MB, ChB Edin. Gave her P1 Med, Misc.99....Told her position—i.e. only one lady doctor's post in Crown Cols. & that filled recently.' RH/MSS.Brit.Emp.r.21, Colonial Office Desk Diary, 1912, 31 January 1912

[81] 'Information as to Colonial Appointments', *Dominions and Colonial Office List*, London, 1939, pp.623–32, p.627

[82] 'Information as to Colonial Appointments', *Colonial Office List*, 1899, p.347

[83] *Colonial Service Recruitment No.3*, p.17. It is interesting, however, that into the 1930s vacancy requests still sometimes expressly stipulated a preference for medical candidates 'unmarried if possible', see NA/822/23/3 Telegram: Governor of Tanganyika to Secretary of State, 25 March 1930

[84] *Miscellaneous No.99*, 1921, p.4; *Colonial Service Recruitment No.3*, p.7

[85] 'John Shircore', *East African Medical Journal*, 30, 1953, pp.355–6, p.355

[86] RHL/MSS.Brit.Emp.r.4, PA Clearkin, *Ramblings and Recollections of a Colonial Doctor 1913–58*, Book I, Durban, 1967, p.16

[87] *Ibid.*

[88] The Liverpool School of Hygiene and Tropical Medicine was to also play its role in training for incipient MOs, but this was not the primary impetus behind its establishment. Indeed, for a very short period (February 1898–August 1900), the Secretary of State stipulated that MOs should attend the London based course for at least two months, *even* if they had attended the Liverpool course. JWW Stephens, W Yorke B Blacklock, *Liverpool School of Tropical Medicine, Historical Record: 1898–1920*, Liverpool, 1920, p.12, p.20

[89] 'Information as to Colonial Appointments', *Colonial Office List*, 1899, p.347

[90] *Miscellaneous No.99*, 1921, p.5

[91] *Ibid.*

[92] From 1930 candidates recruited in Australia or New Zealand could take Diploma of Tropical Medici e (as well as Diploma Public Health) at the Australian Institute of Tropical Medicine (which moved in 1930 from Townsville to Sydney). NA/CO/877/6/13 Furse, 'Report on the Arrangements for the Central Committee for the Appointment of Australian Graduates', 31 July 1929

[93] *Miscellaneous No.407: Primary Courses of Instruction in Tropical Medicine and Hygiene for Officers Selected for Appointment to the Colonial Medical Service*, [6th Ed.], London, 1939, p.1

[94] P Manson-Bahr, *History of the School of Tropical Medicine in London: 1899–1949*, London, 1956, p.51; L Wilkinson and A Hardy, *Prevention and Cure: The London School of Hygiene and Tropical Medicine A 20th Century Quest for Global Public Health*, London, 2001, p.150

[95] *Miscellaneous No.407*, pp.1–2

[96] *African (East) No.1105*, p.6

[97] This was, of course, provided that the candidate embarked at the first available opportunity. *Colonial Service Recruitment No.3*, p.12

[98] LSHTM/GB0809/Manson/09 'Medical Examinations in Connection with the Colonies and Protectorates', 1898–1919 Indeed, Chernin has argued that this was Manson's principal role at the Colonial Office (i.e. more than policy making). E Chernin, 'Sir Patrick Manson: Physician to the Colonial Office, 1897–1912', *Medical History*, 36, 1992, pp.320–31

[99] *Colonial Service Recruitment No.3*, pp.7–8

[100] Ultimately officers would have received two letters of appointment, one from the Colonial Office and another from the colonial government in which they were to serve. KNA/MOH/3/247 Letter of Appointment: Under Secretary of State to P Ross', 14/09/1925; RHL/MSS.Afr.s.1421, Papers of P Rawson, 'Letter of Appointment: Acting Chief Secretary, Uganda to Rawson', 8 February 1922

[101] *Miscellaneous No.441: The Colonial Medical Service, Special Regulations by the Secretary of State for the Colonies*, London, 1934, p.3

[102] In the case of East Africa, *African No.973*

[103] *Miscellaneous No.99*, 1921, p.5

[104] BMA/E/1/41/1 Conditions of officers within the Colonial Medical Service, from 5 November 1919 to 27 April 1926 [My description]

[105] NA/CO/543/1 *East Africa Protectorate Blue Book*, 1901–2; NA/CO/613/1 *Uganda Protectorate Blue Book*, 1901–2

[106] *Miscellaneous No.99*, 1921, p.5

[107] Although there was a note that these were under the process of review. 'Information as to Colonial Appointments', *Dominions and Colonial Office List*, London, 1939, p.627

[108] *Miscellaneous No.99*, 1921, p.5

[109] *Miscellaneous No.99*, 1923, p.5

[110] NA/CO/533/397/6 Compulsory Retirements, 1930; NA/CO/533/415 Moratorium on Leave, 1932; See also BMA/E/1/41/3 *Corrigenda to the Colonial Service Recruitment Series of Memoranda*, 1932

[111] *Colonial Service Recruitment No.3*, p.13

[112] *Ibid.*

[113] *Miscellaneous No.99*, 1921, p.5

114 *Colonial Service Recruitment No.3*, p.16

115 *Miscellaneous No.99*, 1921, p.6; *African (East) No.1103*, p.4; Also KNA/MOH/3/246 N Maclennan, Appointment Letter, 27 November 1926. Later editions of Colonial memoranda for East Africa do not mention the salary supplement for MOHs, so it was most likely stopped in the 1930s. Any supplement that was granted was, furthermore, tied to the position of MOH, as opposed to the possession of the Diploma in Public Health *per se*. NA/CO/850/120/6 AJ O'Brien, Chief Medical Adviser to the Colonial Office to C Hill, [Deputy Secretary, BMA], 23 May 1938

116 *Colonial Service Recruitment No.3*, p.17; See also the sleeping sickness duty allowance. HG Calwell, 'Nineteen Years in the Colonial Medical Service', *The Ulster Medical Journal*, 65 (supplement), 1993, pp.(s)1–(s)42, p.(s)5

117 Outfit allowances were continued for MOs appointed to West Africa, presumably because conditions were regarded as considerably worse in the West. *African (West) No.678: Information for the Use of Candidates for Appointments on the West African Medical Staff*, London, 1930, p.14; Jeffries, *Colonial Empire*, p.120; *African No.973*, p.4

118 *Colonial Service Recruitment No.3*, p.19

119 *African (East) No.1105*, p.4; *Colonial Service Recruitment No.3A*, p.20

120 [My italics] *Colonial Service Recruitment No.3*, p.20

121 Although the relatively salubrious climate of Kenya meant that the maximum tour was raised to thirty-six months. *Ibid.*

122 The period taken travelling to and from leave was not subtracted from this entitlement. *Miscellaneous No.99*, 1921, p.11

123 Under these new leave conditions officers could also receive fourteen days local leave and, subject to official approval, extensions of leave in cases where they were sick or needed the extra time to attend courses of instruction. *African (East) No.1105*, p.4

124 *Colonial Service Recruitment No.3*, p.20

125 After 1934 the upper age limit was raised to fifty-five and the twenty-year service requirement was abolished. *Ibid.*, p.21

126 *Miscellaneous No.99*, 1921, p.12

127 A supplementary pension scheme was provided for cases of forced early retirement. Jeffries, *Colonial Empire*, pp.112–3, p.114

128 *Miscellaneous No.99*, 1921, p.5

129 *African (East) No.1103*, p.4

130 The Watson Committee, 1936

131 *Colonial Service Recruitment No.3*, p.18, p.29

132 *Regulations for His Majesty's Colonial Service*, 1908, pp.12–13; 'Colonial Regulations', *Dominions and Colonial Office List*, London, 1939, p.866

133 *African (East) No.1103*, pp.7–8, quotation, p.8

134 *Ibid.*, p.8. In Kenya, these fees were suspended (to great discontent) during the recession and had still not been restored by 1936. RHL/MSS.Brit.Emp.s.415, Furse Papers, AP Paterson, DMS, Kenya, to Furse, 19 February 1936

135 *African (East) No.1103*, p.6

136 E.g., KNA/MOH/1/685, Annual Confidential Reports, [n.d. *c.*1908–10]

137 *Colonial Service Recruitment No.3A*, p.5

138 Jeffries, *Colonial Empire*, p.153

Chapter 3: Subjective Selection and Recruitment Trends (pp.32-45)

1 *Colonial Service Recruitment No.3: Information Regarding the Colonial Medical Service*, London, 1935 p.10

2 G Evatt, 'Notes on the Organisation of the Colonial Medical Service of the Empire', *BMJ*, ii, 1896, pp.863–4, p.864; [Cmd.939] *Report of the Departmental Committee*, 1920, p.5;

NA/CO/877/6/10 'Recruitment of Candidates for the Home and Colonial Services: Proposal to Hold a Joint Competitive Examination', May 1929

[3] AL Lowell, *Colonial Civil Service: The Selection and Training of Colonial Officials in England, Holland, and France*, London, 1900, p.76.

[4] E Marsh, *A Number of People*, London, 1939, pp.123–4

[5] NA/CO/877/1/18180 Furse to A Hill [Secretary, Universities Bureau of the British Empire], 'Openings for University Men in British Colonies', 23 June 1921. Furthermore, this stress on character was one that was also made by Lord Lugard. Lugard specified in his famous *Dual Mandate in British Tropical Africa*, Hamden, CT, 1965, [5th Ed.], p.139 that the Colonial Service must exclude 'as far as possible the "bounder", the "prig" and the "bookworm"' quoted in H Kuklick, *The Imperial Bureaucrat: The Colonial Administrative Service in the Gold Coast, 1920–1939*, Stanford, CA, 1979, p.20

[6] Volumes 1900, 1901 and 1913 are missing. A Kirk-Greene, 'Not Quite a Gentleman': The Desk Diaries of the Assistant Private Secretary (Appointments) to the Secretary of State for the Colonies 1899–1915', *English Historical Review*, 67, 2002, pp.622–33; p.626

[7] RHL/Mss.Brit.Emp.r.21 Patronage Diary 1903, 15 January 1903; *Ibid.*, 1904, 30 December 1904; *Ibid.*, 1905, 8 August 1905; *Ibid.*, 1908, 6 March 1908; *Ibid.*, 1909, 29 January 1909

[8] C Jeffries, *Partners for Progress: The Men and Women of the Colonial Service*, London, 1949, p.82

[9] R Furse, *Aucuparius: Recollections of a Recruiting Officer*, Oxford, 1962, p.221

[10] *Ibid.*, pp.66–7

[11] F Newbolt, *Appointments Handbook*, 1948, extract 'On the Process of Interviewing' reproduced in A Kirk-Greene, *On Crown Service: A History of HM Colonial and Overseas Civil Services, 1837–1997*, London, 1999, pp. 191–6, p.193

[12] NA/CO/877/15/17 Referees' Statement, (P.7)

[13] Furse, *Aucuparius*, p.223, p.230

[14] M Perham, 'Introduction', in R Heussler, *Yesterday's Rulers: The Making of the British Colonial Service*, New York, NY, 1963, p.xxiv

[15] R Hillary, *The Last Enemy*, London, 1950, p.15

[16] Heussler, *Yesterday's Rulers*, p.41

[17] R Wilkinson, *The Prefects: British Leadership and the Public School Tradition*, Oxford, 1964; JA Mangan (ed.) *'Benefits Bestowed'? Education and British Imperialism*, Manchester, 1988; A Penn, *Targeting Schools: Drill, Militarism and Imperialism*, London, 1999

[18] NA/CO/877/1/37811 Furse, 'Proposal for Holding the Tropical African Services Course at Oxford and Cambridge', 1 April 1920

[19] NA/CO/877/4/11 Memorandum: 'Scholarships from Public Schools to Oxford and Cambridge', 30 May 1927; NA/CO/877/4/16 'Public School's Employment Bureau', 1927–9

[20] Heussler, *Yesterday's Rulers*, p.81

[21] NA/CO/877/1/43122 Minute: Furse, Method of Dealing with Applications for Colonial Employment on the Part of Natives of India', 29 August 1921

[22] NA/CO/877/2/6370 Furse to Falconer, 'Selection of Canadians', 24 April 1922

[23] NA/CO/877/4/15 Minute: Furse, 'Canadian University Graduates of not Pure European Descent', 19 April 1927

[24] NA/CO/877/3/950 Furse to Mr Fennell [University of Toronto], 'Employment of Officers in the Colonial Service of Jewish Origin', 24 January 1924

[25] NA/CO/877/2/56081 Furse to Mr Trustlove [Oxford University Appointments Committee], 'Eyesight Standard of Candidates for Appointment to the Colonial Service', 30 November 1923

[26] Although it is noted that entrance interviews to medical schools often emphasised sport too.

[27] NA/CO/877/3/57672 Minute: Furse, 'Question of the Minimum Age Limits for Candidates for Appointment to Tropical Africa', 6 December 1924

[28] NA/CO/877/4/16 *Public School's Employment Bureau Bulletin No.3A*, July 1929, p.20

[29] NA/CO/850/46/11 'Standard Prescribed Form for Medical Examination for the Colonial Service', 1934

[30] R Havelock Charles, 'Discussion on Special Factors Influencing the Suitability of Europeans for Life in the Tropics', *BMJ*, ii, 1910, pp.869–74, p.870

[31] E.g., K Ordahl Kupperman, 'Fear of Hot Climates in the Anglo-American Experience', *William and Mary Quarterly*, 41, 1984, pp.213-40; D Kennedy, 'The Perils of the Midday Sun: Climatic Anxieties in the Colonial Tropics' in JM MacKenzie, (ed.), *Imperialism and the Natural World*, Manchester, 1990, pp.118–140; M Harrison, '"The Tender Frame of Man": Disease, Climate, and Racial Difference in India and the West Indies, 1760-1860', *Bulletin of the History of Medicine*, 70, 1996, pp.68–93; M Harrison, *Climates and Constitutions: Health, Race, Environment and British Imperialism in India 1600–1850*, New Delhi, 1999

[32] E Shorter, *History of Psychiatry: from the Era of the Asylum to the Age of Prozac*, New York, NY, 2000, p.129

[33] NA/CO/877/4/16 *Public Schools' Employment Bureau Bulletin No.3A*, 1929, p.19

[34] NA/CO/877/4/19 Minute: Furse 'Recruitment of Candidates from Younger Universities', 15 December 1927; Also the rationale behind rejecting candidates with speech impediments on the grounds that 'a disability of this kind arising from some nervous disorder is sometimes liable to become worse in the tropics', NA/CO/877/8/16 Circular Despatch: to All Colonies and Protectorates, 11 July 1932

[35] NA/CO/850/133/1 Governor of Uganda to Secretary of State, 4 November 1938

[36] *Miscellaneous No.488: The Colonial Service, General Conditions of Employment*, London, 1939, p.16

[37] JA Mangan and J Walvin (eds.), *Manliness and Morality: Middle-class Masculinity in Britain and America, 1800–1940*, Manchester, 1987

[38] NA/CO/877/4/11 'Scholarships from Public Schools to Oxford and Cambridge'; RHL/MSS.Brit.Emp.s.415, Furse Papers, 'First Memorandum for the Warren Fisher Committee', 27 April 1929

[39] NA/CO/877/15/17 Referees' Statement, (P.7)

[40] RHL/MSS.Brit.Emp.r.21 Patronage Diary 1905, 24 May 1905

[41] An anecdotal example of this in Kenya (regarding the respect officers should pay to local religious customs) can be found in KNA/MOH/1/1758 Circular: to the Secretariat, 26 January 1910

[42] NA/CO/877/6/11 Furse, 'Notes on the Scheme for Facilitating Recruitment for the Colonial Services from the Australian Universities', 4 September 1928

[43] NA/CO/877/1/37811 Furse, 'Proposal for Holding the Tropical African Services Course at Oxford and Cambridge'

[44] [Cmd.939] *Report of the Departmental Committee*, 1920, p.6

[45] D Cannadine, *Ornamentalism: How the British Saw Their Empire*, Harmondsworth, 2001

[46] See NA/CO/877/4/11 'Scholarships from Public Schools to Oxford and Cambridge'

[47] Newbolt, *Appointments Handbook*, in Kirk-Greene, *On Crown Service*, p.194. In several important ways the *Appointment's Handbook* was an expression of ideas formulated before 1939.

[48] NA/CO/877/3/51477 Minute: Mr Flood, 'Applications for Colonial Appointments from Persons Resident in the Irish Free State', 19 November 1925

[49] NA/CO/877/3/685 Minute: Mr Denniston [? illegible], 'Applications from New Zealanders for Appointments in the Colonial Service', 26 January 1926

[50] RHL/MSS.Brit.Emp.s.415, Furse Papers, 'Note to Colonel Amery on Work of the Appointments Branch,' 19 February 1919

[51] *The East African Standard*, 'A Colonial Office Visitor', 15 January 1936, p.2

[52] D Duckworth, 'On the Education of Medical Practitioners for Colonial Service', A Paper read at the First Inter-colonial Medical Congress, Amsterdam, 1883, pp.1–7, p.5

[53] R Hyam, 'The Colonial Office Mind 1900–1914', *Journal of Imperial and Commonwealth History*, 8, 1979, pp.30–55

[54] NA/CO/877/7/16 Mr Tomlinson, to Secretary, London and National Society for Women's Service, 'Colonial Service Appointments Board, Appointment of Members', 20 January 1932

[55] RHL/MSS.Brit.Emp.s.415, Furse Papers, Furse's Diary [Typescript], 1935–6, 7 February 1936

[56] RHL/MSS.Brit.Emp.s.415, Furse Papers, WH Kauntze to Furse, 6 March 1936

[57] RHL/MSS.Brit.Emp.s.415, Furse Papers, Memorandum: Furse to Milner. In contrast to this tone, from the mid 1920s onwards a concerted effort was made, at least synthetically, to raise the standards of all recruits to the Colonial Services in general, and the medical services specifically. Furse stated in 1927 that the standards of medical recruits had improved enough to allow more 'freedom of choice in the selection of candidates', meaning he no longer had to recruit those he actually felt were not of high standards. RHL/MSS.Brit.Emp.s.415, Furse Papers, Furse, 'Confidential No.38', p.11

[58] 'Information as to Colonial Appointments', *Colonial Office List*, London, 1899, p.347

[59] *Ibid.*, 1908, p.445

[60] Compiled from RHL/Mss.Brit.Emp.r.21 Patronage Diaries 1899, 1902-12, 1914.

[61] Kirk-Greene, *On Crown Service*, p.16

[62] 'Information as to Colonial Appointments', *Dominions and Colonial Office List*, London, 1939, p.623

[63] RHL/MSS.Brit.Emp.s.415, Furse Papers, Memorandum: Furse to Milner

[64] RHL/MSS.Brit.Emp.s.415, Furse Papers, JCC Davidson to Furse, 9 August 1916

[65] RHL/MSS.Brit.Emp.s.415, Furse Papers, Furse, 'Confidential No.38', p.3

[66] *Ibid.*, p.11

[67] RHL/MSS.Brit.Emp.s.415, Furse Papers, 'Note to Colonel Amery on Work of the Appointments Branch,' 19 February 1919

[68] NA/CO/877/1/44273 Minute: 'Appointment of Medical Officers to the Colonial Service', 21 July 1920

[69] KNA/MOH/1/10070 'Retrenchments in 1922'

[70] NA/CO/877/8/18 Furse, 'Progress Report for the Appointments Department, No.2', 10 December 1931, p.8

[71] NA/CO/877/1/6781 Memorandum: Furse to Mr Wood, 'Selection of Canadians', 11 August 1921

[72] 'Indians have not yet shown the fitness to govern themselves, much less others.' NA/CO/877/1/43122 'Applications by Natives of India'. This was interesting as there were Indian doctors in the Indian Medical Service and Syrian and Sudanese doctors in the Sudan Medical Service.

[73] NA/CO/877/8/18 Furse, 'Progress Report for the Appointments Department, No.3', 18 March 1932, p.1

[74] NA/CO/877/16/16 'Colonial Medical Recruitment of Medical Officers', June 1938

[75] A Kirk-Greene, *On Crown Service*, p.77

[76] NA/CO/877/8/18 Furse, 'Progress Report for the Appointments Department, No.1', p.2

[77] *Ibid.*, pp.3–4; p.9

[78] Furse seems to be implying that the Diploma of Tropical Hygiene and Medicine was not absolutely essential for medical candidates during these periods. NA/CO/877/8/18 Furse, 'Progress Report for the Appointments Department, No.2', p.9

[79] NA/CO/877/9/6 Furse, Statement [on the Effects of Retrenchment] to HA Roberts [Cambridge University Appointments Board], 1 February 1932

[80] NA/CO/850/9/1 'Retrenchment: General Summary and Statistics', 1932

[81] NA/CO/877/10/11 Furse, 'Progress Report for the Appointments Department, No.3', p.26

[82] NA/CO/877/16/16 Report: 'Recruitment of Medical Officers for the Colonial Medical Service', [n.d. *c.*1938]

[83] NA/CO/877/16/16 Minute: AJ O'Brien, Chief Medical Adviser to the Colonial Office, 7 June 1938

[84] NA/CO/877/16/16 'Colonial Medical Recruitment of Medical Officers'

[85] *Ibid.*

[86] NA/CO/850/153/18 Draft letter: G Tomlinson to *The Times*, 'Colonial Medical Service, Wartime Recruitment', January 1940

Chapter 4: Identity and Experience I: Practical Reasons for Being a Doctor in East Africa (pp.46-58)

[1] AGH Smart, 'An Impression of Life in the Colonial Medical Service', *St Thomas' Hospital Gazette*, 37, 1939, pp.123–6, p.126

[2] This is a subtle acknowledgment of a complex series of interrelated factors, rather than taking a Marxist stance such as that expounded by Robert Young, which argues for a coercive force from a common context imprinted upon the ideas and actions of historical figures. RM Young, *Darwin's Metaphor: Nature's Place in Victorian Culture*. Cambridge, 1985

[3] One disappointment is that very little personal evidence has been left for participants in the early, formative, era. This is because there were few colonial medical staff during that time, and perhaps also because it was only later that the group came to recognise its comparative historical significance.

[4] DM Haynes, *Imperial Medicine: Patrick Manson and the Conquest of Tropical Disease*, Philadelphia, PA, 2001, p.7, pp.15–18; MJ Peterson, *The Medical Profession in Mid-Victorian London*, Berkeley, CA, 1994, pp.124–6; A Digby, *Making a Medical Living: Doctors and Patients in the English Market for Medicine, 1720–1911*, Cambridge, 2002 [1994], pp.144–7; A Digby, 'A Medical El Dorado? Colonial Medical Incomes and Practice at the Cape', *Social History of Medicine*, 8, 1995, pp.463–79; See also DM Haynes, 'Social Status and Imperial Status: Tropical Medicine and the British Medical Profession in the Nineteenth Century' in D Arnold (ed.), *Warm Climates and Western Medicine: The Emergence of Tropical Medicine, 1600–1900*, Amsterdam, 1996, pp. 208–220

[5] TG Garry, *African Doctor*, London, 1939, p.24

[6] An early survey conducted by James Paget in 1869 of St Bartholomew's Hospital Medical School found that 'for a variety of reasons, not all of them economic, many of these élite entrants had failed to make what was considered a fair living from their profession. Twelve per cent had had only limited success in practice, six per cent had failed entirely, and ten per cent had left the medical profession.' J Paget, 'What becomes of Medical Students?' *St Bartholomew's Hospital Reports*, 5, 1869, p.238 cited in Digby, *Making a Medical Living*, p.161

[7] S Squire Sprigge, *Medicine and the Public*, London, 1905, p.49

[8] Haynes, *Imperial Medicine*, p.18

[9] RHL/MSS.Afr.s.1872/144b HC Trowell, interviews, tape 1B, [n.d. *c*.1984]; see also similar comments for the pre-war period RHL/MSS.Brit.Emp.r.4, PA Clearkin, *Ramblings and Recollections of a Colonial Doctor 1913–58*, Book I, Durban, 1967, pp.14–15

[10] 'Numbers of the Medical Profession', *BMJ*, ii, 1931, pp.418–19, p.418; also 'The Portal of Medicine', *Lancet*, i, 1936, pp.672–3

[11] For information on the growth of medical opportunities for women see TN Bonner, *To the Ends of the Earth: Women's Search for Education in Medicine*, Cambridge, MA, 1992

[12] NA/CO/850/71/9 Minute: AJ O'Brien, 'Colonial Medical Service Recruitment', 8 February 1936; see also NA/CO/877/16/16 Minute: AJ O'Brien, Chief Medical Adviser to the Colonial Office, 7 June 1938

[13] In this case the surge occurred largely because of the Colonial Office's concerted medical recruitment drive coupled with the increased popularity of Empire careers.

[14] RHL/MSS.Afr.s.1872/16 A Boase (compiled, RM Boase), 'Notes on Experiences in Colonial Medical Service in Uganda, 1924–56', 14 February 1983, p.1

[15] P Holden, *Doctors and Other Medical Personnel in the Public Health Services of Africa, 1930–1965*, Oxford, 1984, p.2

[16] RHL/MSS.Brit.Emp.r.4, Clearkin, *Ramblings and Recollections*, Book I, pp.14–15, p.15

[17] RHL/MSS.Afr.s.1653, TF Anderson, *Reminiscences by T Farnworth Anderson*, Book I, Kenya, 1973, p.12

[18] BMA/B/162/1/8 'New Scale of Salaries Proposed by the Colonial Office to be Brought into Effect, 1 April 1920', Dominions Committee Documents, Session 1920–1; NA/CO/543/1 *East Africa Protectorate Blue Book*, 1901–2; NA/613/1 *Uganda Protectorate Blue Book.*, 1901–2; JL Gilks 'The Medical Department and the Health Organization in Kenya, 1909–1933', *East African Medical Journal*, 9, 1932–3, pp.340–54, p.342; Digby, *Making a Medical Living*, p.132

[19] BMA/B/162/1/6 Letter: Drs Henderson, Small and Massey to the BMA Dominions Committee, (Session 1918-19), 16 December 1918

[20] This is indicated by the way official literature sought to justify the salary. *Colonial Service Recruitment No.3: Information Regarding the Colonial Medical Service*, London, 1935, p.13; see also C Jeffries, *The Colonial Empire and its Civil Service*, Cambridge, 1938, p.110

[21] NA/CO/850/12/13 Memorandum: JCS McDouall, [DMSS, Sierra Leone] to Colonial Secretary, 19 October 1931

[22] 'Memorandum of Evidence Placed by the BMA before the Colonial Medical Services Committee (Appointed in November 1919), on 23rd February 1920', *BMJ, Supplement*, 1920, pp.141–3, p.143

[23] A Balfour, 'Vistas and Visions: Some Aspects of the Colonial Medical Services', *Glasgow Medical Journal*, 6, 1924, pp.353–74, p.355

[24] Jeffries, *Colonial Empire*, p.110

[25] Smart, 'An Impression of Life in the Colonial Medical Service', p.123

[26] *Ibid.*, p.125

[27] 'Arthur Bagshawe', *Lancet*, i, 1950, pp.693–4; p.693

[28] RHL/MSS.Afr.s.1872/153a AW Williams, 'Detailed Memoranda on Experiences in the Colonial Medical Service in Uganda and Tanganyika, 1931-1949', [n.d. *c.*1983], p.1

[29] It was due to the 'unhealthiness of the climate' that positions in West African Medical Service were higher paid and on better terms than in other parts of Africa, 'Information as to Colonial Appointments', *Colonial Office List*, London, 1899, pp.346–8, p.347

[30] RHL/MSS.Brit.Emp.s.415, Furse Papers, Memorandum: Furse to Lord Milner, 18 June 1918 [Original italics]

[31] RHL/MSS.Afr.s.1872/16 Boase, 'Notes on Experiences', p.1

[32] Apparently physical examinations for the Indian Medical Service were more stringent too. Clare Wiggins recollected that he applied to the Colonial Medical Service because he was too shortsighted for the Indian Service. CA Wiggins, 'Early Days in British East Africa and Uganda', *East African Medical Journal*, 37, 1960, pp.699–708, p.699

[33] Indian Service and Army Service training was initially conducted at Netley (opened 1863), although after 1902 all army medical training moved to Milbank and after 1905 prospective Indian Medical Service officers went to London School of Tropical Medicine to prepare them for their careers. Similar training was required at Haslar for candidates for the Naval Medical Department. P Manson-Bahr, *History of the School of Tropical Medicine in London: 1899-1949*, London, 1956, p.22

[34] RHL/MSS.Brit.Emp.s.415, Furse Papers, Furse, 'Confidential No.38: Recruitment and Training of Colonial Civil Servants', Colonial Office Conference, 1927, p.11

[35] Balfour, 'Vistas and Visions', p.354

[36] RHL/MSS.Afr.s.1872/75 RS Hennessey, 'Learning About Disease in Uganda: 1929–44 and 1949–55', 1983, p.3; RHL/MSS.Afr.s.1872/82 JK Hunter, 'Detailed Memorandum on Experiences in the Colonial Medical Service in Uganda, 1939–58', [n.d. *c.* 1983], p.3

[37] E.g., JB Purvis, *Handbook to British East Africa and Uganda*, London, 1900; HF Ward and JW Milligan, *Handbook of British East Africa, 1912–13*, London, 1913; *Colonial No.56: Information as to the Conditions and Cost of Living in the Colonies, Protectorates and Mandated Territories*, London, 1930. Sources of further regional information were listed in *Colonial Service Recruitment No.3*, p.14

[38] No source given, quoted in DF Clyde, *History of the Medical Services of Tanganyika*, Dar Es Salaam, 1962, p.104

[39] RHL/MSS.Afr.s.1872/153a Williams, 'Detailed Memoranda', p.1

[40] RHL/MSS.Afr.s.1872/144b Trowell, tape 1B

[41] L Sambon, 'Remarks on the Possibility of the Acclimatisation of Europeans in Tropical Regions', *BMJ*, i, 1897, pp.61–66

[42] Keeping school-age British children in Africa was officially advised against as late as 1936 *Colonial Service Recruitment No.1: The Colonial Service, General Information Regarding Colonial Appointments*, London, 1936, p.52

[43] Kenya Highlands were said to have 'a climate not dissimilar to a fine English summer', *African (East) No.1105: Information for the Use of Candidates to Appointments in the East African Medical Service*, London, 1925, p.6

[44] *Colonial Service Recruitment No.1*, p.8, p.51

[45] Anon, 'The White Man in the Tropics', *BMJ*, ii, 1911, pp.759–60; Anon, 'Medical Science and Colonization', *BMJ*, i, 1905, pp.1002–3

[46] RHL/MSS.Afr.s.1872/33 ACE Cole, 'Memorandum on Experiences in the Colonial Medical Service in Tanganyika, 1939–60', 10 April 1983; RHL/MSS.Afr.s.1872/75 Hennessey, 'Learning About Disease in Uganda', p.4; RHL/MSS.Afr.s.1872/153a Williams, 'Detailed Memoranda', p.1

[47] R Furse, *Aucuparius: Recollections of a Recruiting Officer*, Oxford, 1962, p.62

[48] RHL/MSS.Afr.s.1872/75 Hennessey, 'Learning About Disease in Uganda', 1983, p.2

[49] Harriet Deacon has argued that one of the attractions of the Cape during the early nineteenth century was that doctors could secure greater status and broader professional opportunities there than they could at home. H Deacon, 'Cape Town and 'Country' Doctors in the Cape Colony During the First Half of the Nineteenth Century,' *Social History of Medicine*, 1997, 10, pp.25–52

[50] Jeffries, *Colonial Empire*, p.125

[51] Cannadine, *Ornamentalism*, p. 67

[52] Furse articulated this idea that 'the man with the "country gentleman's" or "yeoman farmer's" background and traditions; the man who had an interest in peoples of a primitive type, their arts and handicrafts and customs, was often particularly suited to the work of the Colonial Service.' NA/CO/877/16/15 'Record of a Meeting of the Public School's Career's Association', 19 May 1938; see also Lord Cranworth, 'The Public School Boy in East Africa', *National Review.*, 336, 1911, pp.992–1000; See also H Kuklick, *The Imperial Bureaucrat: The Colonial Administrative Service in the Gold Coast, 1920–1939*, Stanford, CA, 1979, p.28

[53] RHL/MSS.Afr.s.1872/153a Williams, 'Detailed Memoranda', p.1

[54] D Hall, 'Settlers' Problems in Kenya', *Journal of Royal Society of Arts*, 78, 1930, pp.406–23; E Brodhurst-Hill, *So This is Kenya!*, London, 1936, p.2

[55] Smart, 'An Impression of Life in the Colonial Medical Service', p.125; E Trzebinski, *The Kenya Pioneers: the Frontiersmen of an Adopted Land*, London, 1991 [1985], p.63

[56] Smart, 'An Impression of Life in the Colonial Medical Service', p.125

[57] '...two black silk bow-ties. For dinner wear. Not made up "shyster" ones', A Field, '*Verb. Sap.' On Going to East Africa: British Central Africa, Uganda and Zanzibar and Big Game Shooting in East Africa*, Vol. 2, London, 1906, p.12

[58] NA/CO/877/13/8 Clipping: *The* [Melbourne] *Herald*, 'Empire Careers for Australians', 13 March 1936

[59] Jeffries, *Colonial Empire*, p.125

[60] Cranworth, 'The Public School Boy in East Africa', p.996

[61] Smart, 'An Impression of Life in the Colonial Medical Service', p.125

[62] M Harrison, *Public Health in British India: Anglo-Indian Preventative Medicine 1859–1914*, Cambridge, 1994, p.14

[63] RHL/MSS.Afr.s.1872/153a Williams, 'Detailed Memoranda', p.1

[64] RHL/MSS.Afr.s.1872/84 PW Hutton, 'Memorandum on Service as Physician Specialist, Acting Dean and Honorary Lecturer in Medicine, in Uganda, including Makerere, 1937–1961' [Feb.?] 1983, p.2

[65] 'John Buchanan', *BMJ*, ii, 1976, p.841

[66] NA/CO/877/7/8 'Visit by Major Hutchinson to Scottish Universities and to Liverpool University to Encourage Recruits', February 1930.

[67] NA/CO/877/7/8 Major Hutchinson, 'Report on Visit to Scottish Universities and Liverpool University', 7 April 1930

[68] RHL/MSS.Brit.Emp.s.415, Furse Papers, Memorandum: 'On the Difficulty of Obtaining Candidates for the Colonial Medical Service', March 1931

[69] H Marland, *Medicine and Society in Wakefield and Huddersfield, 1780–1870*, Cambridge, 1987; Peterson, *The Medical Profession in Mid-Victorian London*

[70] A Crowther, 'Life Choices of British Doctors in the Late Nineteenth Century—Consultant or GP?', paper given at the Wellcome Trust Centre for the History of Medicine at UCL, 13 November 2002

[71] D Kennedy, *Islands of White: Settler Society and Culture in Kenya and Southern Rhodesia, 1890–1939*, Durham, NC, 1987

[72] There are too numerous to mention but officers with a medical parent include Arthur Boase, Hugh Calwell, Arthur Cole; Graham Drury, Sidney Hinde, Aubrey Hodges, Alfred Mackie, Philip Manson-Bahr, Douglas Snell, John Shircore, Edwin Trim, Arthur Williams.

[73] RHL/MSS.Afr.s.1872/153a Williams, 'Detailed Memoranda', p.1

[74] 'PEC Manson-Bahr', *BMJ*, 314, 1997, p.609

[75] Harrison, *Public Health in British India*, p.29

[76] 'Arthur Morley', *BMJ*, 295, 1987, p.220

[77] RHL/MSS.Afr.s.1872/33 Cole, 'Memorandum on Experiences'

[78] 'Alfred Mackie', *BMJ*, ii, 1959, p.1262

[79] RHL/MSS.Afr.s.1872/16 Boase, 'Notes on Experiences', p.1

[80] 'John Shircore', *Lancet*, ii, 1953, p.94; 'Herbert Duke', *Who Was Who, 1961–1970*, Vol. VI, 1979 [1972], p.323; DG Crawford, *Roll of the Indian Medical Service, 1615–1930*, London, 1930, p.498

[81] 'Ernest Cook', *BMJ*, i, 1959, pp.1049–50, p.1049

[82] RHL/MSS.Afr.s.1653, Anderson, *Reminiscences*, Book I, p.14

[83] 'Retirement Tribute', [to Albert Owen], *East African Medical Journal*, 11, 1934–5, pp.363–4, p.363

[84] KNA/MOH/3/247 P Ross, P1(Med.), 1925; Although perhaps the Twinings were only related by marriage. Helen Twining was to marry the future Governor of Tanzania. D Bates, *A Gust of Plumes: A Biography of Lord Twining of Godalming and Tanganyika*, London, 1972, p.78

[85] 'William Kauntze', R Trail (ed.), *Munk's Roll*, London, 1968, pp.222–3; p.223; 'Roland Dowdeswell', *BMJ*, ii, 1956, p.305; 'William Ansorge', *Who Was Who, 1897–1916*, Vol. I, 1966 [1920], p.19; 'Arthur Milne', *Who Was Who, 1929–1940*, Vol. III, 1967 [1941], p. 945; WD Foster, 'Robert Moffat and the Beginnings of the Government Medical Service in Uganda', *Medical History*, 13, 1969, pp.237–50, p.237; 'Mary Turton', *BMJ*, ii, 1958, p.1048; 'John Carothers', *BMJ*, 300, 1990, p.1010; 'John Buchanan', *Who Was Who, 1971–1980*, Vol. VII, 1981, p.108; RHL/MSS.Afr.s.1872/84 Hutton, 'Memorandum on Service'

[86] C Wilcocks, *A Tropical Doctor in Africa and London*, unpublished autobiography [Wellcome Library], Surrey, 1977, p.41

[87] RHL/MSS.Afr.s.1872/33 Cole, 'Memorandum on Experiences'

[88] RHL/MSS.Afr.s.1872/9 RE Barrett, 'Memorandum on Experiences in the Colonial Medical Service in East Africa, 1928–55', 18 March 1983

[89] It was directly on this recommendation that Calwell applied (he was later to work, in 1930, in Clearkin's Dar Es Salaam laboratory) RHL/MSS.Afr.s.1872/24 HG Calwell, 'Memorandum on Experiences in the Colonial Medical Service in Tanganyika, 1930–49', 25 April 1983, pp.1–2

[90] 'Arthur Williams', *BMJ*, i, 1958, p.1421

Chapter 5: Identity and Experience II: Ideological Reasons for Being a Doctor in East Africa (pp.59-71)

[1] A Beck, *A History of the British Medical Administration of East Africa: 1900–1950*, Cambridge, MA, 1999 [1970], p.206

[2] Many obituaries speak of firm Christian belief as one of the main guiding lights of MOs. Pat Holden has also noted this common denominator. P Holden, *Doctors and Other Medical Personnel in the Public Health Services of Africa, 1930–1965*, Oxford, 1984, p.1

[3] N Vance, *'The Sinews of the Spirit': The Ideal of Christian Manliness in Victorian Literature and Religious Thought*, Cambridge, 1985

[4] E.g., works by Marryat, Ballantyne and Kingston in the Victorian era, Henty and Stables in the late nineteenth century and Johns (creator of 'Biggles') in the inter-war years. This tradition continued until the mid 1950s, see 'Introduction' in J Richards (ed.), *Imperialism and Juvenile Literature*, Manchester, 1989, pp.1–11

[5] JM MacKenzie, *Propaganda and Empire: the Manipulation of British Public Opinion, 1880–1960*, Manchester, 1997 [1986], pp.199–226

[6] A Warren, 'Popular Manliness: Baden-Powell, Scouting, and the Development of Manly Character', in JA Mangan and J Walvin (eds.), *Manliness and Morality: Middle-Class Masculinity in Britain and America, 1800–1940*, Manchester, 1987, pp.199–219, p.202

[7] E.g., George Allen, Farnworth Anderson, William Ansorge, Robert Archibald, Arthur Bagshawe, Arthur Claypon-Gray, James Hunter, William Kauntze, Archibald Mackinnon, Norman Maclennan, Dawson Milne, Robert Moffat, Arthur Morley and Mary Turton

[8] AD Milne, 'The Rise of the Colonial Medical Service', *Kenya and East African Medical Journal*, 5, 1928–9, pp.50–8, p.50

[9] WD Foster, 'Robert Moffat and the Beginnings of Government Medical Service', *Medical History*, 13, 1969, pp.237–50, p.241

[10] WD Foster, *The Early History of Scientific Medicine in Uganda*, Nairobi, 1970, p.15

[11] RHL/MSS.Afr.s.1872/153a Williams, 'Detailed Memoranda', p.1

[12] 'William Kauntze', Trail (ed.), *Munk's Roll*, p.223

[13] 'William Kauntze', *East African Medical Journal*, 24, 1947, p.425

[14] RHL/MSS.Afr.s.1872/144a HC Trowell, 'Detailed Memorandum on Service as a Medical Officer, Lecturer in Medicine and Specialist Physician in Kenya and Uganda, 1929–57', [n.d. *c*.1984], p.2

[15] RHL/MSS.Afr.s.1872/144b Trowell, tape 1B

[16] E.g., On retirement Clare Wiggins joined the Church Missionary Society and then was ordained an Anglican minister; Marcus Broadbent left the Colonial Medical Service to join the Church Missionary Society in Uganda; Hugh Trowell was also ordained upon retirement and acted as a hospital chaplain; Arthur Brown became a ship's surgeon and then a missionary; Frederick Wright, described as having been 'always a missionary at heart', became a missionary in Tanzania. ('Frederick Wright', *BMJ*, 313, 1996, p.556); Douglas Snell became a churchwarden on retirement.

[17] Beck, *History of British Medical Administration*, pp.53–7

[18] Robert Stones had a wide-ranging missionary career in Nigeria, Egypt, Tanzania and Uganda. See 'Robert Stones', *BMJ*, ii, 1961, pp.966–7

[19] C Jeffries, *The Colonial Empire and its Civil Service*, Cambridge, 1938, p.154

[20] RHL/MSS.Afr.s.1872/9 Barrett, 'Memorandum on Experiences', p.1

[21] NA/CO/877/16/15 'Meeting of the Public School's Career's Association'

[22] MacKenzie, *Propaganda and Empire*

23 These authors built on a late-eighteenth century tradition of African travel writing, e.g., J Bruce, *Travels to Discover the Source of the Nile*, London, 1790 and M Park, *Travel in the Interior Districts of Africa*, London, 1799.

24 P Brantlinger, 'Victorians and Africans: The Genealogy of the Myth of the Dark Continent', *Critical Inquiry*, 1985, 12, pp.166–203, p.176

25 F Driver, *Geography Militant: Cultures of Exploration and Empire*, Oxford, 2001, p.82. See also Driver, Felix and Luciana Martins, *Tropical Visions in an Age of Empire*, Chicago, 2005.

26 Driver, *Geography Militant*, p.82

27 Kirk-Greene created a bibliography of novels which featured, or were by, Colonial Service entrants and has thereby shown the immense influence these novels had in forming and perpetuating an image of a desirable adventurous career (although none of the novels detail a specifically Colonial Medical Service career). A Kirk-Greene, 'The Colonial Service in the Novel' in John Smith (ed.), *Administering Empire: The British Colonial Service in Retrospect*, London, 1999, pp.19–48

28 D Hammond and A Jablow, *The Africa That Never Was: Four Centuries of British Writing About Africa*, New York, NY, 1970; ML Pratt, *Imperial Eyes: Travel Writing and Transculturation*, London, 1992; D Spurr, *The Rhetoric of Empire: Colonial Discourse in Journalism, Travel Writing and Imperial Administration*, Durham, NC, 1993

29 TG August, *The Selling of Empire, British and French Imperialist Propaganda, 1890–1940*, Westport, CT, 1985; T Richards, 'Selling Darkest Africa' in *The Commodity Culture of Victorian England: Advertising and Spectacle, 1851–1914*, Stanford, CA, 1990, pp.119–67; JM MacKenzie (ed.), *Imperialism and Popular Culture*, Manchester, 1993 [1986]; MacKenzie, *Propaganda and Empire*

30 A McKay, *Tibet and the British Raj: The Frontier Cadre, 1904–1947*, Surrey, 1997, p.191

31 Driver, *Geography Militant*, p.126 quoting HM Stanley, *The Congo and the Founding of its Free State*, 2 Vols., London, 1885, Vol. 2, p.266, 230

32 When Kirk-Greene was accepted as a colonial administrator in Nigeria in 1949, the local paper, the *Tunbridge Wells Courier*, ran the story 'Sanders of the River Job for Local Boy'. Kirk-Greene, 'The Colonial Service in the Novel', p.19

33 E Waugh, *Scoop*, Harmondsworth, 2000 [1938], pp.44–5

34 EA Reeves, *Hints to Travellers*, Vol. 1, London, 1935, (11th Ed.), pp.1–2; for a suggested list of what a colonial wife should take see E Bradley, *Dearest Priscilla: Letters to the Wife of a Colonial Civil Servant*, London, 1950, pp.238–9

35 RHL/MSS.Afr.s.1872/144b Trowell, tape 1B

36 E.g.: TH Parke. *Guide to Health in Africa*, London, 1893; H Ziemann, *Hints to Europeans in Tropical Stations Without a Doctor and to Travellers in Warm Climates*, [trans. P Falcke], London, 1910; CJ Ryan, *Health Preservation in West Africa*, London, 1914; *Hints on the Preservation of Health in Tropical Africa*, London, 1943 [1938]

37 A Balfour, 'Vistas and Visions: Some Aspects of the Colonial Medical Services', *Glasgow Medical Journal*, 6, 1924, pp.353–74, p.361; for a literary expression of this combination of game and parasite hunter see A Torrance, *Tracking Down the Enemies of Man*, New York, NY, 1928

38 Curtin, 'The White Man's Grave'; Curtin has analysed the statistics for West Africa and put civilian mortality somewhere between five and seven times higher than the expected death rate at home. Curtin, 'The End of 'White Man's Grave'? p.88

39 JA Carman, *A Medical History of the Colony and Protectorate of Kenya: a Personal Memoir*, London, 1976, p.41

40 McKay, *Tibet and the British Raj*, p.75

41 Smith (ed.), *Administering Empire*, p. ix

42 AGH Smart, 'An Impression of Life in the Colonial Medical Service', *St Thomas' Hospital Gazette*, 37, 1939, p.123

43 R Furse, *Aucuparius: Recollections of a Recruiting Officer*, Oxford, 1962, p.221

44 Balfour, 'Vistas and Visions', p.355

45 *Ibid.*, p.356

[46] NA/CO/877/3/685 Minute: Mr Denniston (? illegible), 'Applications from New Zealanders for Appointments in the Colonial Service', 26 January 1926

[47] NA/CO/877/13/8 'Empire Careers for Australians'

[48] Lord Lloyd, Secretary of State, quoted in C Jeffries, *Partners For Progress: The Men and Women of the Colonial Service*, London, 1949, p.19

[49] Hoppe argues for heroism as part of the appeal of a career in imperial science, KA Hoppe, *Sleeping Sickness Control in British East Africa, 1900–1960*, Westport, CT, 2003, pp.30–42

[50] KNA/MOH/1/9950 J Mitchell to E Northley, Governor EAP4 October 1920

[51] Mckay has drawn attention to this commercial aspect of the Orientalist argument. McKay, *Tibet and the British Raj*, p.206

[52] W Ansorge, *Under the African Sun: A Description of Native Races in Uganda, Sporting Adventures and Other Experiences*, London, 1899, p.3

[53] RHL/MSS.Afr.s.1653, Anderson, *Reminiscences*, Book I, pp.13–14

[54] RHL/MSS.Afr.s.1872/82 Hunter, 'Detailed Memorandum', p.3

[55] RHL/MSS.Afr.s.1872/153a Williams, 'Detailed Memoranda', p.1

[56] RHL/MSS.Afr.s.1872/75 Hennessey, 'Learning About Disease in Uganda', p.1

[57] PH Manson-Bahr and A Alcock, *The Life and Work of Sir Patrick Manson*, London, 1927, p.5, quoted in DM Haynes, *Imperial Medicine: Patrick Manson and the Conquest of Tropical Disease*, Philadelphia, PA, 2001, p.18

[58] A Castellani, *Microbes, Men and Monarchs: A Doctor's Life in Many Lands*, London, 1960, p.29

[59] Smart, 'An Impression of Life in the Colonial Medical Service', p.124

[60] Jeffries, *Colonial Empire*, p.126

[61] *Colonial Service Recruitment No.3: Information Regarding the Colonial Medical Service*, London, 1935, p.16

[62] Smart, 'An Impression of Life in the Colonial Medical Service', p.123

[63] 'Fairfax Bell', *BMJ*, i, 1972, p.450

[64] Also see the comments in this obituary that relate his love of natural history to his choice of career in Africa. 'GDH Carpenter', *Lancet*, i, 1953, pp.300–1, p.300; Perhaps Carpenter was the most serious of all the East African naturalists of the period. On retirement from the Colonial Service he became Professor of Zoology at Oxford (1933–48), served as Vice-President of the Linnean Society, (1935–6); and President of the Royal Entomological Society (1945–6), he also published many books and papers on the subject. 'GDH Carpenter', *BMJ*, i, 1953, pp.406–7

[65] *Ibid.*, p.406; also 'Obituary', *The Times*, 31 January 1953, p.8

[66] 'Arthur Bagshawe', *Lancet*, i, 1950, pp.693–4; 'Enrico Bayon', *BMJ*, ii, 1952, pp.1260–1, p.1261; 'William Lamborn', *BMJ*, ii, 1959, pp.310–1, p. 311; 'Aubrey Hodges', *BMJ*, i, 1946, p.933

[67] Foster, *Early History of Scientific Medicine*, p.15

[68] Ansorge, *Under the African Sun*, 1899

[69] Brockman spent the early part of his career in Somaliland where he authored *Mammals of Somaliland* [n.d.] and *British Somaliland* [n.d.] See 'Ralph Brockman', *Who Was Who, 1951–1960*, Vol. V, 1967 [1961], p.318; 'John Shircore', *Lancet*, ii, 1953, p.94 ; 'Clare Wiggins', *BMJ*, i, 1966, pp.363–4, p.364

[70] NA/CO/877/8/18 Furse, 'Progress Report for the Appointments Department, No.2', pp.9–10

[71] NA/CO/877/16/15 'Meeting of the Public School's Career's Association'; Smart, 'An Impression of Life in the Colonial Medical Service', p.123

[72] The fashion of tropical medical careers to further Empire has been argued particularly by J Farley, *Bilharzia: A History of Imperial Tropical Medicine*, Cambridge, 2003 [1991]; Hoppe, *Sleeping Sickness Control*

[73] NA/CO/877/2/49403 Furse, 'Notes for Proposed Question and Answer in the House of Lords as to the Scheme for the Admission of Canadians to the Colonial Service', 4 June 1923

[74] Balfour, 'Vistas and Visions', pp.369-70

[75] RHL/MSS.Afr.s.1872/82 Hunter, 'Detailed Memorandum', p.3

[76] RHL/MSS.Afr.s.1872/75 Hennessey, 'Learning About Disease in Uganda', p.3

[77] *Ibid.*, pp.3–4

[78] This aspect is stressed in Balfour, 'Vistas and Visions', pp.353–74

[79] A dual appeal also recognised by the Colonial Office See *Colonial Service Recruitment, No.3*, 1935, p.10

[80] 'James Armstrong', *East African Medical Journal*, 13, 1936–7, pp.58–9; 'Robert Cormack', *East African Medical Journal*, 31, 1954, p.186; 'Frederick Corson', *East African Medical Journal*, 25, 1948, pp.18–9, p.18; 'Edward Clarence', *East African Medical Journal*, 14, 1937–8, pp.138–9, p.138; 'Sidney Hinde', *Who Was Who, 1929–1940*, pp.643–4; 'John Bernard Davey', *BMJ*, 3, 1967, p.743

[81] 'Henry Albert Bödeker', *East African Medical Journal*, 17, 1940–1, pp.171–2, p.171; Unusually, Anderson seems to have got the job locally, without having to have returned to London for interview RHL/MSS.Afr.s.1653 Anderson, *Reminiscences*, Book 1, p.20. Tichborne's early history is related in KNA/MOH/1/5513 'Confidential Memorandum on Private Practice by Government Medical Officers in the East Africa Protectorate', 18 June 1909. Although Heard does not appear in the *Colonial Lists*, the *Medical Directory* in 1911 listed him as working in a practice entitled 'MacDonald and Heard'. By 1918 his entries in the *Medical Directory* list him as being a Captain in the East African Medical Service, so it is likely that he joined the service in a temporary capacity to help the war effort.

[82] KNA/MOH/1/5513 W Radford to PMO, 9 July 1909

[83] RHL/MSS.Afr.s.1872/75 Hennessey, 'Learning About Disease in Uganda', p.1

[84] 'The Colonial Medical Services', *BMJ*, ii, 1931, p.21

[85] A Kirk-Greene, *On Crown Service: A History of HM Colonial and Overseas Civil Services, 1837–1997*, London, 1999, p.8

[86] The Overseas Pensioners Association still produces a bi-annual journal for former Colonial Servants. The Corona Club, the official Colonial Service club, closed as recently as 1999.

Chapter 6: The Organisation of the Colonial Medical Service in

East Africa (pp.72-85)

[1] WL/CMAC/PP/HCT/A5 E Bray, *Hugh Trowell: Pioneer Nutritionist*, unpublished biography, 1988, [Chapter 2] p.18

[2] Perhaps the most striking example is Beck's monograph. Despite its title and considerable use as a history of medical policy in the region, this book offers virtually no description of medical duties and the structure of the administration. A Beck, A *History of the British Medical Administration of East Africa: 1900–1950*, Cambridge, MA, 1999 [1970]

[3] J Smith (ed.), *Administering Empire: The British Colonial Service in Retrospect*, London, 1999; EE Sabben-Clare, DJ Bradley and K Kirkwood (eds.), *Health in Tropical Africa During the Colonial Period*, Oxford, 1980. This is a comment on the secondary sources and does not include memoirs by doctors.

[4] 'Organisation of the Colonial Medical Service', *BMJ*, i, 1902, pp.347–8

[5] These similarities were acknowledged at the time. KNA/MOH/1/5517 untitled document [History of British Medical Administration in East Africa], [n.d. *c*.1909]

[6] KNA/MOH/1/7973 J Davey, PMO Tanzania to A Milne, PMO Nairobi, 13 April 1921

[7] Eg, NA/CO/533/231 PMOs' Conference, 1920; See also Beck, *History of British Medical Administration*, pp.183–5

[8] '[A] kind of pyramid' to quote C Jeffries, *Partners for Progress: The Men and Women of the Colonial Service*, London, 1949, p.96

[9] NA/CO/850/12/11 'Seniority', *Colonial Regulations: Being the Regulations for His Majesty's Colonial Service*, London, 1932, pp.95–96

[10] This seems even more fitting when it is remembered that most of the early medical departments were military administrations before they became civil ones. Early debates in the *BMJ* also called for the organisation of the Colonial Medical Service to be based upon the model provided by the Army Medical Services. G Evatt, 'Notes on the Organisation of the Colonial Medical Service of the Empire', *BMJ*, ii, 1896, pp.863–4; CH Eyles, 'The Colonial Medical Service: a Rejoinder', *BMJ*, i, 1897, p.216

[11] Job titles often changed. Throughout this chapter, I use the *earliest* job titles when referring in a general, non-specific, context to a job. In the majority of instances the earliest given job title was the one that was in place for the largest proportion of the period.

[12] Eventually Africans in the European medical establishment in East Africa could obtain full medical degrees. J Iliffe, *East African Doctors: a History of the Modern Profession*, Cambridge, 1999

[13] HG Calwell, 'Nineteen Years in the Colonial Medical Service', *Ulster Medical Journal*, 65 (supplement), 1993, pp.(s)1–(s)42, p.(s)35

[14] *Miscellaneous No.99: Colonial Medical Appointments*, London, 1921 [29th Ed.], p.3; *Colonial Service Recruitment No. 3A: The Colonial Service. Information for the use of Candidates for Appointment to the Colonial Medical Service*, London, 1931, p.5

[15] Such as that created in 1931 for Henry Gordon, as consultant psychiatrist to Mathari Hospital, Kenya.

[16] It was not until 1903 that job titles aside from these two were officially listed for the Uganda Medical Department (the following year for Kenya) NA/CO/613/2 Uganda Blue Book, 1902–3; NA/CO/543/3 East Africa Protectorate Blue Book, 1903–4

[17] *The Dominions Office and Colonial Office List*, London, 1940, pp.366–7; p.491; p.509 NB: The *Colonial Office List* published information from the previous year; information derived from this source is presumed to have occurred during the year *before* the publication date.

[18] JL Gilks, The Medical Department and the Health Organization in Kenya, 1909–1933', *East African Medical Journal*, 9, 1932–3, pp.340–54, p.345; *The Dominions Office and Colonial Office List*, London, 1927, p.453, p.478

[19] For a concise explanation of all of the administrative changes introduced in the 1920s which favoured division of the Medical Departments of East Africa into specialist branches see Kenya, *Annual Medical Report, 1926*, Nairobi, 1927, p.3

[20] For an announcement and explanation of these changes see Kenya, *Annual Medical Report, 1933*, Nairobi, 1935, pp.2–3

[21] NA/CO/612/11 'Changes in Medical Titles', *Uganda Protectorate Government Gazette*, 15 August 1925, p.256; [These changes were formalised in] NA/CO/612/11 'The Public Officers (Change of Titles) Ordinance', 1926', *Uganda Protectorate Government Gazette*, 15 January 1926, p.16; see also NA/CO/542/20 'Medical Officers (Change of Titles) Ordinance', *Kenya Colony Government Gazette*, 24 February 1926, p.281; NA/CO/542/32 'Bill to Provide for the Change of Title of Certain Public Officers, 1934', *Kenya Government Gazette*, 30 January 1934, p.104; See also NA/CO/850/12/13 Circular Despatch: T Stanton to Colonial Governors, November 1932. The first published schedule is *Miscellaneous No.441: The Colonial Medical Service, Special Regulations by the Secretary of State for the Colonies*, London, 1934

[22] *African (East) No.1103: Regulations for the East African Medical Service*, London, 1925, pp.5–6

[23] *The Dominions Office and Colonial Office List*, London, 1926, p.254, p.442, p.459

[24] In theory at least the job title had changed in all territories, but in fact, it did not appear as changed for Tanzania until the following year's *Colonial Office List*. Also NA/CO/542/32 'Bill to Provide for the Change of Title of Certain Public Officers, 1934'

[25] *African (East) No.1103*, p.5

[26] For example, Burke Gaffney wrote of Shircore '[E]ven when he was director, he used to slip into the laboratory'. 'John Owen Shircore', *Lancet*, ii, 1953, p.94

[27] C Jeffries, *The Colonial Empire and its Civil Service*, Cambridge, 1938, p.154

[28] It is worth noting that it took some years for legislative councils to be set up in each colonial dependency — i.e. Kenya in 1905; Uganda in 1920 and Tanzania in 1926. In 1938 the DMS

ceased to be a member of the Executive Council, Kenya. Colony and Protectorate of Kenya, *Annual Medical Report, 1938–9, (Abbreviated)* [n.d. *c.*1940], p.1

[29] G Maclean, 'Medical Administration in the Tropics', *BMJ*, i, 1950, pp.756–61, p.757

[30] This responsibility was exercised via the PMO's Presidency of the Medical Registration Board. *Ibid.*; JA Carman, *A Medical History of the Colony and Protectorate of Kenya: a Personal Memoir*, London, 1976, p.9

[31] KNA/MOH/1/1497 'Medical Building Requirements', PMO to Director Public Works Department, 14 September 1906; 'Uganda Building Requirements, 1907-08', J Will, PMO Uganda, to Superintendent Public Works Department, 21 September 1906; KNA/MOH/1/1633 'New Buildings Needed', Memorandum: A Milne to Director Public Works Department, 29 June 1912

[32] KNA/MOH/1/504 A Milne, PMO Kenya, to C Ainsworth, 16 March 1913

[33] Gilks, 'Proposed Expansion of the Medical Services in Kenya', *Kenya Medical Journal*, 2, 1925–6, pp.318–20, p.319

[34] It was titled Assistant Medical Officer, paid at a higher rate to other MOs. NA/CO/613/1 Uganda Protectorate, Blue Book, 1901–2

[35] Gilks, The Medical Department and the Health Organization', pp.342–3; See also, East Africa Protectorate, *Annual Medical Report, 1913*, 1914, p.12

[36] The history of the deputyships is very complicated. For a detailed examination see A Crozier, *The Colonial Medical Service and the Colonial Identity: Kenya, Uganda and Tanzania Before World War Two*, University College London, PhD, 2005, p.159.

[37] The title Deputy Director of Laboratory Services (DDLS) was never used in Uganda. Laboratory medicine was officially supervised by the DL or, after 1930, the Director of the Human Trypanosomiasis Institute. These positions seemed to be on the same level as the other Deputy Directorships and were basically equivalent to the DDLS used in Tanzania and Kenya.

[38] In 1933 Kenya lost the position of DDLS, and Uganda amalgamated two of its three separate deputy directorships (those of the medical and sanitary services) to form a single undifferentiated job title called DDMS. (*The Dominions Office and Colonial Office List*, London, 1934, pp.387–8; p.462). In 1934 Kenya also abolished separate deputyships in favour of one single general position of DDMS (*Ibid*, 1935, p.342). Tanzania, however, continued until 1936 to have three separate branches headed by three different deputies (*Ibid*, 1937, p.470).

[39] For an explanation of this change occurring after unification in 1934 see Kenya, *Annual Medical Report, 1933*, Nairobi, 1935, p.3.

[40] WD Foster, 'Robert Moffat and the Beginnings of the Government Medical Service in Uganda', *Medical History*, 13, 1969, pp.237–50, pp.247–8. Foster incorrectly claims that Moffat stood down from his position as PMO to that of an 'ordinary Medical Officer'; Government records contradict this and the 1906 *Colonial Office List* shows Moffat as SMO.

[41] In 1910 3 of 58 medical departmental workers were SMOs; in 1920, 11 of 87; in 1930, 27 of 193 and in 1939, 15 of 147

[42] *African (East) No.1103*, p.7. The role of the Indian Sub Assistant Surgeons was very large: see RHL/MSS.Afr.s.1872/9 RE Barrett, 'Memorandum on Experiences in the Colonial Medical Service in East Africa, 1928-55', 1983, p.4

[43] Carman, *Medical History of Kenya*, p.72; RHL/MSS.Afr.s.1872/153a AW Williams, 'Detailed Memoranda on Experiences in the Colonial Medical Service in Uganda and Tanganyika, 1931-1949', [n.d. *c.*1983], p.9

[44] From 1919 in Kenya, MOs were also asked to recommend exactly how long leave for European officials (they had examined) should be. KNA/MOH/1/9410 Circular Despatch: PMO, Kenya to all MOs, 23 August 1919

[45] *African (East) No.1103*, pp.7–8

[46] E.g., David Donald had to work closely with the Public Works Department in planning and establishing a district hospital in Eldama Ravine, Kenya. RHL/MSS.Afr.s.ff.312–321, D

Donald, Sketch Plan of New Hospital, *c*.1900; see also Hodges involvement with hospital building in Uganda RHL/MSS.Afr.s.1782, ADP Hodges, Diaries 1898–1907, 4 April 1899

[47] Via these regulations MOs could 'medically examine any and every person on board any ship arriving at any port of the Protectorate' NA/CO/457/1 'East Africa Plague Regulations, 1899', *East Africa and Uganda Government Gazette*, 1 June 1900, pp.1–4, p.3

[48] This system of government was set up in Tanzania in 1925. J Iliffe, *A Modern History of Tanganyika*, Cambridge, 1994, [1979], pp.320–1; 1921 in Kenya via the Public Health Ordinance. NA/CO/542/15 'Public Health Ordinance, 1921'; 1935 in Uganda. Uganda Protectorate, *Annual Medical Report,1935*, Entebbe, 1936, p.5

[49] For sources see Crozier, *Colonial Medical Officer and Colonial Identity*, PhD, 2005, pp.163–4

[50] Gilks, 'The Medical Department and Health Organization', p.349

[51] AJ Boase, 'Reminiscences of Surgery in Uganda', *East African Medical Journal*, 31, 1954, pp.197–203, p.201

[52] NA/CO/457/4 'Notice', *East Africa and Uganda Government Gazette*, 15 July 1903, p.251; for information on Simpson see RA Baker and RA Bayliss, 'William John Ritchie Simpson (1855–1931): Public Health and Tropical Medicine', *Medical History*, 1987, 31, pp.450–65

[53] For life as a MOH see RR Scott, 'The Growth of a Public Health Service in a Tropical Town', *East African Medical Journal*, 10, 1933–4, pp.130–44; Calwell, 'Nineteen Years in the Colonial Medical Service', esp. pp.(s)2–3

[54] *Colonial Service Recruitment No.3: Information Regarding the Colonial Medical Service*, London, 1935, p.29, p.30, p.35. R Scott, (DMS, Tanzania 1935–45), expressed his conviction while still a Senior Health Officer that 'public health and medicine are one and the same thing' and that the duties of an MO could not be subdivided. Scott, 'The Growth of a Public Health Service in a Tropical Town', p.132

[55] Boase, 'Reminiscences of Surgery', p.197

[56] KNA/MOH/1/9950 Private Secretary, Kenya to J Mitchell, 18 November 1920

[57] Unlike the French Colonial Medical Service which had employed Africans as *aides-medécins* since 1905, the British did not have any systematised training schemes for Africans until after World War One. Iliffe, *East African Doctors*, p.27

[58] Beck, *History of British Medical Administration*, p.147; DF Clyde, *History of the Medical Services of Tanganyika*, Dar Es Salaam, 1962, pp.77–8

[59] W Kauntze, 'Memorandum on Departmental Policy', Uganda Protectorate, *Annual Medical Report, 1934*, Entebbe, 1935, pp.61–4, p.62

[60] This is a list of the main paperwork; there were many more specific forms to fill out for all manner of procedures. FCO/14634 'Organisation of the Medical and Sanitary Services in the British Colonies: Replies to Circular Despatch: 1 February 1913', *Standing Orders for the Medical Department* [Uganda], 1912, pp.6–10. In the later period as bureaucracy increased so did the paperwork.

[61] Boase, 'Reminiscences of Surgery', p.198

[62] Kauntze, 'Memorandum on Departmental Policy', p.64

[63] RHL/MSS.Afr.s.1782, Hodges, Diaries, 27 November 1905; RHL/MSS.Afr.s.1872/153a Williams, 'Detailed Memoranda', p.6(a)

[64] RHL/MSS.Afr.s.1872/82 JK Hunter, 'Duties of [a] District Medical Officer'; 'Duties of a Provincial Medical Officer', 1951

[65] KNA/MOH/1/1287 W Radford to PMO [asking for formalisation of his duties and precise explanation of what they entailed], Nairobi, 1906; KNA/MOH/1/5664 R Small to PMO, Nairobi, 13 January 1910; for examples illustrating the formulation of the job descriptions of the senior positions see KNA/MOH/1/8218 A Milne, 'Duties of the DPMO and DPSO', 12 February 1914

[66] AD Milne 'The Rise of the Colonial Medical Service', *Kenya and East African Medical Journal*, 5, 1928–9, pp.50–8, p.54

[67] NA/CO/533/203 Minute: Bottomley, 24 June 1918

[68] Beck, *History of British Medical Administration*, p.48

[69] RHL/MSS.Afr.s.ff.312–321, D Donald, Letter, 6 October 1900; RHL/MSS.Afr.s.1091, Papers of CJ Baker, Baker to his Father, 23 November 1913

[70] R Ross, 'Some Suggestions for the Improvement of Sanitary and Medical Practice in the Tropics', *BMJ*, ii, 1900, pp.553–4; F Fremantle, 'The Colonial Conference', *BMJ*, i, 1907, p.536; 'The Future of Tropical Medicine', *BMJ*, i, 1909, p.1545

[71] 'Tropical Medicine', *BMJ*, ii, 1912, pp.40–2, p.40; see also 'Sanitary Organization in the Tropics', *BMJ*, ii, 1913, pp.377–9

[72] NA/CO/543/3 East Africa Protectorate Blue Book, 1903–4

[73] KNA/MOH/1/1287 W Radford, 'Correspondence over the Sanitary Condition of Nairobi', 1906

[74] East Africa Protectorate, *Annual Medical Report, 1911*, 1912, p.7, p.12, p.15, p.17, pp.21–9

[75] KNA/MOH/1/1231 'Professor Simpson's Report on Mombassa Sanitation and Other Correspondence', 1913; See also WJ Simpson, *African No.1025: Report on Sanitary Matters in the East Africa Protectorate, Uganda and Zanzibar*, 1915; East Africa Protectorate, *Annual Medical Report, 1913*, 1914, p.18

[76] Beck, *History of British Medical Administration*, p.147; Clyde, *History of the Medical Services of Tanganyika*, p.117; RHL/MSS.Afr.s.2032 WV Kendall, 'Extracts from the Diaries, Letters and Memory of WV Kendall whilst serving in the Colonial Civil Service Uganda Protectorate 1922–1930'

[77] RHL/MSS.Afr.s.1872/9 Barrett, 'Memorandum on Experiences', p.9

[78] *The Colonial Office List*, London, 1920, pp.404–5

[79] RHL/MSS.Afr.s.1872/153a Williams, 'Detailed Memoranda', p.6

[80] NA/CO/737/5 'Establishment of Districts, Proclamation No.1, 1926', *Tanganyika Territory Government Gazette, Supplement*, 5 March 1926, pp.35–6; 'Establishment of Provinces, 1926', *Tanganyika Territory Government Gazette, Supplement*, 5 March 1926, pp.37–8; Carman, *Medical History of Kenya*, pp.33–4

[81] *Ibid.*

[82] This was an enduring feature. RS Ladkin, 'The Medical Officer and Local Government', *Journal of African Administration*, 5, 1953, pp.21–30

[83] RHL/MSS.Afr.s.1653, Anderson, *Reminiscences*, Book I, p.21

[84] The importance of barazas for health propaganda was stressed in Kauntze, 'Memorandum on Departmental Policy', p.63; see also Carman, *Medical History of Kenya*, p.34

[85] RHL/MSS.Afr.s.1872/82 Hunter, 'Detailed Memorandum', p.15

[86] Gilks, 'The Medical Department and Health Organization', p.347

[87] RHL/MSS.Afr.s.1653, Anderson, *Reminiscences*, Book I, p.40

[88] Beck, *History of British Medical Administration*, pp.131–5

[89] Under Gilks leadership, 1920–32, fourteen medical units were established in the reserves and 'over one hundred' dispensaries. Kenya Colony and Protectorate, *Annual Medical Report, 1932*, Nairobi, 1934, pp.1–3, p.2

[90] A Beck, *Medicine,Tradition and Development in Kenya and Tanzania, 1920–1970*, Waltham, MA, 1981, p.15

[91] For a detailed example of a medical safari see JL Gilks, 'A Medical Safari in a Native Reserve', *Kenya Medical Journal*, 1, 1924–5, pp.270–4

[92] RHL/MSS.Afr.s.1872/33 ACE Cole, 'Memorandum on Experiences in the Colonial Medical Service in Tanganyika, 1939–60', 10 April 1983

[93] There were many, e.g., Cole undertook a sleeping sickness survey in 1938. *Ibid.*; Rawson undertook a smallpox investigative safari in Uganda, 1923 RHL/MSS.Afr.s.1421, Papers of PH Rawson, Rawson to PMO, Entebbe, 31 March 1923. Carman was to investigate Yaws at Maseno, Kenya. Carman, *Medical History of Kenya*, p.33

[94] Although the bulk of change occurred after 1920, there were also some earlier moves towards promoting Africans as hospital dispensers, e.g., J Thomson agitated over the issue.

NA/CO/533/210 'Evidence of Dr James Hutcheon Thomson to the East Africa Protectorate Economic Commission', enclosure Northey to Milner, 5 June 1919

[95] GO Ndege, *Health State and Society in Kenya*, Rochester, 2001, p.81; G Keane, 'Review of Native Medical Services for 1924' in Uganda Protectorate, *Annual Medical Report, 1924*, Entebbe, 1925, pp.62–4; WL/CMAC/MS/5677/1 J Davey, Private Papers, 'British Administration in Tanganyika', 1944, p.27

[96] Iliffe, *East African Doctors,* p.103

[97] Maclean, 'Medical Administration in the Tropics', p.757

[98] 'Editorial', *East African Medical Journal*, 9, 1932–3, p.339

[99] Beck, *History of British Medical Administration*, pp.174–5

[100] NA/CO/543/3 East Africa Protectorate Blue Book, 1903–4; Despite a high profile visit to Uganda in 1906 of Robert Koch KNA/MOH/1/5898 'Visit of Dr Koch', 7 June 1906

[101] East Africa Protectorate, *Annual Medical Report, 1915*, 1916, p.9; *The Colonial Office List*, London, 1915, p.403

[102] Clyde, *History of the Medical Services of Tanganyika*, pp.28–32; p.102; Ross in Africa is dealt with in P Cranfield, *Science and Empire: East Coast Fever in Rhodesia and the Transvaal*, History of East Coast Fever, Cambridge, 2002 [1991]

[103] 'Medical Appointments Under the Colonial Office', *BMJ*, ii, 1923, pp.394–6, p.395; 'Tropical Medicine', *BMJ*, ii, 1925, p.235; also 'A Health Department for the Colonial Office', *BMJ*, ii, 1925, p.267

[104] KNA/MOH/1/8093 'Memorandum on Scientific Research in Kenya', December 1924

[105] 'The Colonial Conference', *BMJ*, i, 1927, p.1040.

[106] Beck, *History of British Medical Administration*, pp.183–90

[107] Gilks, 'Proposed Expansion of the Medical Services'

[108] Kauntze, 'Memorandum on Departmental Policy', p.61; East Africa Protectorate, *Annual Medical Report, 1919*, 1920, p.18

Chapter 7: Experiences in the Field (pp.86-101)

[1] RHL/MSS.Afr.s.708 (1), WK Connell, Diary 1924–5, 2 October 1924, pp.23–4

[2] Time was usually given (except in periods of staff shortages) for the candidate to terminate any other employment in which they may have been engaged. *Colonial Service Recruitment No.3: Information Regarding the Colonial Medical Service*, London, 1935, p.8

[3] This same point is made for the Indian Civil Service see DC Potter, 'The Shaping of Young Recruits in the Indian Civil Service', *The Indian Journal of Public Administration*, 23, 1977, pp.875–89

[4] Gilks remembered his 'feeling of helplessness' on being directly posted to a remote station. Gilks, 'Proposed Expansion of the Medical Services in Kenya', *Kenya Medical Journal*, 2, 1925–6, pp.318–20, p.320

[5] For a description of getting settled in a new posting see RHL/MSS.Afr.s.1872/153a Williams, 'Detailed Memoranda', pp.5–6

[6] RHL/MSS.Afr.s.1872/82 Hunter, 'Detailed Memorandum', p.19

[7] R St-Johnston, *Strange Places and Strange Peoples or Life in the Colonial Service*, London, 1936, p.28; Colonial Service doctors were not the only ones to find themselves in this elevated professional position abroad, see JSG Blair, *The Conscript Doctors: Memories of National Service*, Durham, 2001, p.xii

[8] JA Carman, *A Medical History of the Colony and Protectorate of Kenya: a Personal Memoir*, London, 1976, p.39

[9] G Maclean, 'Medical Administration in the Tropics', *BMJ*, i, 1950, pp.756–61, p.756

[10] RHL/MSS.Afr.s.1872/9 Barrett, 'Memorandum on Experiences', p.2

[11] RHL/MSS.Afr.s.1872/82 Hunter, 'Detailed Memorandum', p.5

[12] Carman, *Medical History of Kenya*, p.12

[13] RHL/MSS.Afr.s.1872/33 Cole, 'Memorandum on Experiences'.Although Cole is remembering 1949, the quotation holds true for his experiences during the earlier period.

[14] *Miscellaneous No.99: Colonial Medical Appointments*, London, 1921 [29th Ed.], p.3; this was reiterated in new editions of this pamphlet produced after the Warren Fisher Committee, *Colonial Service Recruitment No.3A: The Colonial Service. Information for the use of Candidates for Appointment to the Colonial Medical Service*, London, 1931, p.6

[15] *Colonial Service Recruitment No.3*, p.35

[16] C Jeffries, *Partners For Progress: The Men and Women of the Colonial Service*, London, 1949, p.66

[17] AJ Boase, 'Reminiscences of Surgery in Uganda', *East African Medical Journal*, 31, 1954, pp.197–203, p.197

[18] RHL/MSS.Afr.s.1872/75 Hennessey, 'Learning About Disease in Uganda', p.5

[19] Especially before 1920. M Worboys, *Science and British Colonial Imperialism: 1895-1940*, University of Sussex, DPhil. Thesis, 1979, p.417

[20] Carman, *Medical History of Kenya*, pp.12–13; RHL/MSS.Afr.s.1872/82 Hunter, 'Detailed Memorandum', p.3

[21] WD Foster, 'Robert Moffat and the Beginnings of Government Medical Service', *Medical History*, 13, 1969, pp.237–50, p.240

[22] Jeffries, *Partners For Progress*, p.118

[23] A Beck, *A History of the British Medical Administration of East Africa: 1900–1950*, Cambridge, MA, 1999 [1970], p.137

[24] Jeffries, *Partners For Progress*, p.65

[25] R Heussler, 'An American Looks at the Colonial Service', *New Commonwealth*, 1960, pp.418–20, p.418

[26] *Colonial Service Recruitment No.3*, p.28

[27] J Iliffe, *East African Doctors: a History of the Modern Profession*, Cambridge, 1999, p.61. Also 'Report on the Uganda Medical School, Mulago for the year 1932', Uganda Protectorate, *Annual Medical Report, 1932*, Entebbe, 1933, pp.68–72

[28] Although some officers naturally felt regret. Bagster Wilson was described as having been 'disappointed' on appointment to public health work (he had wanted to specialise in surgery). RHL/MSS.Afr.s.1872/162(a) M Wilson, 'Memoirs of Service as Entomologist, Health Officer and Medical Officer in Tanganyika, 1933–63' [n.d.]

[29] RHL/MSS.Afr.s.1653, Anderson, *Reminiscences*, Book II, p.86

[30] Maclean, 'Medical Administration in the Tropics', p.757

[31] Jeffries, *Partners For Progress*, p.100

[32] A Beck, 'Problems of British Medical Administration in East Africa Between 1900–1930', *Bulletin for the History of Medicine*, 36, 1962, pp.275–83, p.277

[33] Gilks, 'Proposed Expansion of the Medical Services', p.318

[34] *Ibid.*, Pressure was so great in Tanzania that Davey was called out of sick leave to take up the post of Principal Medical Officer. DF Clyde, *History of the Medical Services of Tanganyika*, Dar Es Salaam, 1962, p.113

[35] Uganda Protectorate, *Annual Medical Report, 1925*, Entebbe, 1926, p.48

[36] See the description of a one day 27 mile hike in HG Calwell, 'Nineteen Years in the Colonial Medical Service', *The Ulster Medical Journal*, 65 (supplement), 1993, pp.(s)1–(s)42, p.(s)8. Also the 90 miles walked in two days by Wiggins. CA Wiggins, 'Early Days in British East Africa and Uganda: Second Tour—1904–1907', *East African Medical Journal*, 37, 1960, pp.780–93, p.782; for a 40 mile walk in Uganda during the 1920s see RHL/MSS.Afr.s.1872/9 Barrett, 'Memorandum on Experiences', p.7

[37] *Colonial Service Recruitment No.3*, p.28

[38] Carman, *Medical History of Kenya*, p.35

[39] RHL/MSS.Afr.s.1378, Papers of BO Wilkin: *Annual Report of Dar Es Salaam*, 1935, p.1

[40] 'Organisation of the Colonial Medical Service', *BMJ*, i, 1902, pp.347–8, p.348

41 Some MOs still clearly made a significant living from private patients in Tanzania. See RHL/MSS.Afr.s.796, C Wilcocks, Diary, 1928–9, 17 May 1929, 1 June 1929

42 KNA/MOH/1/5643A 'Return on question of Private Practice', J Thomson, 27 May 1915; R Spence, 28 May 1915; H Welch, 2 June 1915

43 Wiggins, 'Early Days in British East Africa and Uganda: Second Tour', p.785

44 For an extreme example of only nine months leave in eleven years see *Ibid.*, p.793

45 KNA/MOH/1/5065 'Appointment of Medical Officers: Procedure', 13 March 1912

46 RHL/MSS.Afr.s.1872/9 Barrett, 'Memorandum on Experiences'

47 RHL/MSS.Afr.s.1872/153a Williams, 'Detailed Memoranda', p.14

48 *Ibid.*

49 Kauntze, 'Memorandum on Departmental Policy', p.61

50 RHL/MSS.Afr.s.1091, Papers of CJ Baker, Diary 1904, there are numerous examples of this. A random sample could include 25 January 1904; 12 April 1904, 27 December 1904; also RHL/MSS.Afr.s.1782, Hodges, Diaries

51 CA Wiggins, 'Early Days in British East Africa and Uganda', *East African Medical Journal*, 37, 1960, pp.699–708, p.703; Although he admitted that his district was often shorthanded and when other staff went away, and he could be 'DC. ADC and MO all at once'. *Ibid.*, p.706

52 In fact it was these periods of boredom that encouraged Carpenter towards entomology. 'GDH Carpenter', *BMJ*, i, 1953, pp.406–7, p.406

53 RHL/MSS.Afr.s.1872/9 Barrett, 'Memorandum on Experiences', p.10

54 RHL/MSS.Afr.s.1872/144a HC Trowell, 'Detailed Memorandum on Service as a Medical Officer, Lecturer in Medicine and Specialist Physician in Kenya and Uganda, 1929–57', [n.d. *c.*1984], p.3

55 WL/CMAC/PP/HCT/A5 Bray, *Hugh Trowell: Pioneer Nutritionist*, [Chapter 9] p.8

56 Maclean, 'Medical Administration in the Tropics', p.756

57 RHL/MSS.Afr.s.1872/144b HC Trowell, interviews, tape 1B, [n.d. *c.*1984], p.8; RHL/MSS.Afr.s.1872/82 Hunter, 'Detailed Memorandum', p.5

58 GO Ndege, *Health State and Society in Kenya*, Rochester, 2001; Maryinez Lyons, *The Colonial Disease: A Social History of Sleeping Sickness in Northern Zaire 1900–1940*, Cambridge, 2002 [1992]; RM Packard, *White Plague, Black Labour: Tuberculosis and the Political Economy of Health and Disease in South Africa*, Berkeley, CA, 1989

59 RHL/MSS.Afr.s.702, RAW Procter, 'Random Reminiscences, Mainly Surgical', [n.d.], p.6; see also the account he related of Kikuyu resistance to his public health campaign, p.7

60 RHL/MSS.Afr.s.2032, Kendall, 'Extracts from Diaries, Letters and Memory', p.6

61 Although it is acknowledged that it was in the interests of the British government to suppress reports of resistance and to favour positive accounts of the happy acceptance of western medicine in East Africa. Kenya, *Annual Medical Report, 1938–9, (Abbreviated)*, [n.d. *c.*1940], p.1

62 Kenya, *Annual Medical Report, 1937*, Nairobi, 1938, p.1

63 Furthermore, the danger was apparent to life insurance companies who were sometimes reluctant to offer policies to MOs destined to serve in Africa. Errol Trzebinski, *The Kenya Pioneers: the Frontiersmen of an Adopted Land*, London, 1991 [1985], p.45

64 Calwell, 'Nineteen Years in the Colonial Medical Service', p.(s)13

65 The Medical Department head offices were connected to the telephone exchange in Nairobi in 1909 KNA/MOH/1/5532 A Milne, PMO Nairobi to Superintendent of Telegraphs, 8 July 1909

66 [Re. Kenya] 'It can be stated that Medical Officers are never posted at stations where there is no other European Society.' *Colonial Service Recruitment No.*3, p.28. Similar statements pertaining to Uganda and Tanzania were also made *Ibid.*, pp.30–1, p.35

67 RHL/MSS.Afr.s.1653, Anderson, *Reminiscences*, Book I, p.23

68 Wiggins, 'Early Days in British East Africa and Uganda', p.702

69 KNA/MOH/1/1497 R Small to PMO 1 April 1907

70 'Address by Mr CV Braimbridge', *East African Medical Journal*, 31, 1954, pp.205–8, p.205

71 RHL/MSS.Afr.s.1872/144a Trowell, 'Detailed Memorandum', p.6

72 RHL/MSS.Afr.s.708 (1), WK Connell, Diary 1924–5, 3 October 1924, p.24

73 RHL/MSS.Afr.s.1872/144a Trowell, 'Detailed Memorandum', p.4

74 RHL/MSS.Afr.s.1872/33 Cole, 'Memorandum on Experiences'

75 RHL/MSS.Afr.s.1872/82 Hunter, 'Detailed Memorandum', p.5

76 RHL/MSS.Brit.Emp.r.4, PA Clearkin, *Ramblings and Recollections of a Colonial Doctor 1913–58*, Book I, Durban, 1967, pp.125–6

77 'JF Corson', *Lancet*, ii, 1963, p.1073

78 E.g., Bödeker, Shircore and Ross from Kenya in 1913. East Africa Protectorate, *Annual Medical Report, 1913*, 1914, p.13; or John Goodliffe in 1919. Uganda Protectorate, *Annual Medical Report, 1919*, Entebbe, 1920, p.6

79 RHL/MSS.Afr.s.1782, Hodges, Diaries, 21 April 1900; 15 August 1901

80 RHL/MSS.Afr.s.1872/144b Trowell, tape 1B, p.12; RHL/MSS.Afr.s.1872/82 Hunter, 'Detailed Memorandum', p.22

81 'Alfred Mackie', *BMJ*, ii, 1959, p.1262; 'Neil McLean', *BMJ*, i, 1955, p.917; KNA/MOH/1/4740 R Small to PMO, 31 January 1918; East Africa Protectorate, *Annual Medical Report, 1914*, 1915, p.11; Kenya, *Annual Medical Report, 1928*, Nairobi, 1929, p.56; Kenya, *Annual Medical Report, 1931*, Nairobi, 1932, p.45; Uganda Protectorate, *Annual Medical Report, 1912*, 1913, p.5; Uganda Protectorate, *Annual Medical Report, 1914*, 1915, p.8; Uganda Protectorate, *Annual Medical Report, 1925*, Entebbe, 1926, p.6; Uganda Protectorate, *Annual Medical Report, 1934*, Entebbe, 1935, p.9; C Wilcocks, *A Tropical Doctor in Africa and London*, unpublished autobiography, Surrey, 1977, p.133

82 E.g., James Armstrong, Hugh Baker, Raymond Bury, John Caldwell, Bertham Cherrett, Walter Densham, John Edmond, Alfred Garde, William Heard, Edward Langton, Harold Mann, John O'Connell, Westmore Spence Forbes Tulloch and Karl Uffmann. There were undoubtedly others, this is a list gleaned principally from obituaries which make specific mention of the cause of death.

83 NA/CO/457/6 'Obituary Dr Stoney', *East Africa and Uganda Government Gazette*, 15 November 1905, p.373; NA/CO/457/ 7 'Obituary', *East Africa and Uganda Government Gazette*, 1 July 1907, p.232

84 R Havelock Charles, 'Discussion on Special Factors Influencing the Suitability of Europeans for Life in the Tropics', *BMJ*, ii, 1910, pp.869–74; Crown Agents for the Colonies, *Hints on the Preservation of Health in Tropical Africa*, London, 1943 [1938] See also M Harrison, *Climates and Constitutions: Health, Race, Environment and British Imperialism in India 1600–1850*, New Delhi, 1999

85 'Discussion of the Causes of Invaliding from the Tropics', *BMJ*, ii, 1913, pp.1290–6, p.1290; p.1294

86 RHL/MSS.Afr.s.1872/144a Trowell, 'Detailed Memorandum', p.8; KNA/MOH/1/4740 Case of R Small, January 1918

87 Clyde, *History of the Medical Services of Tanganyika*, pp.99–100

88 RHL/MSS.Brit.Emp.r.4, Clearkin, *Ramblings and Recollections*, Book I, p.110

89 KNA/MOH/1/1468 Commissioner, Entebbe to J Will, PMO, Uganda, 5 September 1905

90 'The East African Medical Staff', *BMJ*, i, 1910, p.177

91 NA/CO/877/2/6370 Furse to R Falconer, 24 April 1922

92 'The chief drawback to the Colonial Medical Service appears to be the uncertainty of promotion', 'The Colonial Medical Service', *BMJ*, i, 1899, p.323

93 RHL/MSS.Afr.s.1872/16 Boase, 'Notes on Experiences', p.2

94 RHL/MSS.Afr.s.1872/82 Hunter, 'Detailed Memorandum', p.10

95 Clyde, *History of the Medical Services of Tanganyika*, p.113

96 RHL/MSS.Afr.s.1653, Anderson, *Reminiscences*, Book I, p.52

97 Chamberlain to Governors of all Colonies, 'Papers Relating to the Investigation of Malaria and Other Tropical Diseases and the Establishment of Schools of Tropical Medicine,' *Parliamentary Papers*, 1903, 44, pp.3–5

[98] RHL/ MSS.Afr.s.796, C Wilcocks, Diary, 1928–9, 4 December 1928; 8 January 1929; 14 January 1929; 2 February 1929

[99] NA/CO/323/1461/13 'Infectious Diseases: Recommendations of East Africa Directors of Medical Services for Standard Form of Weekly Report', 1937.

[100] The Kenya and Uganda branches were formed in 1920, closely followed by the establishment of a branch in Tanzania in 1923. See also TJ Johnson and M Caygill, 'The British Medical Association and its Overseas Branches: A Short History,' *The Journal of Imperial and Commonwealth History*, 1, 1973, pp.304–29

[101] Gilks and Patterson were on the Dominions Committee of the BMA in its discussions over Colonial Office terms and conditions of service in 1936. NA/CO/850/71/13 'Deputation by the BMA, 1936'

[102] BMA/C/1/4 'Annual Reports of UK and Overseas Branches 1930-1937'; BMA/E/1/41 Colonial Medical Services, 1919-1950'; BMA/B/162 'Dominions Committee [originally the Colonial Committee] 1909-1952'

[103] 'Colonial Medical Services: Report of the Departmental Committee', *BMJ*, ii, 1920, pp.448–9; 'Memorandum of Evidence Placed by the BMA Before the Colonial Medical Services Committee, 23 February 1920', *BMJ, Supplement*, 1920, pp.141–3

[104] 'The Colonial Medical Services: Statement by the BMA', *BMJ, Supplement*, 1926, pp.9–10; 'Regulations for the East African Medical Service, Correspondence Between the BMA and the Colonial Office', *BMJ, Supplement*, 1926, pp.27–8; NA/CO/533/662 'East Africa Medical Staff Regulations', 1926–7; Although some MOs felt that the published warning changed things very little. Gilks, 'The Medical Department and Health Organization', p.351

[105] RHL/MSS.Brit.Emp.s.415, Furse Papers, Memorandum: 'On the Difficulty of Obtaining Candidates for the Colonial Medical Service', p.1

[106] The results of a questionnaire submitted to all members of the Kenya Medical Service 'would seem to indicate that no serious dissatisfaction exists in the Kenya Service.' 'British Medical Association', *Kenya Medical Journal*, 1, 1924–5, pp.54–5, p.55

[107] 'European Women and Children in the Tropics', *BMJ*, i, 1931, pp.268–9

[108] E Thomson, 'Physiology, Hygiene and the Entry of Women to the Medical Profession in Edinburgh, c.1869–c.1900', *Studies in the History and Philosophy of Biological and Biomedical Sciences*, 32, pp.105–126

[109] Smart, 'An Impression of Life in the Colonial Medical Service', p.124; Jeffries, *Partners For Progress*, p.152

[110] C Blake, *The Charge of the Parasols: Women's Entry to the Medical Profession*, 1990, p.168; TN Bonner, *To the Ends of the Earth: Women's Search for Education in Medicine*, Cambridge, MA, 1992

[111] The earliest reference I have found to a woman doctor in East Africa was a missionary in Kenya in 1897. 'EM Hooper', *The Medical Directory for 1897*, Vol. 2, 1898, p.1647

[112] 'Muriel Robertson' *Who Was Who, 1971–1980*, Volume VII, 1981, p.676; 'Muriel Robertson', *The Times*, 22 June 1973, p.18

[113] 'Muriel Robertson', Royal Society, *Biographical Memoirs of Fellows of the Royal Society*, Vol. 20, London, 1974, pp.217-47

[114] 'Mary Michael-Shaw', *BMJ*, ii, 1963, p.1343; 'Mary Turton', *BMJ*, ii, 1958, p.1048

[115] Boase, 'Reminiscences of Surgery', p.199

[116] NA/CO/850/14/20 'Women Medical Officers', 1932; NA/CO/850/33/28 'Women Medical Officers', 1933

[117] AR Cook, 'The Medical History of Uganda: Part 2', *East African Medical Journal*, 13, 1936–7, pp.99–110, p.100. This practice (codified by the Contagious Diseases Acts in nineteenth-century England) was much criticised. See J Walkowitz, *Prostitution and Victorian Society: Women, Class and the State*, Cambridge 1980; P Levine, *Prostitution, Race and Politics: Policing Venereal Disease in the British Empire*, London, 2003

[118] NA/CO/381/9 'Kenya: Ladies on Permanent and Pensionable Establishment., Question of Resignation in Event of Marriage', 1928–9

119 NA/CO/850/14/2 'Employment of Women in the Colonial Services', 1932

120 RHL/MSS.Afr.s.796, C Wilcocks, Diary, 1928–9, 13/09/1928; RHL/MSS.Afr.s.1872/162 (a), M Wilson to A Smith, ORDP, 13 February 1983

121 Tanganyika Territory, *Annual Medical Report, 1932*, Dar Es Salaam, 1933, p.22; RHL/MSS.Afr.s.1872/162(a) Wilson, 'Memoirs of Service'

122 RHL/MSS.Afr.s.1872/144b Trowell, tape 1B, p.7; WL/CMAC/PP/HCT/A5 Bray, *Hugh Trowell: Pioneer Nutritionist*, [Chapter 5] p.7

123 RHL/MSS.Afr.s.1653, Anderson, *Reminiscences*, Book I, p.24

124 Quotation from the Moffat Letters, Makerere University Library [no further reference], quoted in W.D. Foster, 'Robert Moffat and the Beginnings of Government Medical Service', p.246

125 RHL/MSS.Afr.s.702, Procter, 'Random Reminiscences', p.4

126 But see Jeffries, *Partners For Progress*, pp.155–8; 'From the Woman's Viewpoint' in A Kirk-Greene, *Glimpses of Empire: A Corona Anthology*, London, 2001, pp.228–77

127 Jeffries, *Partners For Progress*, p.156

128 Lady Cranworth, 'Hints for a Woman in British East Africa' in Lord Cranworth, *A Colony in the Making. Or Sport and Profit in British East Africa*, London, 1912, pp.84–92, p.92

129 RHL/MSS.Afr.s.708 (1), WK Connell, Diary 1924–5, 21 October 1924, p.24

130 For an impressive example of this see the biography of Margaret Trowell, wife of Hugh Trowell and later Head of the School of Art, Makerere College, Uganda. M Trowell, *African Tapestry*, London, 1957

131 After World War Two campaigns began to be directed at including more women in the Colonial Service. See Colonial Office, *Colonial Service Recruitment No. 9: Information Regarding Appointments for Women*, London, 1945, extract reproduced in A Kirk-Greene, *On Crown Service: A History of HM Colonial and Overseas Civil Services, 1837–1997*, London, 1999, pp.196–8

Chapter 8: Medical Recruitment and the Ideals of Empire (pp.102–114)

1 A Kirk-Greene, 'The Colonial Service in the Novel' in John Smith (ed.), *Administering Empire: The British Colonial Service in Retrospect*, London, 1999, pp.19–48, p.41

2 Some of the most famous examples: EW Said, *Orientalism: Western Conceptions of the Orient*, Harmondsworth, 1995 [1978]; E Hobsbawn and T Ranger (eds.), *The Invention of Tradition*, Cambridge 2002 [1983]; D Cannadine, *Ornamentalism: How the British Saw Their Empire*, Harmondsworth, 2001

3 MP Sutphen and B Andrews (eds.), *Medicine and the Colonial Identity*, London, 2003

4 Some important exceptions include work that has been undertaken on the creation of colonial medical subjects. M Vaughan, *Curing Their Ills: Colonial Power and African Illness*, Padstow, 1991; W Anderson, *The Cultivation of Whiteness: Science, Health and Racial Destiny in Australia*, New York, NY, 2003

5 Attendance at Oxbridge, did not necessarily mean that the stereotypical Colonial Officer was academically exceptional. In fact, the more common tendency amongst Colonial Officers was that they were good sporting, practical types more than intellectuals. LA Mills, 'Methods of Appointment and Training in the British and Dutch Colonial Civil Service', *American Political Science Review*, 33, 1939, pp.465–72, p.472

6 P Woodruff, *The Men Who Ruled India: the Guardians*, Vol.2, London, 1963 [1953], pp.75–9

7 DC Potter, *India's Political Administrators 1919–83: From ICS to IAS*, Delhi, 1996 [1986] p.71 quoted in P Marshall, 'The British Experience of Imperial Rule' in J Smith (ed.), *Administering Empire*, pp.1–18, p.5

8 D Hammond and A Jablow, *The Africa That Never Was: Four Centuries of British Writing About Africa*, New York, NY, 1970, p.183

[9] H Kuklick, *The Imperial Bureaucrat: The Colonial Administrative Service in the Gold Coast, 1920–1939*, Stanford, CA, 1979, p.27; A McKay, *Tibet and the British Raj: The Frontier Cadre, 1904–1947*, Surrey, 1997, pp.77–80

[10] B Berman, *Administration and Politics in Colonial Kenya*, Yale University, PhD, 1973, p.95, p.97 cited in D Kennedy, *Islands of White: Settler Society and Culture in Kenya and Southern Rhodesia, 1890–1939*, Durham, NC, 1987, p.73

[11] A Kirk-Greene, *On Crown Service: A History of HM Colonial and Overseas Civil Services, 1837–1997*, London, 1999, p.94; DG Crawford, *Roll of the Indian Medical Service*, 1615–1930, London, 1930, pp.636–55

[12] E.g., Lord Twining, Governor of Tanzania. D Bates, *A Gust of Plumes: A Biography of Lord Twining of Godalming and Tanganyika*, London, 1972, pp.102–5

[13] A Kirk-Greene, 'The Colonial Service in the Novel' in Smith (ed.), *Administering Empire*, pp.19–45, p.41

[14] Cannadine, *Ornamentalism*, pp. 128–30

[15] Harrison has argued that the Indian Medical Service was an essentially conservative group, the ruling classes having become more cautious in their policies since the unrest caused by the mutiny of 1857. M Harrison, *Public Health in British India: Anglo-Indian Preventative Medicine 1859–1914*, Cambridge, 1994, p.5. It should also be noted, however, that some eccentricity was permitted.

[16] JA Mangan, *The Games Ethic and Imperialism: Aspects of the Diffusion of an Ideal*, London, 1998 [1986]

[17] F Driver, *Geography Militant: Cultures of Exploration and Empire*, Oxford, 2001

[18] PA Dunae, 'New Grub Street for Boys', in J Richards (ed.), *Imperialism and Juvenile Literature*, Manchester, 1989, pp.12–33; Edgar Wallace's immensely popular *Sanders of the River* books were said to have been 'immediately and unambiguously recognisable in Britain's popular culture as a symbol for the colonial administrator'. Kirk-Greene, 'The Colonial Service in the Novel', p.19

[19] K Dunn, 'Lights…Camera…Africa: Images of Africa and Africans in Western Popular Films of the 1930s', *African Studies Review*, 39, 1996, pp. 149–75

[20] Vaughan, *Curing Their Ills*, pp.155–79

[21] Oxford and Cambridge predominate as the favoured recruitment sources and the four most frequent places Colonial Administrative Service Officers were schooled were Marlborough, Wellington College, Charterhouse and Winchester. NA/CO/877/16/21 'Colonial Administrative Service: Universities of Successful Candidates 1931–1941 inclusive' and 'Colonial Administrative Service: Schools of Successful Candidates for the Years 1931–1941 inclusive' [n.d. *c.*1942]

[22] E Waugh, *Remote People*, London, 1931, pp.182–3; E Huxley, *White Man's Country: Lord Delamere and the Making of Kenya* (2 Vols.), London, 1953 [1935], pp.248–57

[23] A Kirk-Greene, 'Colonial Service Biographical Data: the Published Sources', *African Research and Documentation*, 46, 1988, pp.2–16, p.2; A handful of complete personnel files were found in the KNA, usually those of officers who were being considered for transfer or retrenchment.

[24] One way of ascertaining social privilege is through analysing schooling. Information of this nature has been found for 125 (roughly a third) of MOs. The data is too crude and patchy to be of much use (it is impossible to know who were scholarship students), but schools mentioned that indicate a high social rank include, Lancing College, Marlborough College, Rugby School, Winchester College, St Paul's School and Robert Gordon's College, Aberdeen

[25] Harrison, *Public Health in British India*, p.29

[26] Marshall, 'The British Experience of Imperial Rule' p.10

[27] Huxley, *White Man's Country*, p.185

[28] E.g., doctors did not have to wear a uniform (apart from the most senior ranks at public events), whereas all Political Officers in Kenya Service were issued a khaki uniform. My thanks to Tony Kirk-Greene for this information.

[29] Kuklick, *The Imperial Bureaucrat*, p.150

[30] *African (East) No.1105: Information for the Use of Candidates to Appointments in the East African Medical Service*, London, 1925, p.8

[31] 'The preponderance of Scotsmen is certainly remarkable.' AR Cook, 'The Medical History of Uganda: Part 1', *East African Medical Journal*, 13, 1936–7, pp.66–81, p.73; the Irish contingent has been less commented upon, but is noteworthy.

[32] MW Dupree, MA Crowther, 'A Profile of the Medical Profession in Scotland in the Early Twentieth Century: The Medical Directory as a Historical Source', *Bulletin of the History of Medicine*, 65, 1991, pp.209–33, p.222

[33] TM Devine, *Scotland's Empire, 1600–1815*, London, 2003; see also M Fry, *The Scottish Empire*, Edinburgh, 2001

[34] DA Dow, 'Some Late Nineteenth-Century Scottish Travellers in Africa', *Proceedings of the Royal Society of Edinburgh.*, 1982, 82A, pp.7–15

[35] A Balfour, 'Vistas and Visions: Some Aspects of the Colonial Medical Services', *Glasgow Medical Journal*, 6, 1924, pp.353–74, p.354

[36] RHL/MSS.Afr.s.1872/82 JK Hunter, 'Detailed Memorandum on Experiences in the Colonial Medical Service in Uganda, 1939–58', [n.d. *c.* 1983], p.22

[37] J Huxley, *Africa View*, London, 1936 [1931], p.152

[38] L Cole, 'Cambridge Medicine and the Medical School in the Twentieth Century' in A Rook (ed.), *Cambridge and its Contribution to Medicine*, 1971, pp.257–84

[39] Colonial Office, 'Report of the Committee Chaired by Sir Warren Fisher', *The System of Appointment in the Colonial Office and the Colonial Services*, London, 1930, p.23

[40] M Weatherall, *Gentlemen, Scientists and Doctors: Medicine at Cambridge, 1800–1940*, Cambridge, 2000, p.163

[41] Dupree and Crowther, 'A Profile of the Medical Profession in Scotland in the Early Twentieth Century', p.221

[42] Muriel Robertson was not medically qualified, but had an MA from Glasgow (1906). She got into the Medical Service having been initially seconded to Africa on a Royal Society Commission. She appears to have slipped through the net with regard to fulfilling certain entrance requirements. This was perhaps fortuitous, as she was later to become one of the most prominent scientists to have had a Colonial Medical Service career.

[43] RHL/MSS.Brit.Emp.s.415, Furse Papers, Memorandum: Furse 'Sources of Supply of Medical Officers 1927–9 (November)', 9 December 1929

[44] Deans of other medical schools were more polarised in their opinions over educational standards. While one (unspecified) Dean complained that the best medical students did not join the Colonial Medical Service, another stated that 'amongst his best students' chose the career. NA/CO/877/7/8 Major Hutchinson, 'Report on visit to Scottish Universities and Liverpool University', 7 April 1930

[45] There was increasing support from the Colonial Office for MOs to gain extra qualifications. NA/CO/850/144/3 'Colonial Medical Service: Financial Recognition of Specialist Qualifications, 1939–41'

[46] RHL/MSS.Brit.Emp.s.415, Furse Papers, Second memorandum for the Warren Fisher Committee, July 1929; K Waddington, *Medical Education at St. Bartholomew's Hospital, 1123–1995*, Suffolk, 2003, p.227

[47] NA/CO/877/4/4 Minute: Furse, [regarding his meeting with Mr Crawford, Secretary, London University Appointments Board], 10 February 1928.

[48] Dupree and Crowther, 'A Profile of the Medical Profession in Scotland in the Early Twentieth Century', p.221

[49] *Miscellaneous No.407: Primary Courses of Instruction in Tropical Medicine and Hygiene for Officers Selected for Appointment to the Colonial Medical Service*, London, 1939, p.1; H Burdett, *Burdett's Hospitals and Charities 1901*, London, 1901, p.240.

[50] RHL/MSS.Brit.Emp.s.415, Furse Papers, Furse, 'Sources of Supply of Medical Officers 1927–9 (November)'

[51] Although it is likely that the 'real' figure is higher, especially as this was a supplementary qualification and many doctors did not regularly update their *Medical Directory* entries. More definitive cross-checking could be obtained by checking the matriculation records at the London and Liverpool School of Tropical Medicine and Hygiene as well as Cambridge and Edinburgh Medical School records.

[52] NA/CO/822/23/1 Memorandum: T Stanton, 11 October 1920

[53] This figure is based upon an average for those officers for whom the information could be obtained. Date of birth was established for 271 (64 per cent) of officers.

[54] 'Information as to Colonial Appointments', in *The Colonial Office List*, London, 1899, pp.346–8, p.347; *Miscellaneous No.99: Colonial Medical Appointments*, London, 1921 [29th Ed.], p.3

[55] 'Information as to Colonial Appointments', *The Colonial Office List*, 1899, pp.346–8, p.347; Also NA/850/71/13, T Stanton to JA Drake, 14 November 1936

[56] E.g., Arthur Boase, John Davies, Clarence Howat, Thomas Lawson, and Alan Maclean all joined Service aged 23

[57] E.g., Ernest Cooke (44); Frank de Smidt (37); Geoffrey Gibbon (37); William Lamborn (40); Walter MacDonald (36)

[58] E.g., William Ansorge (45) or Aubrey Hodges (37)

[59] As doctors supplied the information for *Medical Directory* entries, it is likely that they included all professional experiences, as this added to their public profile.

[60] These figures come to more than 100 per cent as some officers had *both* military and professional experience.

[61] The information calculated for this section is based on *first* retirement dates, as sometimes officers retired and then subsequently rejoined the Service. Appendix 2 lists service dates of individuals.

[62] NA/850/71/13 'Note of a Meeting held in the Colonial Office Between Representatives of the Colonial Office and a Deputation from the Dominions Committee of the BMA, 6 January 1937

[63] C Jeffries, *The Colonial Empire and its Civil Service*, Cambridge, 1938, p.127

[64] Including FRCPsych; FFARCS and FRSTM

[65] Cannadine, *Ornamentalism*, p. 98

Chapter 9: Colonial Medical Communities (pp.115-132)

[1] M Perham, 'Introduction', in R Heussler, *Yesterday's Rulers: The Making of the British Colonial Service*, New York, NY, 1963, p.xx

[2] R Hyam, 'The Colonial Office Mind 1900–1914', *The Journal of Imperial and Commonwealth History*, 8, 1979, pp.30–55

[3] PD Curtin, *The World and the West*, Cambridge, 2000, p.49

[4] McKay has argued that officers in Tibet were fundamentally bound by a sense of duty 'above any consideration for the Tibetans'. McKay, *Tibet and the British Raj: The Frontier Cadre, 1904–1947*, Richmond, Surrey, 1997, p.192. This is not to say that officers never complained, rather they were ultimately constrained in how they could do so.

[5] NA/CO/850/47/4 Lord Crewe, Confidential Circular, 11 January 1909; RHL/Mss.Afr.s.1079, Papers of IC Middleton, 'Memorandum on the Subject of the Acceptance of Business Appointments by Officers of the Crown Services', July 1937

[6] R Furse, *Aucuparius: Recollections of a Recruiting Officer*, Oxford, 1962, p.222

[7] E.g., WJ Simpson, *The Maintenance of Health in the Topics*, London, 1905; RHL/MSS.Afr.s.1782, A Hodges, Diaries 1898–1907, 17 February 1898; RHL/MSS.Afr.s.1872/144b Hugh Trowell, interviews, tape 1B, [n.d. *c.*1984], p.3

[8] Mitchell joined the Colonial Administrative Service in 1912. P Mitchell, 'Forty Years Back' in A Kirk-Greene, *Glimpses of Empire: A Corona Anthology*, London, 2001, pp.278–80, p.279

9 RHL/MSS.Afr.s.1872/153a AW Williams, 'Detailed Memoranda on Experiences in the Colonial Medical Service in Uganda and Tanganyika, 1931-1949', [n.d. c.1983], p.3

10 RHL/MSS.Afr.s.1872/33 ACE Cole, 'Memorandum on Experiences in the Colonial Medical Service in Tanganyika, 1939–60', 10 April 1983; HG Calwell, 'Nineteen Years in the Colonial Medical Service', *The Ulster Medical Journal*, 65 (supplement), 1993, pp.(s)1–(s)42, p.(s)2

11 NA/CO/877/6/10 'Recruitment of Candidates for the Home and Colonial Services: Proposal to Hold a Joint Competitive Examination', c. 5 June 1929

12 This was absolutely typical and references are too numerous to mention. A couple of published examples include: R Scott's assistantship to W Lamborn. RR Scott, 'The Growth of a Public Health Service in a Tropical Town', *East African Medical Journal*, 10, 1933–4, pp.130–44, p.133; C Braimbridge also used to regularly take new recruits under his wing to give them surgical experience. 'Address by Mr CV Braimbridge', *East African Medical Journal*, 31, 1954, pp.205–8, p.207

13 RHL/MSS.Afr.s.1872/33 Cole, 'Memorandum on Experiences'

14 KNA/MOH/1/8020 'Medical Notes to Officers appointed to BEA', 17 July 1920

15 RHL/MSS.Afr.s.1872/153a Williams, 'Detailed Memoranda', p.7

16 KNA/MOH/3/769 Copy of an empty Confidential Report, [n.d. c.1940s]

17 Wiggins immediately on arrival took up the Secretaryship of the Mombassa Club. CA Wiggins, 'Early Days in British East Africa and Uganda', *East African Medical Journal*, 37, 1960, pp.699–708, p.700

18 For a description of typical *boma* see JA Carman, *A Medical History of the Colony and Protectorate of Kenya: a Personal Memoir*, London, London, 1976, p.31; M Trowell, *African Tapestry*, London, 1957, pp.18–20

19 E.g., the priority dispute between Clearkin and Gilks. RHL/MSS.Afr.S.1872/30 Peter Alphonsus Clearkin, 'Tropical Typhus', p.4; Trowell described a bitter personal feud within a small *boma* in Kenya. RHL/MSS.Afr.s.1872/144a HC Trowell, 'Detailed Memorandum on Service as a Medical Officer, Lecturer in Medicine and Specialist Physician in Kenya and Uganda, 1929–57', [n.d. c.1984], p.5

20 WL/CMAC/PP/HCT/A5 E Bray, *Hugh Trowell: Pioneer Nutritionist*, unpublished biography, 1988, p.4; [Chapter 4] p.17; AR Cook, 'The Medical History of Uganda: Part 2', *East African Medical Journal*, 13, 1936–7, pp.99–110, p.100; KNA/MOH/1/1468 Commissioner, Entebbe to J Will, PMO, Uganda, 5 September 1905

21 McKay, *Tibet and the British Raj*, p.205; Also D Kennedy, *Islands of White: Settler Society and Culture in Kenya and Southern Rhodesia, 1890–1939*, Durham, NC, 1987.

22 A Davis, *A Microcosm of Empire (British East Africa)*, Nairobi, [n.d. c.1918], p.67

23 WL/CMAC/PP/PCG/A2 PCC Garnham, Personal Correspondence and Miscellaneous, 1936–44 [untitled, undated notes c.1939]

24 A Kirk-Greene, *The Corona Club: an Introductory History*, London, 1990; A Kirk-Greene, *On Crown Service: A History of HM Colonial and Overseas Civil Services, 1837–1997*, London, 1999, pp.257-8

25 C Jeffries, *The Colonial Empire and its Civil Service*, Cambridge, London, 1938, p.14

26 NA/323/985/4 Circular: LS Amery, 'Osbourne Convalescent Home', 22 February 1927

27 A Kirk-Greene, *Symbol of Authority*, London, 2005

28 Jeffries, *Colonial Empire*, p.125

29 In 1907 the Liverpool School modified and extended the curriculum in line with the precedent established in London, from a 10-week course to a 13-week course. JWW Stephens, W Yorke, and B Blacklock, *Liverpool School of Tropical Medicine, Historical Record: 1898–1920*, Liverpool, 1920, p.38; Also H Power *Tropical Medicine in the Twentieth Century. A History of the Liverpool School of Tropical Medicine*, London, 1999

30 Albert Cook acerbically remembered: 'Our training in specifically tropical diseases at Cambridge and Bart's was nil' Cook, 'The Medical History of Uganda: Part 1', p.77

[31] DM Haynes, *Imperial Medicine: Patrick Manson and the Conquest of Tropical Disease*, Philadelphia, PA, 2001, p.124; It was the London School (not Liverpool) that was seen as the government's brainchild. Although it is acknowledged that other groups attended the tropical medical courses, particularly missionaries, the original intention to establish the London School was the result of a long debate over how the training of Colonial MOs should be conducted. It was, furthermore, politically useful to support colonial scientific endeavour. See M Worboys, *Science and British Colonial Imperialism: 1895-1940*, University of Sussex, DPhil. Thesis, 1979, p.402

[32] A Castellani, *Microbes, Men and Monarchs: A Doctor's Life in Many Lands*, London, 1960, p.28

[33] P Manson-Bahr, *History of the School of Tropical Medicine in London: 1899–1949*, London, 1956, focus on protozoology and helminthology p.7; inclusion of bacteriology p.54

[34] RHL/MSS.Afr.s.1872/9 RE Barrett, 'Memorandum on Experiences in the Colonial Medical Service in East Africa, 1928–55', 1983, p.1; RHL/MSS.Afr.s.1872/153a Williams, 'Detailed Memoranda', p.2

[35] D Duckworth, 'On the Education of Medical Practitioners for Colonial Service', paper read at the First Intercolonial Medical Congress, Amsterdam, 1883, pp.1–7, p.1; P Manson, 'On the Necessity for Special Education in Tropical Medicine,' *Lancet*, ii, 1897, pp. 842–5; also, Manson-Bahr, *History of the School of Tropical Medicine in London*, p.31

[36] Worboys, *Science and British Colonial Imperialism*, pp.191–243

[37] 'Numbers of the Medical Profession', *BMJ*, ii, 1931, pp.414–18, p.418

[38] 'The Association and the Colonies', *BMJ*, i, 1905, p.1394

[39] 'Editorial', *Kenya Medical Journal*, 2, 1925–6, p.299

[40] Past (Colonial Medical Service) Presidents of the Kenya Branch during this period included: Clare Wiggins, John Carman, John Gilks, Henry Gordon, Christopher Wilson, Albert Patterson; of the Uganda Branch: Clare Wiggins (again); Clifford Roberts; of the Tanzanian Branch: John Davey, William Connell

[41] This journal underwent numerous name changes: *Kenya Medical Journal* (1923–4); *Kenya East African Medical Journal* (1924–32); finally the *East African Medical Journal* (1932–present).

[42] Although the *East African Medical Journal* became more generalist in its readership between 1923–c.1945, from the 1950s onwards (and in keeping with growing expectations of specialist journals) it became markedly more technical: containing published papers and book reviews, but very little of its former lively editorial comment or local colour.

[43] 'Christopher Wilson', *BMJ*, i, 1956, p.692

[44] MJ Dobson, M Malowany, K Ombongi and R Snow, 'The Voice of East Africa: The East African Medical Journal at its 75th Anniversary', *Transactions of the Royal Society of Tropical Medicine and Hygiene*, 92, 1998, pp.685–6, p.685

[45] Colonial Medical Service editors were: Christopher Wilson (1923-7); John Carman (Asst. Ed. 1927–45; Ed. 1945–60); John Gilks (1927–30)

[46] E.g., 69 professional journals were listed as being regularly taken in Kenya in 1929. KNA/MOH/1/10274 'Medical Journals for Staff', 1928/9

[47] KNA/MOH/1/402 'Distribution of Sleeping Sickness Bulletin' [n.d. c.1912]

[48] Calwell, 'Nineteen Years in the Colonial Medical Service', p.(s)16

[49] 'The Tropical Diseases Bureau', *BMJ*, i, 1912, p.1149

[50] WL/CMAC/PP/HCT/A5 Bray, *Hugh Trowell: Pioneer Nutritionist*, [Chapter 10], p.9; Charles Wilcocks also commented on the 'quite high' trend amongst MOs to take supplementary qualifications. C Wilcocks, *A Tropical Doctor in Africa and London*, unpublished autobiography, Surrey, 1977, p.128

[51] F Driver, *Geography Militant: Cultures of Exploration and Empire*, Oxford, 2001, e.g. p.51

[52] A glance at the indices of the *Kenya and East African Medical Journal* of the period will reveal an extremely high number of contributions from MOs.

[53] RHL/MSS.Afr.s.1872/82 Hunter, 'Detailed Memorandum', p.12; this was echoed by Farnworth Anderson RHL/MSS.Afr.s.1653, Anderson, *Reminiscences*, Book I, p.58

54 HJO'D Burke Gaffney, 'Forefathers of Tropical Medicine', *East African Medical Journal*, 10, 1933–4, pp.100–114; WD Foster, 'Robert Moffat and the Beginnings of the Government Medical Service in Uganda', *Medical History*, 13, 1969, pp.237–50

55 Charles Wilcocks took an MD based on his research into TB started during his colonial medical career as a port HO in Dar Es Salaam. Wilcocks, *Tropical Doctor*, p.43; Hugh Calwell's interest in sleeping sickness developed in a similar way, see Calwell, 'Nineteen Years in the Colonial Medical Service', pp.(s)5-6

56 There is no space here to mention all the individual contributions made by East African doctors.

57 The examples are numerous, some include: Arthur Bagshawe who became the first Director of the Sleeping Sickness Bureau (later to become the Bureau of Hygiene and Tropical Diseases), and editor of the *Tropical Diseases Bulletin*, and the *Bulletin of Hygiene*; Henry Burke-Gaffney who became Assistant Director of the Bureau of Hygiene and Tropical Diseases in London, becoming its Director in 1961–68; James Corson on leaving Africa went to work for the Bureau of Hygiene and Tropical Diseases, where he remained until 1946; Claud Cole went on to be consultant physician to the Hospital for Tropical Diseases, London as well as consulting physician to the Colonial Office, the Crown Agents and the Overseas Development Administration; Percy Garnham went on to become first a reader in Medical Parasitology at the London School of Hygiene and Tropical Medicine (1947–51) and then a Professor and Director of the Department (1952–68); Ronald Heisch was appointed on his retirement from Kenya, Senior Lecturer in the department of Parasitology at the London School of Hygiene and Tropical Medicine.

58 'Editorial', [Effects of the Climate on the Human Constitution], *K East African Medical Journal*, 8, 1931–2, p.331; DV Latham, 'The White Man in East Africa' *East African Medical Journal*, 9, 1932–3, pp.276–82; M McKinnon, 'Medical Aspects of White Settlement in Kenya', *East African Medical Journal*, 11, 1934–5, pp.376–94; 'Tropical Neurasthenia', *East African Medical Journal*, 12, 1935–6, pp.28–9; A Walter, 'Climate and White Settlement in the East African Highlands', *East African Medical Journal*, 11, 1934–5, pp.210–25

59 This unified perspective of MOs is an interesting contrast to an argument presented by Kuklick. She concluded that the successful administrative officer was someone who held an 'ideological dedication to the conservation of African tradition', H Kuklick, *The Imperial Bureaucrat: The Colonial Administrative Service in the Gold Coast, 1920–1939*, Stanford, CA, 1979, p.43

60 Manson-Bahr, *History of the School of Tropical Medicine in London*, p.29

61 FCO/14634 'Organisation of the Medical and Sanitary Services in the British Colonies: Replies to Circular Despatch: 1 February 1913', *Standing Orders for the Medical Department* [Uganda], Government Press, 1912, p.1

62 Balfour, 'Vistas and Visions'; *Colonial Service Recruitment No.3, Information Regarding the Colonial Medical Service*, 1935, p.11; see also 'Colonial Medical Service', *BMJ*, ii, 1938, pp.546–8, p.546

63 AGH Smart, 'An Impression of Life in the Colonial Medical Service', *St Thomas' Hospital Gazette*, 37, 1939, pp.123–6, p.123; Balfour, 'Vistas and Visions'

64 FCO/14634 'Organisation of the Medical and Sanitary Services in the British Colonies', p.1

65 Carman, *Medical History of Kenya*, p.41

66 SR Bhagwat 'Rupture of Pleura Without Fracture of Ribs Caused by a Buffalo', *BMJ*, i, 1913, p.168

67 NA/CO/612/3 *Uganda Protectorate Government Gazette*, 15 July 1913, p.296

68 RHL/MSS.Afr.s.1872/75 Robert Samuel Hennessey, 'Learning About Disease in Uganda: 1929–44 and 1949–55', 1983, p.8

69 RHL/MSS.Afr.s.1872/16 A Boase (compiled, RM Boase), 'Notes on Experiences in Colonial Medical Service in Uganda, 1924–56', 14 February 1983, p.2.

70 RHL/MSS.Afr.s.1872/82 Hunter, 'Detailed Memorandum', p.23

71 RHL/MSS.Afr.s.1872/153a Williams, 'Detailed Memoranda', p.10

[72] J Huxley, *Africa View*, London, 1936 [1931], p.25

[73] Most prominently, M Vaughan, *Curing Their Ills: Colonial Power and African Illness*, Padstow, 1991.

[74] HB Hinde, 'The 'Black Peril' in British East Africa: A Frank Talk to Women Settlers', *Empire Review*, 1921, pp.193–200

[75] A good summary of these ideas can be found in W Anderson, 'The Third-World Body,' in R Cooter and J Pickstone (eds.), *Medicine in the Twentieth Century*, Amsterdam, 2000, pp.235–45

[76] T Ranger, 'The Invention of Tradition in Colonial Africa' in E Hobsbawn and T Ranger (eds.), *The Invention of Tradition*, Cambridge, 2002 [1983], p.213, p.221

[77] Argued by Cannadine *Ornamentalism*, esp. p.66, p. 122

[78] Quoted without reference in Jeffries, *Partners For Progress*, p.90

[79] A Johansen, *The Kenya I Knew, 1904–1963*, p.48 quoted in E Trzebinski, *The Kenya Pioneers: the Frontiersmen of an Adopted Land*, London, 1991 [1985], pp.103–4

[80] Davis, *Microcosm of Empire*, pp.48–9

[81] Huxley, *Africa View*, p.34

[82] R Heussler, 'An American Looks at the Colonial Service', *New Commonwealth*, 1960, pp.418–20, p.419

[83] Trzebinski, *Kenya Pioneers,* p.101, p.104. The hotel still plays on this colonial image today.

[84] The Gazettes were an important means of keeping widely dispersed communities mutually informed. Calwell, 'Nineteen Years in the Colonial Medical Service', p.(s)13

[85] TFV Buxton, 'A Social Effort in East Africa', *Journal of the Royal African Society*, 39, 1911, pp.342–4; RHL/MSS.Afr.s.1872/33 Cole, 'Memorandum on Experiences'; this point is also made in Kennedy, *Islands of White*, p.189

[86] Lord Cranworth, *A Colony in the Making. Or Sport and Profit in British East Africa*, London, 1912, p.90

[87] T Fuller, 'British Images and Attitudes in Colonial Uganda', *Historian*, 38, 1976, pp.305–18, p.306

[88] Jeffries, *Partners For Progress*, p.158

[89] Lord Cranworth, 'The Public School Boy in East Africa', *National Review.*, 336, 1911, pp.992–1000, p.996

[90] Calwell, 'Nineteen Years in the Colonial Medical Service', p.(s)5, pp.(s)23–4

[91] F Treves, *Uganda for a Holiday*, London, 1910, pp.204–5

[92] Mangan, *The Games Ethic and Imperialism;* JA Mangan (ed.), *The Cultural Bond: Sport, Empire, Society*, London, 1992

[93] 'Clifford Braimbridge, *Lancet*, i, 1964, p.279; 'Edward Clarence', *East African Medical Journal*, 14, 1937–8, pp.138–9, p.139; 'Henry Speldewinde de Boer', *BMJ*, i, 1957, pp.1533–4, p.1533; 'Aubrey Hodges', *East African Medical Journal*, 23, 1946, pp.289–90, p.289; 'Claude Marshall, *East African Medical Journal*, 34, 1957, p.280; 'Arthur Williams', *BMJ*, i, 1958, p.1421; 'Roland Dowdeswell', *BMJ*, ii, 1956, p.305.

[94] Cranworth, *Colony in the Making*, pp.324–42; *Colonial Service Recruitment, No.3*, p.36

[95] H Callaway, 'Dressing for Dinner in the Bush: Rituals of Self-Definition and British Imperial Authority' in R Barnes and JB Eicher (eds.), *Dress and Gender: Making and Meaning in Cultural Contexts*, London, 1992, pp.232–47, p.233

[96] Trowell, *African Tapestry*, pp.22–3

[97] RHL/MSS.Afr.s.1653, Anderson, *Reminiscences*, Book I, p.19

[98] RHL/MSS.Afr.s.1872/82 Hunter, 'Detailed Memorandum', p.4

[99] RHL/MSS.Afr.s.1872/162(a) M Wilson, 'Memoirs of Service as Entomologist, Health Officer and Medical Officer in Tanganyika, 1933–63' [n.d.]

[100] Lady Cranworth, 'Hints for a Woman in British East Africa' in Cranworth, *Colony in the Making,* pp.84–92, p.87

[101] Trzebinski, *Kenya Pioneers*, p.10

[102] E Bradley, *Dearest Priscilla: Letters to the Wife of a Colonial Civil Servant*, London, 1950, p.37

[103] Interview: Heussler with HE Newnham, 6 August 1959; Letter: Newnham to Heussler 2 September 1959 quoted in Heussler, *Yesterday's Rulers*, pp.42–3

[104] Kennedy, *Islands of White*, p.137

[105] RHL/MSS.Afr.s.1653, Anderson, *Reminiscences*, Book I, p.27

[106] Huxley, *Africa View*, p.213

[107] Wiggins, 'Early Days in British East Africa and Uganda', p.708

[108] NA/CO/850/47/4 Lord Crewe, Confidential Circular, 11 January 1909; The drastic change in official attitudes to concubinage that this marked is discussed in Ronald Hyam, 'Concubinage and the Colonial Service: The Crewe Circular (1909)', *The Journal of Imperial and Commonwealth History*, 14, 1986, pp.170-86

[109] A Stoler, 'Making Empire Respectable: The Politics of Race and Sexual Morality in 20th-Century Colonial Cultures' in J Breman, P de Rooy, A Stoler and WF Wertheim (eds.), *Imperial Monkey Business: Racial Supremacy in Social Darwinist Theory and Colonial Practice*, Amsterdam, 1990, pp.35–70; Kuklick, *The Imperial Bureaucrat*, p.122; Hinde, 'The 'Black Peril'', p.195

[110] Mitchell, 'Forty Years Back' p.280

[111] Davis, *Microcosm of Empire*, p.2

[112] Driver has argued conduct was as important as professional work in informing group identity. Driver, *Geography Militant*, pp.63–4

[113] Cranworth, *Colony in the Making*, p.17, p.20

[114] Calwell, 'Nineteen Years in the Colonial Medical Service', p.(s)7

[115] R Surridge, 'Salad Days in Tanganyika' in Kirk-Greene, *Glimpses of Empire*, pp.283–6, p.284

[116] 'Roland Dowdeswell', *BMJ*, ii, 1956, p.305; Mitchell, 'Forty Years Back', p.280; RHL/MSS.Afr.s.1782, ADP Hodges, Diaries 1898–1907, e.g., 19/06/1898 – 12/09/1898

[117] This was an almost universal rite of passage. Explicit references to learning Swahili include: Calwell, 'Nineteen Years in the Colonial Medical Service', p.(s)10; KNA/MOH/1/5409 Swahili Examination to Officers [n.d.]; Officers in Tanzania who passed the Swahili examination were regularly listed in the *Tanganyika Territory Government Gazette*, 'James Henry Bartlett', *East African Medical Journal*, 30, 1953, p.493; 'Enrico Pietro Bayon', *BMJ*, ii, 1952, pp.1260–1, p.1261. In the Colonial Administrative Service officers would not pass probation if they had not achieved a native language examination. Mills, 'Methods of Appointment and Training', p.467

[118] RHL/MSS.Afr.s.1872/153a Williams, 'Detailed Memoranda', p.7

[119] BS Cohn, *Colonialism and its Forms of Knowledge: The British in India*, Princeton, NJ, [1985], pp.16–56

[120] E Brodhurst-Hill, *So This is Kenya!*, London, 1936, p.30

[121] Another name for the Swahili spoken by Europeans was 'Ki-Settler' (a pun on Ki-Swahili). Cook, 'The Medical History of Uganda: Part 1', p.74

[122] Carman, *Medical History of Kenya*, 1976, p.67

[123] Huxley, *Africa View*, p.374

[124] NA/CO/850/120/8 Memorandum for the Colonial Office on the Employment of Refugees (Medical Practitioners), 20 September 1938. See also NA/CO/850/144/1 Memorandum by RR Scott, Tanganyika Territory, 17 April 1939; Brodhurst-Hill, *So This is Kenya!*, p.2; Trzebinski, *Kenya Pioneers*, p.111, p.134

[125] D Cameron, *My Tanganyika Service and Some Nigeria*, London, 1939, p.24

[126] Wiggins, 'Early Days in British East Africa and Uganda', p.701

[127] RHL/MSS.Afr.s.1872/153a Williams, 'Detailed Memoranda', p.3

[128] Although, I would argue, these sub-groups were ultimately defined by their shared colonial experiences over and above individual differences. For similar tropes in a different group of doctors see JSG Blair, *The Conscript Doctors: Memories of National Service*, Durham, 2001

Chapter 10: Conclusion (pp.133-140)

[1] C Jeffries, *Partners For Progress: The Men and Women of the Colonial Service*, London, 1949, p.101

[2] This has been done elsewhere. See DF Clyde, *History of the Medical Services of Tanganyika*, Dar Es Salaam, 1962; A Beck, *A History of the British Medical Administration of East Africa: 1900–1950*, Cambridge, MA, 1999 [1970]; JA Carman, *A Medical History of the Colony and Protectorate of Kenya: a Personal Memoir*, London, 1976; WD Foster, *The Early History of Scientific Medicine in Uganda*, Nairobi, 1970; O Ransford, *Bid the Sickness Cease: Disease in the History of Black Africa*, London, 1983

[3] Not least because sovereignty and borders changed during the early colonial period.

[4] Some of this information can be gleaned from H Power, *Tropical Medicine in the Twentieth Century. A History of the Liverpool School of Tropical Medicine*, London, 1999; L Wilkinson and A Hardy, *Prevention and Cure: The London School of Hygiene and Tropical Medicine A 20th Century Quest for Global Public Health*, London, 2001

[5] This has been partly done by W Eckart, *Medizin und Kolinialimperialismus, Deutschland, 1884– 1945*, München,1997; Foster, *Early History of Scientific Medicine in Uganda*

[6] As has been done by: J Farley, *Bilharzia: A History of Imperial Tropical Medicine*, Cambridge, 2003 [1991]; DM Haynes, *Imperial Medicine: Patrick Manson and the Conquest of Tropical Disease*, Pennsylvania, 2001

[7] For 75 case studies of individual careers, see A Crozier, *The Colonial Medical Officer and the Colonial Identity: Kenya, Uganda and Tanzania before World War Two*, University College London, PhD thesis, 2005, Appendix 5.

[8] These histories have been told amply well elsewhere. J Iliffe, *East African Doctors: a History of the Modern Profession*, Cambridge, 1999; EE Sabben-Clare, DJ Bradley and K Kirkwood (eds.), *Health in Tropical Africa During the Colonial Period*, Oxford,1980; KA Hoppe, *Sleeping Sickness Control in British East Africa, 1900–1960*, Westport, CT, 2003; M Dobson, M Malowany and R Snow, 'Roll Back Malaria: The History of Malaria and its Control in Twentieth Century East Africa', *Wellcome Trust Review*, 8, 1999, pp.54–7; M Dobson, M Malowany and D Stapleton (eds.), 'Dealing with Malaria in the Last 60 Years: Aims, Methods and Results', *Parassitologia*, 2, 2000; Randall Packard examines the history of malaria control in a wider context. R Packard, "No Other Logical Choice': Global Malaria Eradication and the Politics of International Health', *Parassitologia* 40, 1998, pp. 217–30

[9] M Vaughan, *Curing Their Ills: Colonial Power and African Illness*, Padstow, 1991; D Arnold, *Colonizing the Body: State Medicine and Epidemic Disease in Nineteenth-Century India*, California, CA, 1993

[10] Beck, *History of British Medical Administration*, p.149

[11] C Jeffries, *Partners For Progress*, p.19

[12] P Holden, *Doctors and Other Medical Personnel in the Public Health Services of Africa, 1930–1965*, Oxford, 1984, p.6

[13] *Ibid.*, p.10

[14] In 1943 Furse submitted a scheme for post-war Colonial Service training, endorsed by the Duke of Devonshire.

[15] For post war developments see LA Mills 'Methods of Appointment and Training in the British and Dutch Colonial Civil Service', *American Political Science Review*, 33, 1939, pp.465–72

[16] Jeffries, *Partners For Progress*, p.81, p.21

[17] A Kirk-Greene, *A Biographical Dictionary of the British Colonial Service, 1939–1966*, London, 1991, p.vi

[18] A Kirk-Greene, *On Crown Service: A History of HM Colonial and Overseas Civil Services, 1837– 1997*, London, 1999, p.47

[19] *Organization of the Colonial Service*, 1946, Parliamentary Papers, Col. No. 197, reproduced in *Ibid.*, pp. 202–9, p.203

[20] C Dundas, Governor of Uganda, Dispatch to the Colonial Office and Ugandan Provincial Administration on Postwar Africa, May 1942, reproduced in *Ibid.*, pp. 216–9, p.218

[21] Jeffries, *Partners For Progress*, p.20

[22] 'The Colonial Medical Services', *BMJ*, ii, 1931, p.21

[23] RHL/MSS.Afr.s.1872/82 JK Hunter, 'Notices on District Medical Work in Uganda', 1951

[24] J Currie, 'Present Day Difficulties of a Young Officer in the Tropics', Reprinted from *The Colonial Services Club Magazine*, Cambridge, [n.d. *c.*1932], pp.1–8, p.1

[25] Although subsequent histories argued that medical and scientific progress were in fact used to advance colonial aims. E.g., M Worboys, *Science and British Colonial Imperialism: 1895-1940*, University of Sussex, DPhil. Thesis, 1979; AW Crosby, *Ecological Imperialism: the Biological Expansion of Europe, 900–1900*, Cambridge, 2004 [1986]; R Macleod and M Lewis (eds.), *Disease Medicine and Empire: Perspectives on Western Medicine and the Experience of European Expansion*, New York, NY, 1988; Vaughan, *Curing Their Ills*; M Lyons, *The Colonial Disease: A Social History of Sleeping Sickness in Northern Zaire 1900–1940*, Cambridge, 2002 [1992]; Arnold, *Colonizing the Body*

[26] E.g., William Barnetson, Fairfax Bell, Ronald Heisch, Douglas Snell

[27] E.g., Philip Bell (became DMS, Nyasaland); Stanley Branch (became Chief M and HO, St Vincent); Kenneth Edmundson (became Chief MO, Gibraltar and DMS, Seychelles); George Maclean (became DMS, Trinidad)

[28] E.g., Arthur Bagshawe (became the first Director of the Sleeping Sickness Bureau, later to become the Bureau of Hygiene and Tropical Diseases); Henry Burke-Gaffney (became Assistant Director of the Bureau of Hygiene and Tropical Diseases in London, becoming its director in 1961); Percy Garnham (Reader in Medical Parasitology at the LSH&TM (1947–51) and then Professor and Director of the Department (1952–68)

[29] E.g., John Buchanan (became the last Chief Medical Adviser to the Colonial Office in 1960); Claud Cole (became consulting physician to the Colonial Office, the Crown Agents and the Overseas Development Administration); William Kauntze (became first, Assistant (1941) and later, Chief (1944–7) Medical Adviser to the Colonial Office).

[30] E.g., Clifford Braimbridge (retired Kenya); Albert Paterson (retired Kenya); Arthur Williams (retired Kenya); Edwin Trim (retired Uganda)

[31] As is evidenced by the number of ex-Colonial Officers who wrote histories of their Colonial experiences (or about the Service in general): e.g., Carman; Clark; Clyde; Foster; Gelfand; Kirk-Greene; Ransford; Schram

[32] AD Milne, 'The Rise of the Colonial Medical Service', *East African Medical Journal*, 5, 1928-9, pp.50-8, p.50

[33] Manson-Bahr served in Tanzania, 1939–40, Tanzania, 1946–8, Kenya 1953–62. He became a senior lecturer in clinical tropical medicine, London School of Hygiene and Tropical Medicine.

[34] M Trowell, *African Tapestry*, London, 1957, p.16

[35] 'Robert Hennessey', *BMJ*, 299, 1989, pp.176–7, p.176

[36] RHL/MSS.Afr.s.1872/75 RS Hennessey, 'Learning About Disease in Uganda: 1929–44 and 1949–55', 1983, p.1

[37] E Trzebinski, *The Kenya Pioneers: the Frontiersmen of an Adopted Land*, London, 1991 [1985], p.31

Bibliography

Primary Sources

Rhodes House Library, Oxford

RHL/MSS.Afr.s.1653 Theodore Farnworth Anderson, *Reminiscences by T. Farnworth Anderson*, Book I, Limuru, Kenya, 1973

RHL/MSS.Afr.s.1091 Papers of Clement John Baker, 1901–28

RHL/MSS.Brit.Emp.r.4 Peter Alphonsus Clearkin, *Ramblings and Recollections of a Colonial Doctor 1913–58*, Book I, Durban, 1967

RHL/MSS.Afr.s.708 (1) Papers of William Kerr Connell, Diary 1924–5

RHL/MSS.Afr.r.97 Papers of John Bernard Davey, 1909–10

RHL/MSS.Afr.s.313-15 Papers of Henry Speldewinde De Boer, *c.*1929

RHL/MSS.Afr.s.ff.312–321 Papers of David Donald, 1900

RHL/MSS.Afr.s.1269 Papers of George Samuel Hale, 1946

RHL/MSS.Afr.s.1782 Aubrey Dallas Percival Hodges, Diaries 1898–1907

RHL/MSS.Afr.s.2032 William V Kendall, 'Extracts from the Diaries, Letters and Memory of WV Kendall whilst Serving in the Colonial Civil Service Uganda Protectorate 1922–30'

RHL/MSS.Afr.s.1079 Papers of Ian Cameron Middleton

RHL/MSS.Afr.s.702 Robert Arthur Welsford Procter, 'Random Reminiscences, Mainly Surgical', [n.d.]

RHL/MSS.Afr.s.1094 & MSS.Afr.s.1421 Papers of Philip Hugh Rawson, 1922–39

RHL/MSS.Afr.s.796 Diary of Charles Wilcocks, 1928–9

RHL/MSS.Afr.s.1378 Papers of Bertrand Osborne Wilkin, 1932–62

RHL/MSS.Afr.s.1519 Papers of William Arthur Young

RHL/MSS.Brit.Emp.s.415 Papers of Ralph Furse

RHL/MSS.Brit.Emp.r.21 Desk Diaries of the Assistant Private Secretary (Appointments) to the Secretary of State for the Colonies 1899–1915

RHL/MSS.Afr.s.1872/9 Raymond Edward Barrett, 'Memorandum on Experiences in the Colonial Medical Service in East Africa, 1928–55', 18th March 1983

RHL/MSS.Afr.s.1872/16 Arthur Boase (compiled by his wife, R.M. Boase), 'Notes on Experiences in Colonial Medical Service in Uganda, 1924–56', 14th February 1983

RHL/MSS.Afr.s.1872/24 Hugh Gault Calwell, 'Memorandum on Experiences in the Colonial Medical Service in Tanganyika, 1930–49', 25th April 1983

RHL/MSS.Afr.s.1872/33 Arthur Claud Ely Cole, 'Memorandum on Experiences in the Colonial Medical Service in Tanganyika, 1939–60', April 1983

RHL/MSS.Afr.s.1872/75 Robert Samuel Hennessey, 'Memorandum on Experiences in the Colonial Medical Service in Uganda, 1929–55'

RHL/MSS.Afr.s.1872/82 James Kellock Hunter, 'Detailed Memorandum on Experiences in the Colonial Medical Service in Uganda, 1939–58', [n.d. c. 1983]

RHL/MSS.Afr.s.1872/84 Philip William Hutton, 'Memorandum on Service as Physician Specialist, Acting Dean and Honorary Lecturer in Medicine, in Uganda, including Makerere, 1937–1961' [Feb?] 1983

RHL/MSS.Afr.s.1872/144b Hugh Carey Trowell, typescript of interviews conducted by his daughter, Tape 1B, [n.d. *c*.1984]

RHL/MSS.Afr.s.1872/153a Arthur Warriner Williams, 'Detailed Memoranda on Experiences in the Colonial Medical Service in Uganda and Tanganyika, 1931-1949', [n.d. *c*.1983]

RHL/MSS.Afr.s.1872/162(a) Margaret Wilson, 'Memoirs of Service as Entomologist, Health Officer and Medical Officer in Tanganyika, 1933–63' [n.d.]

Kenya National Archives, Nairobi

KNA/MOH/1 Archives of the Ministry of Health
KNA/MOH/3 Archives of the Ministry of Health

National Archive, Kew

NA/CO/429 Patronage: Original Correspondence, 1867–19
NA/CO/457 East Africa and Uganda: Government Gazettes, 1899–1907
NA/CO/519 East Africa and Uganda: Original Correspondence, 1904–5
NA/CO/533 Kenya: Original Correspondence, 1905–51
NA/CO/536 Uganda: Original Correspondence, 1905–51
NA/CO/542 Kenya: Government Gazettes, 1908–75
NA/CO/543 Kenya: Miscellanea, 1901–46
NA/CO/612 Uganda: Government Gazettes, 1908–73
NA/CO/613 Uganda: Miscellanea, 1901–45
NA/CO/691 Tanganyika: Original Correspondence, 1916–51
NA/CO/726 Tanganyika: Miscellanea, 1921–48
NA/CO/737 Tanganyika: Government Gazettes, 1919–64
NA/CO/822 East Africa: Original Correspondence, 1905–51
NA/CO/850 Colonial Office Personnel: Original Correspondence, 1932–52
NA/CO/877 Colonial Office Appointments: Original Correspondence, 1920–52
NA/CO/885 War and Colonial Department, Colonial Office: Subjects Affecting Colonies Generally, Confidential Print, 1839–1936

British Medical Association Archives, London

BMA/B/162 Dominions Committee [Originally the Colonial Committee]
BMA/C/1/4 Annual Reports of UK and Overseas Branches 1930-37
BMA/E/1/41 Colonial Medical Services, 1919–50

Contemporary Medical Archives Centre, Wellcome Trust, London

WL/CMAC/PP/HCT/A5 Elizabeth Bray, *Hugh Trowell: Pioneer Nutritionist*, unpublished biography, London, 1988

WL/CMAC/MS/5677 Private Papers of John Davey, 'British Administration in Tanganyika', 1944

WL/CMAC/PP/PCG/A2 Percy Claude Cyril Garnham, Personal Correspondence and Miscellaneous, 1936–44

WL/CMAC/MS/3353–3355 Papers of Robert Ernest McConnell, *c.*1909–10

Foreign and Commonwealth Office, London

FCO/14634 'Organisation of the Medical and Sanitary Services in the British Colonies: Replies to Circular Despatch: 1st February 1913', *Standing Orders for the Medical Department* [Uganda], Government Press, 1912

FCO/East African Staff Lists, 1914-15, 1921

London School of Hygiene and Tropical Medicine, London

LSHTM/GBO809 Papers of Aubrey Dallas Percival Hodges, 1898–06

LSHTM/[no further class mark] Papers of Geoffrey Douglas Hale Carpenter, 1913–30

Official Publications

Annual Medical Reports of East Africa Protectorate (later Kenya), 1911–1939

Annual Medical Reports of Tanganyika Territory, 1921–1939

Annual Medical Reports of Uganda Protectorate, 1912-1939

Anon 'Papers Relating to the Investigation of Malaria and Other Tropical Diseases and the Establishment of Schools of Tropical Medicine,' *Parliamentary Papers*, 1903, 44, pp.3–5

Cmd.939 *Report of the Departmental Committee Appointed by the Secretary of State for the Colonies to Enquire into the Colonial Medical Services*, London, HMSO, 1920

Cmd. 2883 *Report of the Lovat Committee on the Colonial Scientific and Research Service*, 1927

Colonial Office *Regulations for His Majesty's Colonial Service*, London, HMSO, 1908,

Colonial Office [William J Simpson] African No.1025: *Report on Sanitary Matters in the East Africa Protectorate, Uganda and Zanzibar*, London, The Colonial Office, 1915

Colonial Office *Miscellaneous No.99: Colonial Medical Appointments*, London, The Colonial Office, 1921 (twenty–ninth edition)

Colonial Office *African (East) No.1103: Regulations for the East African Medical Service*, London, The Colonial Office, 1925

Colonial Office *African (West) No.678: Information for the Use of Candidates for Appointments on the West African Medical Staff*, London, The Colonial Office, 1930

Colonial Office *Colonial No.56: Information as to the Conditions and Cost of Living in the Colonies, Protectorates and Mandated Territories*, London, HMSO, 1930

Colonial Office 'Report of the Committee Chaired by Sir Warren Fisher', *The System of Appointment in the Colonial Office and the Colonial Services*, London, HMSO, 1930

Colonial Office *Colonial Service Recruitment No.3A: The Colonial Service. Information for the use of Candidates for Appointment to the Colonial Medical Service*, London, The Colonial Office, 1931

Colonial Office *Miscellaneous No.441: The Colonial Medical Service, Special Regulations by the Secretary of State for the Colonies*, London, The Colonial Office, 1934

Colonial Office *Colonial Service Recruitment, No.3: Information Regarding the Colonial Medical Service*, London, The Colonial Office, 1935

Colonial Office *African No.973: Regulations for the Employment of Officers in the East African Dependencies*, London, The Colonial Office, 1935

Colonial Office *Colonial Service Recruitment No.1: The Colonial Service, General Information Regarding Colonial Appointments*, London, The Colonial Office, 1936

Colonial Office *Miscellaneous No.407: Primary Courses of Instruction in Tropical Medicine and Hygiene for Officers Selected for Appointment to the Colonial Medical Service*, (sixth edition), London, The Colonial Office, 1939

Colonial Office *Miscellaneous No.488: The Colonial Service, General Conditions of Employment*, London, The Colonial Office, 1939

Published Primary Sources (including works by participants)

Anon 'Medical Appointments in the Colonies', *British Medical Journal*, i, 1891, p.770

Anon 'Instruction in Tropical Diseases,' *British Medical Journal*, i, 1895, p.771

Anon 'The Colonial Medical Service: A Rejoinder,' *British Medical Journal*, i, 1897, p.216

Anon 'The Colonial Medical Service', *British Medical Journal*, i, 1899, p.323

Anon 'Correspondence: The Colonial Medical Service', *British Medical Journal*, ii, 1899, pp.1479–80

Anon 'Organisation of the Colonial Medical Service', *British Medical Journal*, i, 1902, pp.347–8

Anon 'Medical Science and Colonization', *British Medical Journal*, i, 1905, pp.1002–3

Anon 'Medical Appointments in the Colonies', *British Medical Journal*, ii, 1905, pp.585–8

Anon 'The Association and the Colonies', *British Medical Journal*, i, 1905, p.1394

Anon 'The Future of Tropical Medicine' (Report of the Society of Tropical Medicine and Hygiene), *British Medical Journal*, i, 1909, p.1545

Anon 'The East African Medical Staff', *British Medical Journal*, i, 1910, p.177

Anon 'The White Man in the Tropics', *British Medical Journal*, ii, 1911, pp.759–60

Anon 'The Tropical Diseases Bureau', *The British Medical Journal*, i, 1912, p.1149

Anon 'Medical Notes in Parliament: Tropical Medicine', *British Medical Journal*, ii, 1912, pp.40–2

Anon 'Sanitary Organization in the Tropics', *British Medical Journal*, ii, 1913, pp.377–9

Anon 'Discussion of the Causes of Invaliding from the Tropics', *British Medical Journal*, ii, 1913, pp.1290–6

Anon 'Memorandum of Evidence Placed by the British Medical Association before the Colonial Medical Services Committee (Appointed in November 1919, by the Secretary of State for the Colonies), on 23rd February 1920', *Supplement to the British Medical Journal*, 1920, pp.141–3

Anon 'Colonial Medical Services: Report of the Departmental Committee', *British Medical Journal*, ii, 1920, pp.448–9

Anon 'The Future of Research in Tropical Medicine', *British Medical Journal*, i, 1921, pp.388–9

Anon 'Medical Appointments Under the Colonial Office', *British Medical Journal*, ii, 1923, pp.394–6

Anon 'British Medical Association', *The Kenya Medical Journal*, 1, 1924–5, pp.54–5, p.55

Anon 'Medical Notes in Parliament: Tropical Medicine', *British Medical Journal*, ii, 1925, p.235

Anon 'A Health Department for the Colonial Office', *British Medical Journal*, ii, 1925, p.267

Anon 'The Colonial Medical Services: Statement by the British Medical Association', *Supplement to the British Medical Journal*, 1926, pp.9–10

Anon 'Regulations for the East African Medical Service, Correspondence Between the British Medical Association and the Colonial Office', *Supplement to the British Medical Journal*, 1926, pp.27–8

Anon 'The Colonial Conference', *British Medical Journal*, i, 1927, p.1040

Anon 'European Women and Children in the Tropics' [Report on a Discussion held at the Royal Society of Medicine], *British Medical Journal*, i, 1931, pp.268–9

Anon 'Numbers of the Medical Profession', *British Medical Journal*, ii, 1931, pp.418–19

Anon 'Editorial', Kenya and East African Medical Journal, 8, 1931–2, p.331

Anon 'Editorial', *The East African Medical Journal*, 9, 1932–3, p.339

Anon 'Correspondence: Tropical Neurasthenia', *East African Medical Journal*, 12, 1935–6, pp.28–9

Anon 'A Colonial Office Visitor', *The East African Standard*, 15th January 1936, p.2

Anon 'The Portal of Medicine', *The Lancet*, i, 1936, pp.672–3

Anon 'Colonial Medical Service', *British Medical Journal*, ii, 1938, pp.546–8

Anon 'Medical Practice Overseas', *British Medical Journal*, ii, 1939, pp.540–4

Ansorge, William John *Under the African Sun: A Description of Native Races in Uganda, Sporting Adventures and Other Experiences*, London, William Heinemann, 1899

Archer, Geoffrey *Personal and Historical Memoirs of an East African Administrator*, London, Oliver and Boyd Ltd., 1963

Bell, Hesketh *Glimpses of a Governor's Life*, London, Sampson, Low, Marston and Co. Ltd., [n.d.]

Balfour, Andrew 'Vistas and Visions: Some Aspects of the Colonial Medical Services', *Glasgow Medical Journal*, 6, 1924, pp.353–74

Bertram, Sir Anton *The Colonial Service*, Cambridge University Press, 1930

Bhagwat, Sakharam Ramachandra 'Rupture of Pleura Without Fracture of Ribs Caused by a Buffalo', *British Medical Journal*, i, 1913, p.168

Boase, Arthur J 'Reminiscences of Surgery in Uganda', *The East African Medical Journal*, 31, 1954, pp.197–203

Bödeker, HA 'Some Sidelights on Early Medical History in East Africa', *The East African Medical Journal*, 12, 1935–36, pp.100–7

Bradley, Emily *Dearest Priscilla: Letters to the Wife of a Colonial Civil Servant*, London, Max Parish, 1950

Braimbridge, Clifford V 'Address by Mr C.V. Braimbridge', *The East African Medical Journal*, 31, 1954, pp.205–8

Brodhurst-Hill, Evelyn *So, This is Kenya!* London and Glasgow, Blackie and Son Ltd., 1936

Burdett, Henry *Burdett's Hospitals and Charities 1901*, London, The Scientific Press Ltd., 1901

Burdett, Henry *Burdett's Hospitals and Charities 1911*, London, The Scientific Press Ltd., 1911

Burke Gaffney, HJOD 'Forefathers of Tropical Medicine', *East African Medical Journal*, 10, 1933–4, pp.100–114

Burke-Gaffney, HJOD 'The History of Medicine in the African Countries', *Medical History*, 12, 1968, pp.31–41

Buxton, TF Victor 'A Social Effort in East Africa', *Journal of the Royal African Society*, 39, 1911, pp.342–4

Calwell, Hugh Gault 'Nineteen Years in the Colonial Medical Service', *The Ulster Medical Journal*, 65 (supplement), April 1993, pp. s1–s42

Cameron, Donald *My Tanganyika Service and Some Nigeria*, London, George Allen and Unwin, 1939

Carman, John A *A Medial History of the Colony and Protectorate of Kenya: A Personal Memoir*, London, Rex Collings, 1976

Carpenter, Geoffrey Douglas Hale *A Naturalist on Lake Victoria*, London, Fisher and Unwin Ltd., 1920

Carpenter, Geoffrey Douglas Hale *A Naturalist in East Africa*, Oxford, The Clarendon Press, 1925

Castellani, Aldo *Microbes, Men and Monarchs: A Doctor's Life in Many Lands*, London, Victor Gollancz Ltd., 1960

Charles, R Havelock 'Discussion on Special Factors Influencing the Suitability of Europeans for Life in the Tropics', *British Medical Journal*, ii, 1910, pp.869–74

Cook, Albert R 'The Medical History of Uganda: Part 1', *The East African Medical Journal*, 13, 1936–7, pp.66–81

Cook, Albert R 'The Medical History of Uganda: Part 2', *The East African Medical Journal*, 13, 1936–7, pp.99–110

Cook, Albert R *Uganda Memories, 1897–1940*, Kampala, Uganda Society, 1945

Cook, Ernest Neville *Doctors in Africa*, London, Church Missionary Society, [n.d. c.1918]

Cranworth, Lord 'The Public School Boy in East Africa', *National Review*, 336, 1911, pp.992–1000

Cranworth, Lord *A Colony in the Making. Or Sport and Profit in British East Africa*, London, Macmillan and Co., 1912

Cross, D Kerr *Health in Africa: A Medical Handbook for European Travellers and Residents, Embracing a Study of Malarial Fever as it is Found in British Central Africa*, London, James Nisbet & Co., Ltd., 1897

Crown Agents for the Colonies *Hints on the Preservation of Health in Tropical Africa*, London, The Crown Agents for the Colonies, 1943 (first published, 1938)

Currie, James 'Present Day Difficulties of a Young Officer in the Tropics', Reprinted from *The Colonial Services Club Magazine*, Cambridge, [n.d. *c.*1932], pp.1–8

Davis, Alexander *A Microcosm of Empire (British East Africa)*, Nairobi, Mombasa and London, The Caxton (BEA) Printing and Publishing Co., Ltd., [n.d. *c.*1918]

Duckworth, Dyce 'On the Education of Medical Practitioners for Colonial Service', A Paper read at the First Inter-colonial Medical Congress, held at Amsterdam, September 1883, pp.1–7

Edge, Granville 'The Contents of Colonial Medical Reports', *East African Medical Journal*, 14, 1937–8, pp.146–7

Evatt, George 'Notes on the Organisation of the Colonial Medical Service of the Empire', *British Medical Journal*, ii, 1896, pp.863–4

Eyles, CH 'The Colonial Medical Service: a Rejoinder', *British Medical Journal*, i, 1897, p.216

Field, Alan *'Verb. Sap.' On Going to East Africa: British Central Africa, Uganda and Zanzibar and Big Game Shooting in East Africa*, Vols.1 & 2, London, John Bale, Sons & Danielsson Ltd., 1906

Fremantle, Francis 'The Colonial Conference', *British Medical Journal*, i, 1907, p.536

Furse, Ralph *Aucuparius: Recollections of a Recruiting Officer*, London, Oxford University Press, 1962

Garnham, Percy Cecil Claude 'Britain's Contribution to Tropical Medicine 1868–1968', *The Practitioner*, 201, 1968, pp.153–61

Garry, T Gerald *African Doctor*, London, The Book Club, 1939

Gilks, John Langton 'A Medical Safari in a Native Reserve', *The Kenya Medical Journal*, 1, 1924–5, pp.270–4

Gilks, John Langton 'Proposed Expansion of the Medical Services in Kenya', *The Kenya Medical Journal*, 2, 1925–6, pp.318–20

Gilks, John Langton 'The Medical Department and the Health Organization in Kenya, 1909–1933', *The East African Medical Journal*, 9, 1932–3, pp.340–54

Gregory, JR *Under the Sun (A Memoir of Dr RW Burkitt, of Kenya)*, Nairobi, The English Press Ltd., 1951

Hailey, Lord *An African Survey: a Study of Problems Arising in Africa South of the Sahara*, Oxford University Press, 1938

Hall, Sir Daniel 'Settlers' Problems in Kenya', *Journal of the Royal Society of Arts*, 78, 1930, pp.406–23

Hinde, Hildegarde Beatrice 'The 'Black Peril' in British East Africa: A Frank Talk to Women Settlers', *Empire Review*, 1921, pp.193–200

Huxley, Elspeth *White Man's Country: Lord Delamere and the Making of Kenya*, (2 Vols), New York and Washington, Praeger, 1968 (first published, 1935)

Huxley, Julian *Africa View*, London Chatto and Windus, 1936 (first published, 1931)

Jeffries, Charles *The Colonial Empire and its Civil Service*, Cambridge University Press, 1938,

Jeffries, Charles *Partners For Progress: The Men and Women of the Colonial Service*, London, George C Harrap, 1949

Ladkin, R.S 'The Medical Officer and Local Government', *Journal of African Administration*, 5, 1953, pp.21–30

Latham, DV 'The White Man in East Africa' *East African Medical Journal*, 9, 1932–3, pp.276–82

Leys, Norman Maclean *Kenya*, London, The Hogarth Press, 1924

Lowell, Lawrence *Colonial Civil Service: The Selection and Training of Colonial Officials in England, Holland, and France*, London, Macmillan & Co. Ltd., 1900

Maclean, George 'Medical Administration in the Tropics', *British Medical Journal*, i, 1950, pp.756–61

Manson, Patrick 'On the Necessity for Special Education in Tropical Medicine,' *Lancet*, 2nd October 1897, pp. 842–5

Marsh, Edward *A Number of People*, London, Heinemann, 1939

McKinnon, Murdoch 'Medical Aspects of White Settlement in Kenya', *East African Medical Journal*, 11, 1934–5, pp.376–94

Mills, Lennox A 'Methods of Appointment and Training in the British and Dutch Colonial Civil Service', *American Political Science Review*, 33, 1939, pp.465–72

Milne, Arthur Dawson 'The Rise of the Colonial Medical Service', *Kenya and East African Medical Journal*, 5, 1928–9, pp.50–8

Mitchell, Sir Philip 'Forty Years Back' in Anthony Kirk-Greene, *Glimpses of Empire: A Corona Anthology*, London and New York, I.B. Tauris, 2001, pp.278–80

Nash, TAM *A Zoo Without Bars: Life in the East African Bush 1927–1932*, Tunbridge Wells, Wayte Binding, 1984

Parke, Thomas Heazle *Guide to Health in Africa*, London, Sampson Low, Marston & Company Ltd., 1893

Parkinson, Cosmo *The Colonial Office From Within, 1909–1945*, London, Faber and Faber Ltd., 1947

Purvis, John B *Handbook to British East Africa and Uganda*, London, Swan Sonnenschein & Co. Ltd., 1900

Reeves, E A *Hints to Travellers,* Vol. 1, Royal Geographical Society, 1935 (11th edition)

Ross, Ronald 'Some Suggestions for the Improvement of Sanitary and Medical Practice in the Tropics', *British Medical Journal*, ii, 1900, pp.553–4

Ryan, Charles J *Health Preservation in West Africa*, London, John Bale, Sons & Danielsson, Ltd., 1914

Sambon, Luigi 'Remarks on the Possibility of the Acclimatisation of Europeans in Tropical Regions', *British Medical Journal*, i 1897, pp.61–6

Scott. Ralph Roylance 'The Growth of a Public Health Service in a Tropical Town', *The East African Medical Journal*, 10, 1933–4, pp.130–44

Simpson, WJ *The Maintenance of Health in the Topics*, London, John Bale and Danielsson, ltd., 1905

Smart, AGH 'An Impression of Life in the Colonial Medical Service', *St. Thomas's Hospital Gazette*, 37, 1939, pp.123–6

Squire Sprigge, Samuel *Medicine and the Public*, London, William Heinemann, 1905

Stephens, JWW, Yorke, Warrington and Blacklock, Breadalbane (compilers), *Liverpool School of Tropical Medicine, Historical Record: 1898–1920*, Liverpool University Press, 1920

Stirrett, AP *Medical Book for the Treatment of Diseases in West Africa*, Nigeria, The Niger Press, 1931

Stirling, Leader *Tanzania Doctor*, Christopher Hurst and Co., 1977

St-Johnston, Sir Reginald *Strange Places and Strange Peoples or Life in the Colonial Service*, London, Hutchinson and Co., Ltd., 1936

Surridge, Rex 'Salad Days in Tanganyika' in Anthony Kirk-Greene, *Glimpses of Empire: A Corona Anthology*, London and New York, I.B. Tauris, 2001, pp.283–6

Taylor, Stephen and Gadsden, Phyllis, *Shadows in the Sun*, London, George G Harrap and Co. Ltd., 1949

Torrance, Arthur *Tracking Down the Enemies of Man*, New York, J. H. Sears & Company Inc., 1928

Treves, Sir Frederick *Uganda for a Holiday*, London, Smith Elder, 1910

Trowell, Margaret *African Tapestry*, London, Faber and Faber, 1957

Walter, A 'Climate and White Settlement in the East African Highlands', *East African Medical Journal*, 11, 1934–5, pp.210–25

Ward HF and Milligan JW (compilers), *Handbook of British East Africa, 1912–13*, London, Sifton Praed and Co. Ltd. and Nairobi, The Caxton (BEA) Printing and Publishing Company Ltd., 1913 (second impression)

Waugh, Evelyn *Remote People*, London, Duckworth, 1931

Waugh, Evelyn *Scoop*, Harmondsworth, Middlesex, Penguin Books, 2000 (first published, 1938)

Wiggins, Clare Aveling 'Early Days in British East Africa and Uganda', *The East African Medical Journal*, 37, 1960, pp.699–708

Wiggins, Clare Aveling 'Early Days in British East Africa and Uganda: Second Tour—1904–1907', *The East African Medical Journal*, 37, 1960, pp.780–93

Wilcocks, Charles *A Tropical Doctor in Africa and London*, unpublished autobiography, Leatherhead, Surrey, 1977

Wilson, Christopher *Before the Dawn in Kenya: An Authentic Account of Life in East Africa when it was Under African Rule*, Nairobi, The English Press Ltd., 1953 (first published, 1952)

Wilson, Christopher *Kenya's Warning: The Challenge to White Supremacy in Our British Colony*, Nairobi, The English Press Ltd., 1954

Ziemann, Hans *Hints to Europeans in Tropical Stations Without a Doctor and to Travellers in Warm Climates*, translated by Pauline Falcke, London, John Bale, Sons & Danielsson, Ltd., 1910

Other Biographical Sources

The Medical Directory: 1893–1940
The Medical Register: 1893–1940
The Colonial Office List: 1899–1940
The East African Medical Service Staff List: 1922– 33
Colonial Medical Service Staff List: 1936–39
Who was Who: 1897–1980
Crawford, DG *Roll of the Indian Medical Service,* 1615–1930, London, W. Thacker & Co., 1930
Drew, Robert *Commissioned Officers in the Medical Services of the British Army, 1660– 1960,* London, The Wellcome Historical Medical Library, 1968
Kirk-Greene, Anthony *A Biographical Dictionary of the British Colonial Service, 1939– 1966,* London, Hans Zell Publishers, 1991
Royal Society *Biographical Memoirs of Fellows of the Royal Society,* Vol. 20, 1974
Schram, Ralph *Heroes of Health Care in Africa,* unpublished folio, Isle of Wight, 1997
Trail, Richard (ed.), *Munk's Roll or Lives of the Fellows of the Royal College of Physicians of London,* London, Royal College of Physicians, 1968

Secondary Sources

Anderson, David M and Killingray, David (eds.), *Policing the Empire: Government, Authority and Control: 1830-1940,* Manchester University Press, 1991
Anderson, Warwick 'Climates of Opinion: Acclimatization in Nineteenth Century France and England', *Victorian Studies,* 35, 1992, pp.135–57
Anderson, Warwick 'Immunities of Empire: Race, Disease, and the New Tropical Medicine, 1900–1920', *Bulletin for the History of Medicine,* 70, 1996, pp.94–118
Anderson, Warwick 'The Trespass Speaks: White Masculinity and Colonial Breakdown', *American Historical Review,* 102, 1997, pp.1343–70
Anderson, Warwick *The Cultivation of Whiteness: Science, Health and Racial Destiny in Australia,* New York, Basic Books, 2003
Arnold, David 'Medical Priorities and Practice in Nineteenth-Century British India', *South Asia Research,* 5, 1985, pp.167–85
Arnold, David (ed.) *Imperial Medicine and Indigenous Societies,* Manchester University Press, 1988
Arnold, David *Colonizing the Body: State Medicine and Epidemic Disease in Nineteenth-Century India,* University of California Press, 1993
Arnold, David (ed.) *Warm Climates and Western Medicine: The Emergence of Tropical Medicine, 1600–1900,* Amsterdam, Rodopi, 1996
August, Thomas G *The Selling of Empire, British and French Imperialist Propaganda, 1890–1940,* Westport Connecticut, Greenwood Press, 1985
Baker, Colin 'The Government Medical Service in Malawi: an Administrative History, 1891–1974', *Medical History,* 20, 1976, pp.296–311
Baker, RA and Bayliss, RA 'William John Ritchie Simpson (1855–1931): Public Health and Tropical Medicine', *Medical History,* 1987, 31, pp.450–65

Bates, Darrell *A Gust of Plumes: A Biography of Lord Twining of Godalming and Tanganyika*, London, Hodder and Stoughton, 1972

Bayoumi, A *The History of the Sudan Health Services*, Nairobi, Kenya Literature Bureau, 1979

Beck, Ann 'Problems of British Medical Administration in East Africa between 1900–1930' *Bulletin of the History of Medicine*, 36, 1962, pp.275–83

Beck, Ann 'Native Medical Services in British East Africa and Native Patterns of Society' in *Verhandlungen des XX Internationalen Kongresses für Geschichte der Medizin, Berlin, 22–27 August 1966*, Hildesheim, Georg Olms Verlagsbuchhandlung, 1968, pp.870–75

Beck, Ann *A History of the British Medical Administration of East Africa: 1900–1950*, Cambridge, Massachusetts, Harvard University Press, 1999 (first published, 1970)

Beck, Ann 'The Role of Medicine in German East Africa', *Bulletin of the History of Medicine*, 45, 1971, pp.170–8

Beck, Ann 'Medical Administration and Medical Research in Developing Countries: Remarks on Their History in Colonial East Africa', *Bulletin of the History of Medicine*, 46, 1972, pp.349–58

Beck, Ann 'The State and Medical Research: British Government Policy Toward Tropical Medicine in East Africa', *Proceedings of the XXIII International Congress of the History of Medicine, London, 2–9 September 1972*, London, Wellcome Institute for the History of Medicine, 1974, pp.488–93

Bell, Heather *Frontiers of Medicine in the Anglo-Egyptian Sudan, 1899–1940*, Oxford, Clarendon Press, 1999

Berman, Bruce *Administration and Politics in Colonial Kenya*, PhD. Thesis, Yale University, 1973

Berman, Bruce and Lonsdale, John *Unhappy Valley: Conflict in Kenya and Africa, Book 1: State and Class*, London, Nairobi, Athens, James Currey, Heinemann, Kenya, Ohio University Press, 1992

Bhugra, Dinesh and Littlewood, Roland (eds.) *Colonialism and Psychiatry*, New Delhi, Oxford University Press, 2001

Blair, John SG *The Conscript Doctors: Memories of National Service*, Durham, The Pentland Press, 2001

Blake, Catriona *The Charge of the Parasols: Women's Entry to the Medical Profession*, London, Women's Press, 1990

Blunt, Alison *Travel, Gender and Imperialism: Mary Kingsley and West Africa*, London, The Guilford Press, 1994

Boahen, A Adu (ed.) *Africa Under Colonial Domination 1880–1935*, General History of Africa, Vol. VII, California, James Currey, 1990

Bonner, Thomas Neville *To the Ends of the Earth: Women's Search for Education in Medicine*, Cambridge, Mass., Harvard University Press, 1992

Bonner, Thomas Neville *Becoming a Physician, Medical Education in Britain, France, Germany and the United States, 1750–1945*, Baltimore & London, Johns Hopkins University Press, 2000 (first published, 1995)

Boyd, JS 'Fifty Years of Tropical Medicine', *British Medical Journal*, i, 1950, pp.37–43

Bradley, James, Crowther, Anne and Dupree, Marguerite 'Mobility and Selection in Scottish Medical Education 1858-1886' *Medical History* 40, 1996, pp.1–24

Brantlinger, Patrick 'Victorians and Africans: The Genealogy of the Myth of the Dark Continent', *Critical Inquiry*, 12, 1985, pp.166–203

British Empire and Commonwealth Museum, *Voices and Echoes: A Catalogue of Oral History Holdings of the British Empire and Commonwealth Museum*, Bristol, British Empire and Commonwealth Museum, 1999 (first published, 1998)

Brown, Spencer H 'British Army Surgeons Commissioned 1840–1909 with West Indian/West African Service: A Prosopographical Evaluation' *Medical History*, 37, 1993, pp.411–31

Bull, Mary *The Medical Services of Uganda 1954–5*, Report 20, Oxford Development Records Project, Rhodes House Library, Oxford, [n.d. *c.*198?]

Bull, Mary *The Medical Services of Tanganyika 1955*, Report 21, Oxford Development Records Project, Rhodes House Library, Oxford, [n.d. *c.*198?]

Bynum, William F *Science and the Practice of Medicine in the Nineteenth Century*, Cambridge University Press, 1994

Bynum, William F and Overy, Caroline *The Beast in the Mosquito: the Correspondence of Ronald Ross and Patrick Manson*, Amsterdam, Rodopi, 1998

Callaway, Helen 'Dressing for Dinner in the Bush: Rituals of Self-Definition and British Imperial Authority' in Ruth Barnes and Joanne B Eicher (eds), *Dress and Gender: Making and Meaning in Cultural Contexts*, Berg, 1992, pp.232–47

Cannadine, David *Ornamentalism: How the British Saw Their Empire*, London, Allen Lane, The Penguin Press, 2001

Chernin, Eli 'The Early British and American Journals of Tropical Medicine and Hygiene: an Informal Survey', *Medical History*, 36, 1992, pp.70–83

Chernin, Eli 'Sir Patrick Manson: Physician to the Colonial Office, 1897–1912', *Medical History*, 36, 1992, pp.320–31

Clyde, David F *History of the Medical Services of Tanganyika*, Dar Es Salaam, Government Press, 1962

Cohn, Bernard S *Colonialism and its Forms of Knowledge: The British in India*, Princeton University Press, 1996 (first published, 1985)

Cole, Leslie 'Cambridge Medicine and the Medical School in the Twentieth Century' in Arthur Rook (ed.), *Cambridge and its Contribution to Medicine: Proceedings of the Seventh British Congress on the History of Medicine, University of Cambridge, 10–13 September 1969*, London, Wellcome Institute of the History of Medicine, 1971, pp.257–84

Collingham, EM *Imperial Bodies: the Physical Experience of the Raj*, Bodmin, Cornwall, Polity Press, 2001

Colls, Robert *Identity of England*, Oxford University Press, 2002

Cooter, Roger and Pickstone, John *Medicine in the Twentieth Century*, Amsterdam, Harwood Academic Publishers, 2000

Cranefield Paul F *Science and Empire: East Coast Fever in Rhodesia and the Transvaal, History of East Coast Fever* Cambridge University Press, 2002 (first published, 1991)

Crawford, DG *A History of the Indian Medical Service, 1600–1913*, London, Thacker and Co., 1914

Crosby, Alfred W *Ecological Imperialism: the Biological Expansion of Europe, 900–1900*, Cambridge University Press, 2004 (first published, 1986)

Crowther, Anne and Dupree, Marguerite 'The Invisible GP: The Careers of Scottish Medical Students in the Late Nineteenth Century', *Bulletin of the History of Medicine*, 70, 1996, pp.387-413

Crozier, Anna *The Colonial Medical Service and the Colonial Identity: Kenya, Uganda and Tanzania Before World War Two*, University College London, PhD, 2005

Crozier, Anna 'Sensationalising Africa: British Medical Impressions of Sub-Saharan Africa 1890-1939,' *Journal of Imperial and Commonwealth History*, 35, 2007, pp.393–415

Cunningham, Andrew and Andrews, Bridie (eds.) *Western Medicine as Contested Knowledge*, Manchester University Press, 1997

Curtin, Philip 'The White Man's Grave: Image and Reality, 1780–1850', *Journal of British Studies*, 1, 1961, pp.94–110

Curtin, Philip *The Image of Africa: British Ideas and Action, 1780–1850*, Madison, University of Wisconsin Press, 1964

Curtin, Philip 'Medical Knowledge and Urban Planning in Tropical Africa', *American Historical Review*, 90, 1985, pp.594–613

Curtin, Philip *Death by Migration: Europe's Encounter with the Tropical World in the Nineteenth Century*, Cambridge University Press, 1995 (first published, 1989)

Curtin, Philip 'The End of 'White Man's Grave'? Nineteenth-Century Mortality in West Africa', *The Journal of Interdisciplinary History*, 21, 1990, pp.63–88

Curtin, Philip *Disease and Empire: the Health of European Troops in the Conquest of Africa*, Cambridge University Press, 1998

Curtin, Philip *The World and the West: The European Challenge and the Overseas Response in the Age of Empire*, Cambridge University Press, 2000

Deacon, Harriet 'Cape Town and 'Country' Doctors in the Cape Colony During the First Half of the Nineteenth Century,' *Social History of Medicine*, 1997, 10, pp.25–52

De Breton, Elisabeth *The Up-Country Child*, Surrey, R.W. Simpson & Co. Ltd., 1951

Delaporte, François *The History of Yellow Fever: an Essay on the Birth of Tropical Medicine*, Cambridge, MA, MIT Press, 1991 (first published, 1989)

Devine, Thomas M *Scotland's Empire, 1600–1815*, London, Allen Lane, 2003

Dewey, Clive *Anglo-Indian Attitudes: The Mind of the Indian Civil Service*, London, The Hambledon Press, 1993

Digby, Anne *Making a Medical Living; Doctors and Patients in the English Market for Medicine, 1720–1911*, Cambridge University Press, 1994

Digby, Anne 'A Medical El Dorado? Colonial Medical Incomes and Practice at the Cape', *Social History of Medicine*, 8, 1995, pp.463–79

Dobson, Mary, Malowany, Maureen, Ombongi, Kenneth and Snow, Robert 'The Voice of East Africa: The East African Medical Journal at its 75th Anniversary', *Transactions of the Royal Society of Tropical Medicine and Hygiene*, 92, 1998, pp.685–6

Dobson, Mary, Malowany, Maureen and Snow, Robert 'Roll Back Malaria: The History of Malaria and its Control in Twentieth Century East Africa', *Wellcome Trust Review*, 8, 1999, pp.54–7

Dobson, Mary, Malowany, Maureen and Stapleton, Darwin (eds.), 'Dealing with Malaria in the Last 60 Years: Aims, Methods and Results', *Parassitologia*, 42, 2000

Douglas, Mary Purity and Danger: an Analysis of Concepts of Pollution, London, Routledge, 1966

Dow, Derek A 'Some Late Nineteenth-Century Scottish Travellers in Africa', *Proceedings of the Royal Society of Edinburgh*, 82A, 1982, pp.7–15

Driver, Felix *Geography Militant: Cultures of Exploration and Empire*, Oxford, Blackwell Publishers, 2001

Driver, Felix and Luciana Martins, *Tropical Visions in an Age of Empire*, University of Chicago Press, 2005

Dubow, Saul (ed.) *Science and Society in Southern Africa*, Manchester University Press, 2000,

Dunn, Kevin 'Lights...Camera...Africa: Images of Africa and Africans in Western Popular Films of the 1930s', *African Studies Review*, 39, 1996, pp. 149–75

Dupree, Marguerite and Crowther, Anne 'A Profile of the Medical Profession in Scotland in the Early Twentieth Century: The Medical Directory as a Historical Source', *Bulletin of the History of Medicine*, 65, 1991, pp.209–33

Eckart, Wolfgang *Medizin und Kolonialimperialismus, Deutschland, 1884–1945*, Paderborn, München, Wein, Zurich, Ferdinand Schöningh, 1997

Echenberg, Myron *Black Death, White Medicine: Bubonic Plague and the Politics of Public Health in Colonial Senegal, 1914–1945*, Portsmouth, NH, Heinemann, Oxford, James Currey, Cape Town, David Philips, 2002

Farley, John *Bilharzia: A History of Imperial Tropical Medicine*, Cambridge University Press, 2003 (first published, 1991)

Feierman, Steven 'Struggles for Control: The Social Roots of Health and Healing in Modern Africa', *African Studies Review*, 28, 1985, pp.73–147

Feierman, Steven and Janzen, John M (eds.) *The Social Basis of Health and Healing in Africa*, University of California Press, 1992

Ferguson, Ed *Colonialism, Health and Medicine in Tanganyika, 1885–1961*, Unpublished Research Paper, University of Dar Es Salaam, 1974

Foster, WD 'Robert Moffat and the Beginnings of the Government Medical Service in Uganda', *Medical History*, 13, 1969, pp.237–50

Foster, WD *The Early History of Scientific Medicine in Uganda*, Nairobi, East Africa Literature Bureau, 1970

Foucault, Michel *Discipline and Punish: The Birth of the Prison*, trans. Alan Sheridan, New York, Vintage, 1977

Fry, Michael *The Scottish Empire*, East Linton, Edinburgh, Tuckwell Press, 2001

Fuller, Thomas 'British Images and Attitudes in Colonial Uganda', *The Historian*, 38, 1976, pp.305–18

Gelfand, Michael *Tropical Victory: An Account of the Influence of Medicine on the History of Southern Rhodesia, 1900–1923*, Cape Town, Juta, 1953

Gordon, David 'A Sword of Empire? Medicine and Colonialism at King William's Town, Xhosaland, 1856–91' in Mary P Sutphen and Bridie Andrews (eds.), *Medicine and the Colonial Identity*, London, Routledge, 2003, pp.41–60

Hall, Catherine Civilising *Subjects: Metropole and Colony in the English Imagination, 1830–1867*, Cambridge, Polity Press, 2002

Hall, Stuart "Who Needs Identity" in Stuart Hall and Paul du Gay (eds), *Questions of Cultural Identity*, London, Sage Books, 1996, pp.1–17

Hammond, Dorothy and Jablow, Alta *The Africa That Never Was: Four Centuries of British Writing About Africa*, New York, Twayne Publishers Inc., 1970

Harrison, Mark 'Tropical Medicine in Nineteenth-Century India', *British Journal for the History of Science*, 25, 1992, pp.299–318

Harrison, Mark *Public Health in British India: Anglo-Indian Preventative Medicine 1859–1914,* Cambridge University Press, 1994

Harrison, Mark '"The Tender Frame of Man": Disease, Climate, and Racial Difference in India and the West Indies, 1760-1860', *Bulletin of the History of Medicine,* 70, 1996 pp.68–93

Harrison, Mark *Climates and Constitutions: Health, Race, Environment and British Imperialism in India 1600–1850*, New Delhi, Oxford University Press, 1999

Hartwig, GW and Paterson, KD *Disease in African History: An Introductory Survey and Case Studies*, Durham DC, Duke University Press, 1978

Haynes, Douglas M *Imperial Medicine: Patrick Manson and the Conquest of Tropical Disease*, University of Pennsylvania Press, 2001

Headrick, Daniel R *The Tools of Empire: Technology and European Imperialism in the Nineteenth Century*, Oxford University Press, 1981

Helly, Dorothy O "Informed Opinion' on Tropical Africa in Great Britain, 1860–1890', *African Affairs*, 68, 1969, pp.195–217

Heussler, Robert 'An American Looks at the Colonial Service', *New Commonwealth*, July 1960, pp.418–20

Heussler Robert 'Why Study the Colonial Service?', *Corona*, 13, 1961, pp.165–8

Heussler Robert *Yesterday's Rulers: The Making of the British Colonial Service*, New York, Syracuse University Press, 1963

Hicks, Andrew 'Forty Years of the British Medical Association (Kenya Branch)', *The East African Medical Journal*, 38, 1961, pp.43–53

Hillary, Richard *The Last Enemy*, London, Macmillan and Co. Ltd., 1950

Hobsbawn, Eric and Ranger, Terence (eds.) *The Invention of Tradition*, Cambridge University Press, 2002 (first published, 1983)

Holden, Pat *Doctors and Other Medical Personnel in the Public Health Services of Africa, 1930–1965*, A Report for the ODRP, Rhodes House Library, Oxford, 1984

Hoppe, Kirk Arden *Sleeping Sickness Control in British East Africa, 1900–1960*, Westport Connecticut, Praeger, 2003

Hyam, Ronald 'The Colonial Office Mind 1900–1914', *The Journal of Imperial and Commonwealth History*, 8, 1979, pp.30–55

Hyam, Ronald 'Concubinage and the Colonial Service: The Crewe Circular (1909)', *Journal of Imperial and Commonwealth History*, 14, 1986, pp.170-86

Iliffe, John *A Modern History of Tanganyika*, Cambridge University Press, 1994, (first published, 1979)

Iliffe, John *Africans: The History of a Continent*, Cambridge University Press, 1998 (first published, 1995)

Iliffe, John *East African Doctors: a History of the Modern Profession*, Cambridge University Press, 1999

Inden, Ronald B *Imagining India*, London, Hurst and Co., 2000 (first published, 1990)

Johnson, Terence J and Caygill, Marjorie 'The British Medical Association and its Overseas Branches: A Short History,' *Journal of Imperial and Commonwealth History*, 1, 1973, pp.304–29

Jones, HJE 'Recruitment for the Colonial Service', *Corona*, 3, 1951, pp.212–14

Kennedy, Dane *Islands of White: Settler Society and Culture in Kenya and Southern Rhodesia, 1890–1939*, Durham, Duke University Press, 1987

Kennedy, Dane 'The Perils of the Midday Sun: Climatic Anxieties in the Colonial Tropics' in John M MacKenzie, (ed.), *Imperialism and the Natural World*, Manchester University Press, 1990

Kennedy, Dane *The Magic Mountains: Hill Stations of the British Raj*, Berkeley and Los Angeles, University of California Press, 1996

Kennedy, Dane *Britain and Empire, 1880–1945*, London, Longman, 2002

Kirk-Greene, Anthony 'Bureaucratic Cadres in a Traditional Milieu' in JS Coleman (ed.), *Education and Political Development*, Princeton University Press, 1965, pp.372–407

Kirk-Greene, Anthony 'The New African Administrator', *Journal of Modern African Studies*, 10, 1972, pp.93–107

Kirk-Greene, Anthony 'Taking Canada into Partnership in the 'White Man's Burden': The British Colonial Service and the Dominions Selection Scheme of 1923', *Canadian Journal of African Studies*, 15, 1981, pp.33-54

Kirk-Greene, Anthony 'Colonial Service Biographical Data: the Published Sources', *African Research and Documentation*, 46, 1988, pp.2–16

Kirk-Greene, Anthony *The Corona Club: an Introductory History*, London, [s.n.], 1990

Kirk-Greene, Anthony *On Crown Service: A History of HM Colonial and Overseas Civil Services, 1837–1997*, London, I.B. Tauris, 1999

Kirk-Greene, Anthony 'The Colonial Service in the Novel' in John Smith (ed.), *Administering Empire: The British Colonial Service in Retrospect*, University of London Press, 1999, pp.19–48

Kirk-Greene, Anthony *Britain's Imperial Administrators, 1858-1966*, London, Macmillan, 2000

Kirk-Greene, Anthony *Glimpses of Empire: A Corona Anthology*, London and New York, I.B. Tauris, 2001

Kirk-Greene, Anthony 'Not Quite a Gentleman': The Desk Diaries of the Assistant Private Secretary (Appointments) to the Secretary of State for the Colonies 1899–1915', *English Historical Review*, 67, 2002, pp.622–33

Kirk-Greene, Anthony *Symbol of Authority*, London, IB Tauris, 2005

Kuklick, Henrika *The Imperial Bureaucrat: The Colonial Administrative Service in the Gold Coast, 1920–1939*, Stanford, California, Hoover Institution Press, 1979

Kupperman, Karen Ordahl 'Fear of Hot Climates in the Anglo-American Experience', *William and Mary Quarterly*, 41, 1984, pp.213-40

Lasker, Judith N 'The Role of Health Services in Colonial Rule: the Case of the Ivory Coast', *Culture, Medicine and Psychiatry*, 1, 1977, pp.277-97

Lemaine, Gerard, Macleod, Roy, Mulkay, Michael and Weingart, Peter (eds.) *Perspectives on the Emergence of Scientific Disciplines*, Paris, Maison des Sciences de l'homme, 1976

Livingstone, David N 'Human Acclimatization: Perspectives on a Contested Field of Inquiry in Science, Medicine and Geography', *History of Science*, 25, 1987, pp.359–94

Lyons, Maryinez 'Sleeping Sickness, Colonial Medicine and Imperialism: Some Connections in the Belgian Congo', in Roy Macleod and Milton Lewis (eds.), *Disease, Medicine and Empire: Perspectives on Western Medicine and the Experience of European Expansion*, New York, Routledge, 1988, pp.242–56

Lyons, Maryinez *The Colonial Disease: A Social History of Sleeping Sickness in Northern Zaire 1900–1940*, Cambridge University Press, 2002 (First published, 1992)

Mackenzie, John *Propaganda and Empire: The Manipulation of British Public Opinion, 1860–1960*, Manchester University Press, 1997 (first published, 1984)

MacKenzie, John M (ed.), *Imperialism and Popular Culture*, Manchester University Press, 1993 (first published, 1986)

Macleod, Roy (ed.) *Government and Expertise: Specialists, Administrators and Professionals 1860–1919*, Cambridge University Press, 1983

Macleod, Roy and Lewis, Milton (eds.) *Disease, Medicine and Empire: Perspectives on Western Medicine and the Experience of European Expansion*, New York, Routledge, 1988

Macleod, Roy 'The 'Practical Man': Myth and Metaphor in Anglo-Australian Science', *Australian Cultural History*, 8, 1989, pp.24–49

Mandler, Peter 'Against 'Englishness': English Culture and the Limits to Rural Nostalgia, 1850–1940', *Transactions of the Royal Historical Society*, 7, 1997, pp.155–75

Mangan, James Anthony *The Games Ethic and Imperialism: Aspects of the Diffusion of an Ideal*, London, Frank Cass, 1998 (first published, 1986)

Mangan, James Anthony and Walvin, James (eds.) *Manliness and Morality: Middle-class Masculinity in Britain and America, 1800–1940*, Manchester University Press, 1987

Mangan, James Anthony (ed.) *'Benefits Bestowed'? Education and British Imperialism*, Manchester University Press, 1988

Mangan, James Anthony (ed.), *The Cultural Bond: Sport, Empire, Society*, London, Frank Cass, 1992

Manson-Bahr, Philip H. and Alcock, A *The Life and Work of Sir Patrick Manson*, London, Cassell, 1927

Manson-Bahr, Philip *History of the School of Tropical Medicine in London: 1899–1949*, London, H.K. Lewis & Co. Ltd., 1956

Manson-Bahr, Philip 'The March of Tropical Medicine and Hygiene During the Last Fifty Years', *Transactions of the Royal Society of Tropical Medicine and Hygiene*, 52, 1958, pp.482–99

Manson-Bahr, Philip *Patrick Manson*, Edinburgh, Thomas Nelson & Son Ltd., 1962

Marks, Shula 'What is Colonial about Colonial Medicine? And What has Happened to Imperialism and Health?', *Social History of Medicine*, 10, 1997, pp.205–19

Marland, Hilary *Medicine and Society in Wakefield and Huddersfield, 1780–1870*, Cambridge University Press, 1987

McClintock, Anne *Imperial Leather: Race, Gender and Sexuality in the Colonial Conquest*, New York, London, Routledge, 1995

McCulloch, Jock *Colonial Psychiatry and The African Mind*, Cambridge University Press, 1995

McKay, Alex *Tibet and the British Raj: The Frontier Cadre, 1904–1947*, Richmond, Surrey, Curzon Press, 1997

Ndege, George Odour *Health State and Society in Kenya*, University of Rochester Press, 2001

Nsekela, A J and Nhonoli, AM *Health Services and Society in Mainland Tanzania: a Historical Overview 'Tumetoka Mbali'*, Kenya, East African Literature Bureau, 1976

Packard, Randall M *White Plague, Black Labour: Tuberculosis and the Political Economy of Health and Disease in South Africa*, Berkeley, University of California Press, 1989

Packard, Randall M 'No Other Logical Choice': Global Malaria Eradication and the Politics of International Health', *Parassitologia* 40, 1998, pp. 217–30

Penn, Alan *Targeting Schools: Drill, Militarism and Imperialism*, London, Woburn Press, 1999

Peterson, Jeanne M 'Gentlemen and Medical Men: The Problem of Professional Recruitment', *Bulletin of the History of Medicine*, 58 1984, pp.457–73

Peterson, Jeanne M *The Medical Profession in Mid-Victorian London*, Berkeley, University of California Press, 1994

Potter, David C 'Manpower Shortage and the End of Colonialism: the Case of the Indian Civil Service', *Modern Asian Studies*, 7, 1973, pp.47–73

Potter, David C 'The Shaping of Young Recruits in the Indian Civil Service', *The Indian Journal of Public Administration*, 23, 1977, pp.875–89

Potter, David C *India's Political Administrators 1919–83: From ICS to IAS*, Delhi, Oxford University Press, 1996 (first published, 1986)

Power, Helen 'The Calcutta School of Tropical Medicine: Institutionalising Medical Research in the Periphery', *Medical History*, 40, 1996, pp.197–214

Power, Helen *Tropical Medicine in the Twentieth Century. A History of the Liverpool School of Tropical Medicine*, London, Kegan Paul International, 1999

Pratt, Mary Louise 'Killed by Science': Travel Narrative and Ethnographic Writing' in Jonathan Hall and Ackbar Abbas (eds.) *Literature and Anthropology*, 1986, pp.197–229

Pratt, Mary Louise *Imperial Eyes: Travel Writing and Transculturation*, London, Routledge, 1992

Ranger, Terence 'Godly Medicine: the Ambiguities of Mission Medicine in Southeast Tanzania, 1900–45', *Social Science and Medicine*, 15B, 1981, pp.261–78

Ranger, Terence 'The Invention of Tradition in Colonial Africa' in Eric Hobsbawn and Terence Ranger (eds.), *The Invention of Tradition*, Cambridge University Press, 2002 (first published, 1983), pp.211–62

Ranger, Terence and Slack, Paul (eds.) *Epidemics and Ideas: Essays on the Historical Perception of Pestilence*, Cambridge University Press, 1992

Ransford, Oliver *Bid the Sickness Cease: Disease in the History of Black Africa*, London, John Murray, 1983

Richards, Jeffrey (ed.) *Imperialism and Juvenile Literature*, Manchester University Press, 1989

Richards, Thomas 'Selling Darkest Africa' in idem. *The Commodity Culture of Victorian England: Advertising and Spectacle, 1851–1914*, Stanford University Press, 1990, pp.119–67

Rook, Arthur (ed.) *Cambridge and its Contribution to Medicine: Proceedings of the Seventh British Congress on the History of Medicine, University of Cambridge, 10–13 September 1969*, London, Wellcome Institute of the History of Medicine, 1971

Ryan, James R, *Picturing Empire: Photography and Visualization of the British Empire*, London, Reaktion Books, 1997

Sabben-Clare, EE, Bradley, DJ and Kirkwood, K (eds.) *Health in Tropical Africa During the Colonial Period*, Oxford, Clarendon Press, 1980

Sahlins, Marshall 'Goodbye to Tristes Tropes: Ethnography in the Context of Modern World History, *The Journal of Modern History*, 65, 1993, pp.1–25

Sahlins, Marshall *Culture in Practice: Selected Essays*, New York, Zone Books, 2000

Said, Edward W *Orientalism: Western Conceptions of the Orient*, Harmondsworth, Penguin Books, 1995 (first published, 1978)

Schram, Ralph *A History of the Nigerian Health Services*, Ibadan University Press, 1971

Squires, HC *The Sudan Medical Service, an Experiment in Social Medicine*, London, William Heinemann, 1958

Shorter, Edward *History of Psychiatry: from the Era of the Asylum to the Age of Prozac*, New York, John Wiley, 2000

Smith, John (ed.) *Administering Empire: The British Colonial Service in Retrospect*, University of London Press, 1999

Spurr, David *The Rhetoric of Empire: Colonial Discourse in Journalism, Travel Writing and Imperial Administration*, Durham and London, Duke University Press, 1993

Stepan, Nancy Leys *Picturing Tropical Nature*, London, Reaktion Books Ltd., 2001

Stoler, Ann 'Making Empire Respectable: The Politics of Race and Sexual Morality in 20th-Century Colonial Cultures' in Jan Breman, Piet de Rooy,

Ann Stoler and Wim F. Wertheim (eds.), *Imperial Monkey Business: Racial Supremacy in Social Darwinist Theory and Colonial Practice*, Amsterdam, VU University Press, 1990, pp.35–70

Sutphen, Mary P and Andrews, Bridie (eds.) *Medicine and the Colonial Identity*, London and New York, Routledge, 2003

Swanson, MW 'The Sanitation Syndrome: The Bubonic Plague and Urban Native Policy in the Cape Colony, 1900–1909', *Journal of African History*, 18, 1977, pp.387–410

Tolmie, Penny *Medicine and Public Health in British Tropical Africa: Documents*, Report 16, Oxford Development Records Project, Rhodes House Library, Oxford, 1986

Thomson, Elaine 'Physiology, Hygiene and the Entry of Women to the Medical Profession in Edinburgh, c.1869–c.1900', *Studies in History and Philosophy of Biological and Biomedical Sciences*, 32, pp.105–126

Tidrick, Kathryn *Empire and the English Character*, London, I.B. Tauris, 1990

Titmuss, Richard; Abel-Smith, Brian; Macdonald, George; Williams, Arthur W Wood, Christopher H *The Health Services of Tanganyika: A Report to the Government*, London, Pitman Medical Publishing Co. Ltd., 1964

Trzebinski, Errol *The Kenya Pioneers: the Frontiersmen of an Adopted Land*, London, Mandarin Paperbacks, 1991 (first published, William Heinemann Ltd., 1985)

Vance, Norman *'The Sinews of the Spirit': The Ideal of Christian Manliness in Victorian Literature and Religious Thought*, Cambridge University Press, 1985

Van Heyningen, EB "Agents of Empire': The Medical Profession in the Cape Colony, 1880-1910', *Medical History*, 33,1989, pp.450–71

Vaughan, Megan *Curing Their Ills: Colonial Power and African Illness*, Padstow, Polity Press, 1991

Vaughan, Megan 'Healing and Curing: Issues in the Social History and Anthropology of Medicine in Africa', *Social History of Medicine*, 7, 1994, pp.283–95

Waddington, Keir *Medical Education at St. Bartholomew's Hospital, 1123–1995*, Woodbridge, Suffolk, Rochester, NY, Boydell Press, 2003

Walkowitz, Judith *Prostitution and Victorian Society: Women, Class and the State*, Cambridge University Press, 1980

Warren, Allen 'Popular Manliness: Baden-Powell, Scouting, and the Development of Manly Character', in James Anthony Mangan and James Walvin (eds.), *Manliness and Morality: Middle-Class Masculinity in Britain and America, 1800–1940*, Manchester University Press, 1987, pp.199–219

Watkins, Dorothy *The English Revolution in Social Medicine, 1889–1911*, University of London, PhD. Thesis, 1984

Wear, Andrew 'Perceptions of Health and New Environments in the Early English Settlement of North America: Ideals and Reality' in International Congress on the Great Maritime Discoveries and World Health, 1991: Lisbon, Portugal. *The Great Maritime Discoveries and World Health: Proceedings of the First International Congress on the Great Maritime Discoveries and World Health held in Lisbon on 10–13 September 1990* Lisbon: Escola Nacional de Saúde Pública, 1991, pp.273–8

Weatherall, Mark *Gentlemen, Scientists and Doctors: Medicine at Cambridge, 1800–1940*, Cambridge, The Boydell Press, 2000

West, GP (ed.) *A History of the Overseas Veterinary Services*, London, British Veterinary Association, 1973

Wilkinson, Lise and Hardy, Anne *Prevention and Cure: The London School of Hygiene and Tropical Medicine A 20th Century Quest for Global Public Health*, London, Kegan Paul, 2001

Wilkinson, Rupert *The Prefects: British Leadership and the Public School Tradition*, London, Oxford University Press, 1964

Woodruff, Philip *The Men who Ruled India: the Guardians* Vol.2, London Jonathan Cape, 1963 (first published, 1953)

Worboys, Michael 'The Emergence of Tropical Medicine: A Study in the Establishment of a Scientific Speciality', in Gerald Lemaine, Roy Macleod, Michael Mulkay and Peter Weingart (eds.), *Perspectives on the Emergence of Scientific Disciplines*, Paris, Maison des Sciences de l'Homme, 1976, pp.75–98

Worboys, Michael *Science and British Colonial Imperialism: 1895-1940*, University of Sussex, DPhil. Thesis, 1979

Worboys, Michael 'Manson Ross and Colonial Medical Policy: Tropical Medicine in London and Liverpool, 1899–1914', in Roy Macleod and Milton Lewis (eds.), *Disease Medicine and Empire: Perspectives on Western Medicine and the Experiences of European Expansion*, New York, Routledge, 1988, pp.21–37

Worboys, Michael 'The Discovery of Colonial Malnutrition Between the Wars' in David Arnold (ed.), *Imperial Medicine and Indigenous Societies*, Manchester University Press, 1988, pp.208–225

Worboys, Michael 'Tropical Diseases' in William Bynum and Roy Porter (eds.), *Companion Encyclopaedia of the History of Medicine*, London, Routledge, 1993, pp.512–536

Worboys, Michael 'The Comparative History of Sleeping Sickness in East and Central Africa, 1900–1914', *History of Science*, 32, 1994, pp.89–102

Worboys, Michael 'Colonial Medicine' in Roger Cooter and John Pickstone (eds.), *Medicine in the Twentieth Century*, Amsterdam, Harwood Academic Publishers, 2000, pp.67–80

Young, Robert M *Darwin's Metaphor: Nature's Place in Victorian Culture*, Cambridge University Press, 1985

Index